Radiologic Word Book

Barbara De Lorenzo

Springhouse Word Book Series

Springhouse Corporation
Springhouse, Pennsylvania

Springhouse Corporation
1111 Bethlehem Pike
Springhouse, Pennsylvania 19477

Printed in the United States of America

Library of Congress Catalog Card Number: 89-043328

ISBN: 0-87434-421-2

SWB 5-010891

To my aunt and uncle
Ann Tomassi
and
Bernard Tomassi

Acknowledgments

To Harry Benson, Phyllis Leggoe, Lynn Borders, and David Murphy for their help publishing this book.

I am also especially grateful to my family and friends for their support, particularly my parents, Mary De Lorenzo and Michael De Lorenzo, and my good friends, Marion Labanec and Steve Labanec.

Barbara De Lorcnzo

Preface

This word book is designed to provide a comprehensive terminology reference in the field of radiology, related radiation, oncology, and nuclear medicine.

The format of this text is simple and designed to provide a quick terminology reference. It is in strict alphabetical style based on letter sequence, disregarding spaces, hyphens, or numbers appearing the beginning or the middle of the entry.

Note that indentations are used in the following manner. The abbreviation for the lead word appearing in an indented entry is always placed after the word to allow for quick retrieval of the indented entry. A comma denotes the beginning of the indented entry. In the event that there is no comma, the entry indented is read as it appears in the text, as follows:

seed
    array, s. (reads-seed array)
    125 I s. (reads-125 I seed)
    radon s. implantation (reads-radon seed implantation)

This book contains thousands of entries, including terminology related to radiographic/roentgenographic examinations, radiation oncology, clinical radiation, diagnostic scanning procedures, scanners, radioactive agents, radiopaque media, radionuclides (radioisotopes), therapeutic applications, radiological diagnoses, scintigraphic techniques, related instrumentation, and anatomy.

No tables or appendices appear in this book since it is in strict alphabetical style. In keeping with this style, you will find a list of muscles, veins, arteries, and bones in alphabetical order under the appropriate heading (also in Latin when needed).

Many related medical terms have been included for the convenience of the user and to ensure an accurate reflection of the rapidly expanding scope of diagnostic radiology.

I hope that the material presented will save you time, contribute to your professional growth, and serve you well.

Barbara De Lorenzo
Medical Transcriptionist
Toms River, New Jersey

A

A (mass number/ampere)
Abbokinase
Abbott butterfly set
Abbott-Miller (Miller-Abbott) tube
Abbott-Rawson tube
abdomen
  apertures, a.
  fascia of a.
abutting
abdominal
  aorta, a.
  aortic aneurysm, a.
  aortic plexus, a.
  aortography, a.
  panniculus, a.
  ring, a.
  viscera, a.
  wall, a.
abdominoperineal resection (APR)
abducens
abduction
abductor
aberrant
  renal vasculature, a.
  right subclavian artery, a.
  thyroid, a.
ablation
  dose, a.
abnormal situs
abortion
  threatened a.
  incomplete a.
  inevitable a.
  missed a.
Abrams' biopsy needle
abruptio placentae
Abrodil
abruption
abscess
absent
  perfusion, a.
  haustral pattern, a.
absorbable carrier
absorbed
  dose, a.
absorber
absorptiometry
absorption
  coefficient, a.
  dose, a.
  edges, a.
  equivalent thickness (AET), a.
  line, a.
abut
Ac (actinium)
ac (alternating current)
acalculous acute cholecystitis
acanthosis nigricans
ACAT (automated computerized axial tomography)
AC (acromioclavicular)
  joint, AC
accelerated
  fractionation, a.
  treatment, a.
accelerating
  magnetic flux, a.
  tube, a.
accelerator
  linear a.
accessory
  epiphysis, a.
  hemiazygos vein, a.
  muscles, a.
  nerve, a.
  obturator nerve, a.
  olivary nuclei, a.
  ossification center, a.

Additional Entries ______________________

____

____

accessory *(continued)*
pancreatic duct, a.
processes, a.
pudendal artery, a.
sinuses of nose, a.
spleen, a.
thyroid glands, a.
accumulation
acenocoumarol
acetabular
angle of Caffey, a.
cup, a.
fossa, a.
notch, a.
prosthesis, a.
acetabulum
sunken a.
acetanilidoiminodiacetic acid
acetrizoate
acetrizoic acid
acetylcholine (ACh)
induced cardiac arrest, a.
acetylcysteine
Achilles
bursa, A.
jerk, A.
reflex, A.
tendon, A.
achlorhydria
apepsia, a.
achondrogenous
achondroplasia
achondroplastic dwarf
Ackrad H/S catheter
acorn-tipped catheter
acoustic
couplant, a.
coupling medium, a.
enhancement, a.
impedance, a.
interface, a.
meatus, a.

acoustic *(continued)*
neurinoma, a.
shadowing, a.
window, a.
acquired
A-V fistula, a.
fistula, a.
heart block, a.
hydrocephalus, a.
immune deficiency syndrome (AIDS), a.
parenchymal lesion, a.
spinal fusion, a.
acquisition time
acridine orange
acrocephalosyndactyly
acrodysostosis
acromegaly
acromial angle
acromioclavicular (AC) joint
acromion
scapulae, a. of
acromiothoracic artery
acro-osteolitis
acrylic cement
acrylic cylinder
actinic
light rays, a.
radiation, a.
rays, a.
actinium (Ac)
series, a.
actinokymography
action potential
Acuson computed sonography
acute
abdominal series, a.
communicating hydrocephalus, a.
disseminated encephalomyelitis, a.
flexion fracture, a.

Additional Entries

acute *(continued)*
tubular necrosis, a. (ATN)
acyanotic tetralogy
ADAC digital angiography system
ADAC EXL-22 DP (Mitsubishi) accelerator
Adamkiewicz, artery of (anterior radicular)
Adam's apple
A/D converter (analogue-to-digital)
a' demeure, catheter
adenomatosis coli
Addison's plane
adduction (to draw toward)
acquisition time, a.
activation of nuclides, a.
cross section, a.
activity callibrator, a.
adductor
adenocystic carcinoma
adenoid
adenoidal hypertrophy
adenoma
adenomatoid malformation
adenomatous polyp
adenopathy
adhesive capsulitis
adiabatic demagnetization
adipose
capsule, a.
tissue, a.
aditus ad antrum
adjacent
field, a.
tissue, a.
adjoining lesion
adminiculum lineae albae
adnexa
adrenal (s)
arteriogram, a.

adrenal (s) *(continued)*
calcification, a.
cyst, a.
gland, a.
hemorrhage, a.
leukodystrophy, a.
lesion, a.
Marchand's a's.
mass, a.
tumor, a.
adrenocortical insufficiency
adrenocorticotropic
adrenogram
adrenoleukodystrophy
Adrian-Crooks cassette
adult polycystic disease
adult respiratory distress syndrome (ARDS)
adynamic ileus
Aeby's muscle
AECL Brachytron afterloader
AECL Therac 25 accelerator
aeration
aerogram
aerosol
bronchography, a.
imaging, a.
lung imaging, a.
aerosolized solution
AET (absorption equivalent thickness)
afferent
arteriolar constriction, a.
arteriole, a.
glomerular artery, a.
loop, a.
nerve, a.
vessel, a.
view, a.
afterbirth
afterloading
technique, a.

Additional Entries

Ag (silver)
agammaglobulinemia
agenesis
    corpus callosum, a. of
aganglionosis
agger
    nasi, a.
    perpendicularis, a.
    valvae venae, a.
aggregated lymphatic nodules
AgI (silver iodide)
agminated follicles (a/k/a clustered follicles)'
AIDS (acquired immune deficiency syndrome)
air
    activated, a.
    bronchogram, a.
    cells, a.
    contrast barium enema, a.
    contrast radiography, a.
    contrast study, a.
    crescent sign, a.
    cystogram, a.
    dried Romanovsky's stained smears, a.
    embolism, a.
    ethmoidal a. cells
    fluid level, a.
    gap, a.
    intraperitoneal a.
    ionization, a.
    kerma rate constant, a.
    leak, a.
    mastoid a. cells
    sacrum, a. of
    space disease, a.
    study, a.
    trapping, a.
    tube, a.
airway disease
Akerlund spiral type diaphragm
akinetic
Al (aluminum)
ala (pl. alae)
    alba medialis, a.
    cinerea, a.
    magna ossis sphenoidalis, a.
    major ossis sphenoidalis, a.
    minor ossis sphenoidalis, a.
    nasi, a.
    ossis ilii, a.
    parva ossis sphenoidalis, a.
Albers-Schonberg disease
Albert position
Albright Butler syndrome
Albright hereditary osteodystrophy
albumin
    iodinated I 125 serum, a.
    iodinated I 131 serum, a.
    radioiodinated (125 I; 131 I) serum, a.
    technetium (Tc 99m) aggregated, a.
Alcock's canal
alcoholic hyaline fibrosis
alcoholic cardiomyopathy
algebraic reconstruction technique (ART)
algorithm
alignment
alimentary
    canal, a.
    tract, a.
A-line
aliquot
alkaptonuria

Additional Entries

allantoic vessels
allantois
allograft
Aloka
    linear scanner, A.
    sector scanner, A.
    ultrasound, A.
alopecia
alpha
    -1–antitrypsin, a.
    decay, a.
    fetoprotein, a.
    occipital, a.
    particles, a.
    radiation, a.
    ray, a.
    threshold, a.
    wave, a.
Alpha Cradle mold
Alpha Cradle mold-maker kit
Alpha Cradle repositioning device
Alpha-Omega Services, Inc.
Alphazurine
Altmann-Gersh method
aluminum (Al)
    ion, a.
    ion contamination of radiopharmaceuticals, a.
    nicotinate, a.
aluminum marker
alveolar
    arch, a.
    arteries, a.
    capillary membrane, a.
    concentration. a.
    crest, a.
    edema, a.
    hypoxia, a.
    nerves, a.
    point, a.
    process of maxilla, a.

alveolar *(continued)*
    proteinosis, a.
    sac, a.
    sarcoid, a.
alveoli
alveolus
    dental a.
    pulmonary a.
Am (americum)
amacrine cell
amebic abscess
amelogenesis imperfecta
American Edwards Corporation
American Heyer Schulte Corporation
americum (Am)
Amersham Corporation
Amersham-Buchler GmHt & Company
amine
aminocaproic acid
aminohippurate sodium
p-aminohippuric acid (PAH)
aminophylline
Amipaque
    myelography, A.
ammeter
ammonia detoxicant
ammonium
    molybdate Mo-99, a.
    thiosulfate, a.
Ammon's
    filaments, A.
    fissure, A.
    horn, A.
    operation, A.
amniography
amnion
amniotic
    cavity, a.
    fluid, a.

Additional Entries ______________________

____

____

A-mode (amplitide mode)
amorphous calcifications
ampere (a. or amp.)
amphiarthroses
Amplatz
dilator, A.
injector, A.
needle, A.
amplitude (A mode) imaging
amplitude modulation (A mode)
ampulla
ductus deferens, a. of
gallbladder a.
Henle's a.
lacrimal a.
Lieberkuhn's a.
phrenic a.
rectal a.
semicircular canal, a. of
uterine tube, a. of
Vater, a. of
amygdala
amygdaloid nucleus
amyloid
amyloidosis
amyoplasia congenita
anal
canal, a.
fascia, a.
fissure, a.
membrane, a.
valves, a.
verge, a.
analogue-to-digital (A/D) converter
analytic reconstruction
anaphylactic shock
anasarca
anastamosis (anastamoses-pl.)
Billroth II a.
anatomic barrier
anatomical marker
anatomical position
anazolene sodium
Anderson-Haynes pyeloplasty
android pelvic contour
anechoic
structure, a.
anconaeus muscle
Anderson-Haynes pyeloplasty
anemia
anencephaly
aneurysm
atherosclerotic a.
fusiform a.
leaking a.
multiple a.
mycotic a.
needle, a.
ruptured a.
saccular a.
syphilitic a.
traumatic a.
vein of Galen, a. of
aneurysmal
bone cyst, a.
dilatation, a.
Anger
camera, A.
scintillation camera, A.
tomographic scanner, A.
angioblasts
angiocardiography
angiocath
Angio-Conray
angiocardiography
bolus effect, a.
deconvolution analysis, a.
first-pass radionuclide a.

Additional Entries

angiocardiography *(continued)*
 pulmonary embolism, a.
 shunt quantification by a.
angiodysplasia
 colonic a.
Angiografin
angiogram
angiographic catheter
angiography
 balloon a.
 intravenous a.
 renal a.
 selective a.
 selective adrenal a.
angioma
Angiomat 3000 ClearVu syringe
angiomyolipoma
angioneurotic edema
angioplasty
Angiovist 282, 292, 370
angle
 acromial a.
 alpha a.
 axial a.
 beta a.
 board, a.
 Bohlet a. of
 Caffcy, a. of
 cardiophrenic a.
 cardiodiaphragmatic a.
 cavity a.
 cerebellopontine a.
 costophrenic a.
 costovertebral a.
 filtration a.
 infrasternal a.
 iridocorneal a.
 kappa a.
 line a.
 mandibular a.

angle *(continued)*
 meter a.
 obtuse a.
 optic point a.
 pontine a.
 pubis, a. of
 radiocarpal a.
 sacrovertebral a.
 scatter, a. of
 sternoclavicular a.
 sternum, a. of
 subpubic a.
 subscapular a.
 true a.
 urethrovesical a.
 vertebrophrenic a.
 vesicourethral a.
 visual a.
 Y a.
Angle's classification
angstrom (A)
Angstrom unit (A.U.)
angular
 artery, a.
 branch, a.
 frequency, a.
 gyrus, a.
 momentum, a.
 movement, a.
 sampling range, a.
 vein, a.
angulation
angulus
anion
 gap, a.
aniridia
anisotrophy
anisotropic
ankle mortise
ankylosed tooth
ankylosing
 spondylitis, a.

Additional Entries

ankylosis
ankylotic spondylitis
annihilation
    peak, a.
    photons, a.
    radiation, a.
annular
    ankle, a. ligament of
    lesion, a.
    ligament, a.
    pancreas, a.
    phased array, a.
    radius, a. ligament of
    wrist, a. ligament of
annulus
    bulging, a.
    fibrosus, a.
    inguinalis abdominis, a.
    ovalis, a.
    tendineus communis, a.
anococcygeal
    body, a.
    nerves, a.
    raphe, a.
anode
    angle, a.
    body capacity, a.
    diameter, a.
    heating, a.
    heat storage capacity, a.
    heel effect, a.
    mass, a.
    material, a.
    ray, a.
    rotation speed, a.
anomalad
anomalous
    chordae tendinae, a.
    insertion, a.
    muscle bundle, a.
    venous return, a.
anomaly
anorectal
    malformation, a.
    ring, a.
anoxia
anoxic encephalopathy
anoxynaphthonate sodium
ansa
    cervicalis, a.
    hypoglossi, a.
    lenticularis, a.
    subclavia a.
    vitellina, a.
antebrachial
    cutaneous nerve, a.
    fascia, a.
    vein, a.
antecubital
    fossa, a.
    vein, a.
antegrade
    blood flow, a.
    femoral catheterization, a.
    pyelography, a.
    ureteral shunt, a.
    ureteral stent, a.
anterior
    annular ligament, a.
    arch of atlas, a.
    axillary line ,a. (AAL)
    basis bundle, a.
    capsular dislocation, a.
    cerebral artery, a.
    choroidal artery, a.
    circumflex artery, a.
    clinoid process, a.
    communicating artery, a.
    condyloid foramen, a.
    costotransverse ligament, a.
    crural nerve, a.
    depth, a.

Additional Entries

anterior *(continued)*
exenteration, a.
fibromuscular stroma, a.
horn, a.
humeral circumflex artery, a.
inferior space, a.
inferior tibiofibular ligament, a.
intercostal arteries, a.
interosseous artery, a.
interosseous nerve, a.
jugular vein, a.
ligament of knee, a.
ligament of wrist, a.
peroneal artery, a.
pilar of fauces, a.
pituitary hyperfunction, a.
pituitary hypofunction, a.
pulmonary nerves, a.
radioulnar ligament, a.
reverberation artifact, a.
segmental artery, a.
superior dental nerve, a.
superior space, a.
talotibial ligament, a.
temporal artery, a.
tibial artery, a.
tibial nerve a.
tonsillar pillar, a.
urethra, a.
anterofundal placenta
anteroposterior (AP)
oblique view, a.
mantle field simulator film, a.
projection, a.
anteversion
Anthron catheter
anthropoid pelvic contour
anthropological line
anthropomorphic phantom
antibodies
radiolabeled a.
anticathode
anticholinergic
antigenic
antihelix
antimony (Sb)
antiparticle
antitrachitic ray
antral
gastritis, a.
antrum
gastric a.
greater curvature of a.
Highmore, a. of
mastoid a.
maxillary a.
pyloric a.
tympanic a.
anuric
anus
imperforate a.
Ao (aorta)
aorta (Ao)
abdominal a.
arch of a.
ascendens, a.
ascending a.
coarctation of a.
descending a.
thoracalis, a.
thoracic a.
transverse a.
aortae
dorsal a.
primitive a.
ventral a.
aortic
aneurysm, a.
arch, a.
atresia, a.
bifurcation, a.

Additional Entries

aortic *(continued)*
- bodies, a.
- cusp, a.
- dissection, a.
- flush pigtail catheter, a.
- flush straight catheter, a.
- glands, a.
- hiatus, a.
- insufficiency, a.
- isthmus, a.
- knob, a.
- knuckle, a.
- lymph nodes, a.
- opening of heart, a.
- ostia, a.
- plexus, a.
- pulmonic window, a.
- receptors, a.
- semilunar valves, a.
- septum, a.
- sinuses, a.
- spindle, a.
- stenosis, a.
- supply, a.
- valve, a.
- vestibule, a.
- window, a.

aorticorenal ganglion

aortofemoral
- arterial runoff, a.
- bypass graft, a.
- runoff, a.

aortogram

aortography
- adrenal a.
- abdominal a.
- catheter a.
- thoracic a.
- needle a.
- aortic arch a.
- aortic peripheral a.
- translumbar a.
- intravenous a.

AP (anteroposterior) projection

aperture

apex (pl.apices)
- cordis, a.
- fibula, a. of
- heart, a. of
- linguae, a.
- nose, a. of
- ossis sacri, a.
- prostatae, a.
- pulmonis, a.

aphthous ulcer

apical
- cap, a.
- disease, a.
- granuloma, a.
- lordotic view, a.
- segments, a.
- view, a.

apices (pl. of apex)

apocrine glands

aponeurosis
- abdominal a.
- bicipital a.
- epicranial a.
- external oblique a.
- lumbocostal a.
- lumbar a.
- palatine a.
- palmar a.
- palmaris a.
- pharyngeal a.
- plantar a.
- plantaris a.

apophyseal
- joint disease, a.

apoptosis

appendicolith

appendicular
- artery, a.
- skeleton, a.

appendix

Additional Entries

appendix *(continued)*
- auricular a.
- ensiform a.
- epididymis, a. of
- perforated a.
- ruptured a.
- suppurative a.
- testis, a.
- vermiform a.
- xiphoid a.

apple-core like lesion
apposition
appositional
- field, a.
- portal, a.

approximate
APR (abdominoperineal resection)
apron
AP simulation film
aqueduct
- cerebral a.
- cochlea, a. of
- fallopian a.
- Fallopius, a. of
- stenosis, a.
- Sylvius, a. of

aqueductal stenosis
aqueous humor
Ar (argon)
arachnoid
- cyst, a.
- granulations, a.
- mater, a.

arachnoidea
- encephali, a.
- spinalis, a.

arachnoiditis
Aran-Duchenne atrophy
Arantius
- bodies, a.
- nodules, a.

arbor

arbor *(continued)*
- bronchialis, a.
- vitae cerebelli, a.

Arcelin's view
arc
- Buhler, a. of
- Burkow, a. of
- Riolan, a. of
- therapy, a.

Arcelin's view
arch (s)
- abdominothoracic a.
- alveolar a.
- aorta, a. of
- aortic a.
- aortogram, a.
- atlas, a. of
- axillary a.
- branchial a.
- carotid a.
- carpal a.
- coracoacromial a.
- Corti, a. of
- costal a.
- crural a.
- dental a.
- double aortic a.
- fauces, a. of
- foot, a. of
- glossopalatinc a.
- hemal a.
- hyoid a.
- jugular a.
- lingual a.
- lumbocostal a.
- malar a.
- mandibular a.
- maxillary a.
- nasal a.
- neural a.
- oral a.
- palatal a.
- palatomaxillary a.

Additional Entries ______

arch (s) *(continued)*
- palmar a.
- palpebral a.
- passive lingual a.
- pharyngeal a.
- pharyngopalatine a.
- plantar a.
- postaural a.
- pulmonary a.
- pubic a.
- residual dental a.
- right aortic a.
- stationary lingual a.
- superciliary a.
- supraorbital a.
- tendinous a.
- venous dorsal a.
- vertebral a.
- visceral a.
- volar a.
- zygomatic a.

arcuate
- artery, a.
- fibers, a.
- ligaments, a.
- line of ilium, a.
- nucleus, a.
- popliteal ligament, a.

arcus
- adiposus, a.
- aortae a.
- cartilaginous cricoideae a.
- glossopalatinus a.
- juvenilis, a.
- lumbocostalis lateralis (Halleri) a.
- parieto-occipitalis a.
- pharyngopalatinus a.
- senilis, a.
- volaris profundus a.
- volaris superficialis a.

arclofenin

ARDS (adult respiratory distress syndrome)

areola (pl.areolae)
- bone, a. of
- Chaussier's a.
- mammary gland, a. of
- nipple, a. of
- umbilical a.

areolar
- glands, a.

arginine

argon (Ar)
- laser, a.

Armanni-Ebstein lesion

Arnold's
- bodies, A.
- canal, A.
- ganglion, A.
- nerve, A.

Arnold-Chiari malformation

Arnold-Chiari II

array
- linear a.
- processor, a.

arrectores pilorum muscle

Arrhenius plot

arsenic (As)

ART (algebraic reconstruction device)

arteria
- alveolaris inferior, a.
- alveolaris superior posterior, a.
- angularis, a.
- anonyma, a.
- arcuata, a.
- auditiva interna, a.
- auricularis posterior, a.
- auricularis profunda, a.
- axillaris, a.
- basilaris, a.
- brachialis, a.
- buccinatoria, a.

Additional Entries

arteria *(continued)*
- bulbi urethrae, a.
- canalis pterygoidei, a.
- carotis communis, a.
- carotis externa, a.
- carotis interna, a.
- centralis retinae, a.
- cerebelli inferior anterior
- cerebelli inferior posterior, a.
- cerebelli superior, a.
- cerebri anterior, a.
- cerebri media, a.
- cerebri posterior, a.
- cervicalis ascendens, a.
- cervicalis profunda, a.
- cervicalis superficialis, a.
- choroidea anterior, a.
- circumflexa femoris lateralis, a.
- circumflexa femoris medialis, a.
- circumflexa humeri anterior, a.
- circumflexa humeri posterior, a.
- circumflexa ilium profunda, a.
- circumflexa ilium superficialis, a.
- circumflexa scapulae, a.
- coeliaca, a.
- colica dextra, a.
- colica media, a.
- colica sinistra, a.
- collateralis ulnaris inferior, a.
- collateralis ulnaris superior, a.
- comitans nervi ischiadici, a.
- communicans anterior cerebri, a.

arteria *(continued)*
- communicans posterior cerebri, a.
- coronaria dextra, a.
- coronaria sinistra, a.
- cystica, a.
- dorsalis hallucis, a.
- dorsalis nasi, a.
- dorsalis pedis, a.
- dorsalis penis, a.
- epigastrica inferior, a.
- epigastrica superficialis, a.
- epigastrica superior, a.
- femoralis, a.
- frontalis, a.
- gastrica dextra, a.
- gastrica sinistra, a.
- gastroduodenalis, a.
- gastroepiploica dextra, a.
- gastroepiploica sinistra, a.
- genus media, a.
- glutaea inferior, a.
- glutaea ramus iliacus, a.
- glutaea ramus lumbalis, a.
- glutaea superior, a.
- haemorrhoidalis inferior, a.
- haemorrhoidalis media, a.
- haemorrhoidalis superior, a.
- hepatica, a.
- hepatica communis, a.
- hepatica propria, a.
- hypogastrica, a.
- ileocolica, a.
- iliaca externa, a.
- iliolumbalis, a.
- infraorbitalis, a.

Additional Entries

arteria *(continued)*
innominata, a.
interossea communis, a.
interossea dorsalis, a.
interossea recurrens, a.
interossea volaris, a.
labialis inferior, a.
labialis superior, a.
lacrimalis, a.
laryngea inferior, a.
laryngea superior, a.
lienalis, a.
lingualis, a.
lingualis ramus hyoideus, a.
malleolaris anterior lateralis, a.
malleolaris anterior medialis, a.
malleolaris posterior medialis, a.
mammaria interna, a.
mammaria rami intercostales, a.
mammaria perforantes, a.
mammaria sternales, a.
masseterica, a.
maxillaris externa, a.
maxillaris interna, a.
maxillaris interna ramus meningeus, a.
maxillaris interna ramus accessorius, a.
maxillaris ramus tonsillaris, a.
meningea anterior, a.
meningea media, a.
mesenterica inferior, a.
mesenterica superior, a.
musculophrenica, a.
nutricia fibulae, aa.

arteria *(continued)*
nutricia humeri, aa.
nutricia tibiae, aa.
obturatoria, a.
occipitalis, a.
occipitalis rami musculares, aa.
occipitalis ramus auricularis, a.
occipitalis ramus descendens, a.
occipitalis ramus meningeus, a.
ophthalmica, a.
palatina ascendens, a.
palatina descendens, a.
pancreatica magna, a.
pancreaticoduodenalis inferior, a.
pancreaticoduodenalis superior, a.
perforans prima femoris, a.
perforans secunda femoris, a.
perforans tertia femoris, a.
pericardiacophrenica, a.
perinealis, a.
peronea, a.
peronea ramus calcaneus lateralis, a.
peronea ramus communicans, a.
peronea ramus perforans, a.
pharyngea ascendens, a.
pharyngea rami pharyngei, aa.
plantaris lateralis, a.
plantaris medialis, a.
poplitea, a.

Additional Entries

arteria *(continued)*
princeps cervicis, a.
princeps hallucis, a.
princeps pollicis, a.
profunda brachii, a.
profunda femoris, a.
profunda linguae, a.
profunda penis, a.
pudenda externae, a.
pudenda interna, a.
pudenda superficialis, a.
pulmonalis, a.
pulmonalis ramus dextra, a.
pulmonalis ramus sinister, a.
radialis, a.
radialis rami musculares, aa.
radialis rami perforantes, aa.
radialis ramus carpeus dorsalis, a.
radialis ramus volaris, a.
radialis ramus volaris superficialis, a.
recurrens radialis, a.
recurrens tibialis anterior, a.
recurrens tibialis posterior, a.
recurrens ulnaris anterior, a.
recurrens ulnaris posterior, a.
sacralis lateralis, a.
sacralis media, a.
sacralis mediana, a.
sphenopalatina, a.
spinalis anterior, a.
spinalis posterior, a.
sternocleidomastoidea, a.

arteria *(continued)*
stylomastoidea, a.
subclavia, a.
sublingualis, a.
submentalis, a.
subscapularis, a.
supraorbitalis, a.
tarsea lateralis, a.
tarseae mediales, a.
temporalis media, a.
temporalis superficialis, a.
temporalis superficialis rami auriculares anteriores, aa.
temporalis superficialis ramus frontalis, a.
temporalis superficialis ramus parietalis, a.
thoracalis lateralis, a.
thoracalis suprema, a.
thoracoacromialis, a.
thoracodorsalis, a.
thyreoidea ima, a.
thyreoidea inferior, a.
thyreoidea inferior rami aesophagei, aa.
thyreoidea superior, a.
thyreoidea superior ramus cricothyreoideus, a.
thyreoidea superior ramus hyoideus, a.
thyreoidea superior sternocleidomastoideus, a.
tibialis anterior, a.
tibialis anterior rami musculares, aa.
tibialis posterior, a.
tibialis posterior rami calcanei mediales, aa.
tibialis posterior ramus communicans, a.

Additional Entries

arteria *(continued)*
transversa colli, a.
transversa colli ramus ascendens, a.
transversa colli ramus descendens, a.
transversa faciei, a.
transversa scapulae, a.
tympanica anterior, a.
tympanica inferior, a.
ulnaris, a.
ulnaris rami musculares, aa.
ulnaris ramus carpeus dorsalis, a.
urethralis, a.
uterina, a.
vaginalis, a.
vertebralis, a.
vertebralis rami spinales, aa.
vertebraalis ramus meningeus, a.
vesicalis inferior, a.
vesicalis medialis, a.
vesicalis superior, a.
volaris indicis radialis, a.

arterial
cutdown, a.
groove, a.
line, a.
malformation, a.
occlusion, a.
puncture needle, a.
trauma, a.

arteriogram

arteriograph

arteriography
adrenal a.
aortic arch a.
brachial a.
bronchial a.

arteriography *(continued)*
celiac a.
C02 a.
common carotid a.
coronary a.
dorsal pancreatic a.
external carotid a.
gastroduodenal a.
hepatic a.
inferior mesenteric a.
inferior phrenic a.
internal carotid a.
interosseous a.
intravenous a.
left gastric a.
lumbar a.
nonselective a.
pulmonary a.
selective a.
splenic a.
subclavian a.
subselective a.
superior mesenteric a.
transthoracic a.
umbilical a.
venous a.
vertebral a.

arteriola

arteriolar
narrowing, a.
nephrosclerosis, a.
sclerosis, a.

arteriole
afferent a.
efferent a.
glomerular a.
postglomerular a.
precapillary a.
preglomerular a.
straight a.

arteriosclerosis
cerebral a.
coronary a.

Additional Entries

arteriosclerosis *(continued)*
- hyaline a.
- hypertensive a.
- intimal a.
- Monckeberg's a.
- nodular a.
- obliterans a.
- peripheral a.
- presenile a.
- senile a.

arteriosclerotic
- cardiovascular disease, a. (ASCVD)
- occlusive disease, a. (AOD)

arteriovenous
- aneurysm, a.
- first degree a. block
- fissure, a.
- fistula, a.
- leaking, a.
- malformation, a. (AVM)
- nicking, a.
- shunt, a.

arteritis
- brachiocephalic a.
- coronary a.
- cranial a.
- giant cell a.
- Horton's a.
- rheumatic a.
- Takayasu's a.
- temporal a.
- tuberculous a.

artery
- acetabular a.
- acromial a.
- acromiothoracic a.
- alar a.
- alveolar a.
- angular a.
- aortic a.
- appendicular a.

artery *(continued)*
- arciform a.
- arcuate a.
- auditory a.
- auricular a.
- axillary a.
- azygos a.
- basilar a.
- brachial a.
- bronchial a.
- buccal a.
- buccinator a.
- calcaneal a.
- calcarine a.
- caroticotympanic a.
- carotid a.
- carpal a.
- cavernous a.
- cecal a.
- celiac a.
- central a.
- cerebellar a.
- cervical a.
- choroid a.
- ciliary a.
- circumflex a.
- colic a.
- collateral a.
- common carotid a.
- communicating a.
- conjunctival a.
- coronary a.
- cortical a.
- costocervical a.
- cricothyroid a.
- crural a.
- cystic a.
- deferential a.
- dental a.
- digital a.
- diploic a.
- dorsal a.
- epigastric a.

Additional Entries ______________________

artery *(continued)*
episcleral a.
esophageal a.
ethmoidal a.
external carotid a.
femoral a.
frontal a.
gastric a.
gastroduodenal a.
gastroepiploic a.
genicular a.
gluteal a.
hemorrhoidal a.
hepatic a.
humeral a.
hypophyseal a.
ileal a.
ileocolic a.
iliac a.
iliolumbar a.
inferior dental a.
inferior hemorrhoidal a.
inferior mesenteric a.
inferior pancreatic a.
infraorbital a.
infrascapular a.
innominate a.
interocstal a.
interlobar a.
internal carotid a.
interosseous a.
interventricular a.
intestinal a.
jejunal a.
labial a.
lacrimal a.
laryngeal a.
lateral nasal a.
lateral striate a.
lenticular a.
lenticulostriate a.
lienal a.
lingual a.

artery *(continued)*
lumbar a.
macular a.
malleolar a.
mammary a.
mandibular a.
marginal a.
masseteric a.
mastoid a.
maxillary a.
medial striate a.
median a.
mediastinal a.
medullary a.
meningeal a.
mental a.
mesenteric a.
metacarpal a.
musculophrenic a.
nutrient a.
obturator a.
occipital a.
ophthalmic a.
ovarian a.
palatine a.
palmar a.
palpebral a.
pancrfeatic a.
pancreaticoduodenal a.
perforating a.
pericardiocophrenic a.
perineal a.
peroneal a.
pharyngeal a.
phrenic a.
plantar a.
pontine a.
poplieal a.
principal a.
pubic a.
pudendal a.
pulmonary a.
pyloric a.

Additional Entries ______________________________

artery *(continued)*
- quadriceps a.
- radial a.
- radicular a.
- ranine a.
- recurrent a.
- renal a.
- sacral a.
- scapular a.
- scrotal a.
- septal a.
- sigmoid a.
- somatic a.
- spermatic a.
- sphenopalatine a.
- spinal a.
- spiral a.
- splanchnic a.
- splenic a.
- stapedial a.
- sternal a.
- sternocleidomastoid a.
- sternomastoid a.
- striate a.
- stylomastoid a.
- subclavian a.
- subcostal a.
- sublingual a.
- submental a.
- subscapular a.
- sulcal a.
- supraorbital a.
- suprarenal a.
- sural a.
- tarsal a.
- temporal a.
- terminal a.
- testicular a.
- thoracic a.
- thoracoacromial a.
- thoracodorsal a.
- thymic a.
- thyrocervical a.

artery *(continued)*
- thyroid a.
- tibial a.
- tonsillar a.
- transverse a.
- tympanic a.
- ulnar a.
- umbilical a.
- urethral a.
- uterine a.
- vaginal a.
- vertebral a.
- vesical a.
- volar a.
- zygomatico-orbital a.

arthritic
- degenerative changes, a.
- ridging, a.
- spur, a.

arthritis
- atrophic a.
- cricoarytenoid a.
- deformans, a.
- gouty a.
- hypertrophic a.
- juvenile a.
- Lyme a.
- psoriatic a.
- rheumatoid a.
- suppurative a.
- tuberculous a.

articular
- arteries, a.
- capsules, a.
- cartilage, a.
- disk, a.
- lamella, a.
- meniscus, a.
- process, a.
- tubercle, a.

arthrogram

articulation

arteriovenous

Additional Entries ____________________

____

____

arteriovenous *(continued)*
aneurysm, a.
fistula, a.
arthritis
septic a.
arthrography
arthrogryposis
multiplex congenita, a.
arthropathy
articular
cartilage, a.
facet, a.
articulating arm (manual) scanning
artifact
artifactual contamination
artificial radioactive isotopes
aryepiglottic fold
arytenoid
cartilage, a.
glands, a.
swelling, a.
asbestosis
A-scan (amplitude mode)
ascending
aorta, a.
cervical artery, a.
colon, a.
frontal convolution, a.
limb of Henle's loop, a.
lumbar vein, a.
oblique muscle, a.
palatine artery, a.
parietal convolution, a.
pharyngeal artery, a.
ramus of ischium, a.
ramus of os pubis, a.
ascites
abdominal a.
bloody a.
chylous a.
exudative a.
fatty a.

ascites *(continued)*
hemorrhagic a.
massive a.
hydremic a.
milky a.
transudative a.
As (arsenic)
ascitic
fluid, a.
aseptic
conditions, a.
necrosis, a.
precautions, a.
process, a.
technique, a.
ASD (atrial septal defect)
ASHD (arteriosclerotic heart disease)
aspergillosis
aural a.
pneumonary a.
pneumonic a.
asphyxiating thoracic dysplasia
asphyxiating thoracic dystrophy
aspirating needle
aspiration
biopsy, a.
bronchography, a.
cytology, a.
meconium a.
needle a.
pneumonia, a.
vacuum a.
asplenia
functional a.
aster ray
asterion
Astler-Coller lesions
astragalus
astral ray
astroblastoma

Additional Entries

astrocytoma
glioblastoma multiforme, a.
grade 1, grade 2, grade 3, grade 4, a.
asymmetric wash-in
asymmetrical
articular facet, a.
pattern, a.
skull, a.
vessels, a.
asymmetry
asystole
atavistic epiphyses
ataxic
atelectasis
bibasilar a.
congenital a.
lobar a.
lobular a.
lung base, a. of
patchy a.
platelike a.
postoperative a.
primary a.
secondary a.
segmental a.
subsegmental a.
atelectatic
AtheroCath catheter
atheroma
atheromatous emboli
atherosclerosis
obliterans, a.
atherosclerotic
deposit, a.
cardiovascular disease, a. (ASCVD)
ectasia, a.
atlantoaxial articulation
atlantooccipital
articulation, a.
fusion, a.
atlantooccipital *(continued)*
membrane, a.
atlas
ATN (acute tubular necrosis)
aTNM (autopsy staging)
atomic
accelerator, a.
number, a.
structure, a.
weight, a.
atomizer
atony
uterine a.
atresia
anal a.
aortic a.
aural a.
biliary a.
choanal a.
duodenal a.
esophageal a.
follicular a.
foramen of Luschka, a. of
foramen of Magendie, a. of
intestinal a.
mitral a.
ostium, a. of
prepyloric a.
pulmonary a.
tricuspid a.
atresic
atretic
follicles, a.
atria
atrial
canal, a.
left a. hypertrophy (LAH)
myxoma, a.
paroxysmal a. tachycardia, (PAT)

Additional Entries

atrial *(continued)*
premature contractions, a.
septal defect, a. (ASD)
ventricular shunt, a.
atrioventricular
bundle of His, a.
canal, a.
node, a.
opening, a.
atrium
common a.
dextrum, a.
heart, a. of
left a.
nasal fossa, a. of
right a.
sinistrum, a.
atrophic
changes, a.
gastritis, chronic a.
mucosal changes, a.
pyelonephritis, a.
skin changes, a.
atrophied
atrophoderma
atrophy
acute yellow a.
Aran-Duchenne a.
arthritic a.
bone a.
degenerative a.
diffuse central a.
diffuse cortical a.
eccentric a.
epithelial a.
facial a.
focal central a.
focal cortical a.
healed yellow a.
Leber's optic a.
lobar a.

atrophy *(continued)*
myelopathic a.
muscular a.
physiologic a.
progressive neuropathic a.
spinal muscular a.
subacute yellow a.
yellow a.
attenuation
coefficient, a.
process, a.
valve, a.
attic
atypical
findings, a.
pneumonia, a.
Au (gold)
colloid, 198 Au
grains, 198 Au
irradiation, 198 Au
isotope seed, 198 Au
ophthalmic applicator, 198 Au
audio signal
auditory
artery, a.
canal, a.
cartilaginous portion of a. tube
cushion of a. tube
external a. canal
external a. meatus
internal a. canal
internal a. meatus
isthmus of a. tube
meatus, a.
nerve, a.
osseous portion of a. tube
ossicles, a.
pharyngeal ostium of a. tube

Additional Entries

auditory *(continued)*
pit, a.
plate, a.
teeth of Huschke, a.
tonsil of a. tube
tube, a.
veins, a.
vesicle, a.
Auerbach's
ganglia, A.
plexus, A.
Auger electron
augmentation
mammoplasty, a.
auricle
heart, a. of (left/right)
auricula (pl. auriculae)
dextra, a.
ear, a. of
cartilage of a.
ligaments of a.
muscle of a.
nerves of a.
vessels of a.
heart, a. of
sinistra, a.
auricular
appendix, a.
artery, a.
beats, premature a.
fibrillation, a.
flutter, a.
line, a.
lymph nodes, a.
nerve, a.
surface of ilium, a.
tubercle of Darwin, a.
vein, a.
auriculoventricular groove
auris
externa, a.
interna, a.
auris *(continued)*
media, a.
auscultation
triangle of a.
Austin-Moore prosthesis
autoclave tape
autogenous
blood clot, a.
bone graft, a.
vein graft, a.
autologous
blood clot, a.
bone graft, a.
bone marrow transplant, a.
embolic media, a.
platelets, a.
automated computerized axial tomography (ACAT)
automatic
collimator, a.
injector, a.
autonephrectomy
autonomic
ganglia of nerves, a.
nervous system, a.
autopsy staging (aTNM)
autoradiography
autoreimplantation
autotomography
autotransformer
autotransplanted splenic tissue
Auvard weighted retractor
avascular
necrosis, a.
space, a.
tissue, a.
avascularization
average
gradient, a.
life, a.

Additional Entries

average *(continued)*
lifetime, a.
target absorbed dose, a.
AVM (arteriovenous malformation)
Avogadro's number
A-V shunting
avulsed
avulsion
chip, a.
fracture, a.
nerve a.
phrenic a.
traumatic a.
AW (atomic weight)
axes of pelvis
axial
computerized a. tomography (CAT)
fashion, a.
filament, a.
length scan, a.
multi-echo a.
plane, a.
position, a.
scan, a.
sections, a.
skeleton, a.
spermatozoon, a.
view, a.
axilla (pl. axillae)
fascia of a.
axillary
adenopathy, a.
arch, a.
artery, a.
contents, a.
line, a.
lymph nodes, a.
nerve, a.
node, a.
pathway, a.
sheath, a.
axillary *(continued)*
vein, a.
view, a.
axiobuccal
axiobuccocervical
axiobuccogingival
axiobuccolingual
axiocervical
axiodistal
axiodistocervical
axiodistogingival
axiodistoincisal
axiodisto-occlusal
axioencephalographic chair
axiogingival
axioincisal
axiolabial
axiolabiogingival
axiolabiolingual
axiolateral position
axiolingual
axiolinguocervical
axiolinguogingival
axiolinguo-occlusal
Axiom DG catheter
axiomesial
axiomesiocervical
axiomesiodistal
axiomesiogingival
axiomesioincisal
axiomesio-occlusal
axis (pl. axes)
basibregmatic a.
basicranial a.
basifacial a.
binauricular a.
celiac a.
cephalocaudal a.
cylinders, a.
deviation, a.
dorsoventral a.
electrical a. of heart
eye, a. of

Additional Entries

axis (pl. axes) *(continued)*
- facial a.
- frontal a.
- heart, a. of
- lens, a. of
- neural a.
- optic a.
- process, a.
- renal a.
- sagittal a. of eye
- thoracic a.
- thyroid a.
- vertebral a.
- visual a.

axon

axon *(continued)*
- giant a.
- naked a.
- unmyelinated a.

axonal

azotemia

azygography

azygos
- arteries, a.
- continuation of inferior vena cava, a.
- hemi a. system
- node, a.
- uvulae muscle, a.
- vein, a.

Additional Entries

B

B (boron)
Ba (barium)
Babcock needle
back
  bones, b.
  leak, b.
  muscles, b.
  pressure atrophy, b.
  projection, b.
backflow
background
  count rate, b.
  slow wave activity, b.
  subtraction technique, b.
back pressure atrophy
backscattered electrons
backscatter
  factor, b.
  view, b.
Baehr-Lohlein lesion
bag
  colostomy b.
  ileostomy b.
  testicular b.
bagassosis
Bailey and Cushing grading
 system
Baillarger
  band, B.
  lines, B.
Baker cyst
balanopreputial region
balanopreputial sulcus
Balkan nephropathy
ball and socket joint
balloon
  angioplasty, b.
  catheter, b.
  catheter occlusion tech-
   nique, b.

balloon *(continued)*
  French shaft, b.
  intra-aortic b. pump
  pump, b.
  technique, b.
  tipped catheter, b.
  tuboplasty, b.
ball-shaped head
Bamberger's area
band
  absorption b.
  amniotic b.
  anogenital b.
  atrioventricular b.
  auriculoventricular b.
  axis b.
  Baillarger b.
  broad adhesive b.
  gap, b.
  Gennari b.
  Giacomini b.
  His' b.
  iliotibial b.
  moderator b.
  omental b.
  omental adhesive b.
  retention b.
bar
  arch b.
  Erich arch b.
  formation, b.
  hyoid b.
  labial b.
  lingual b.
  magnet, b.
  median b.
  occlusal rest b.
  palatal b.
  sternal b.
Bard bioptic gun

Additional Entries ______________________________

____

____

Bard ureteral dilating balloon
bare area of liver
bare orbit
barium (Ba)
- air contrast b. enema
- aspiration, b.
- carbonate, b.
- column, b.
- cyanoplatinate, b.
- double contrast b. enema
- enema, b.(BE)
- full column b. enema
- meal, b.
- reflux of b.
- residual b.
- retained b.
- retrograde flow of b.
- single contrast b. enema
- sulfate, b.
- swallow, b.
- transit time of b.

Barlow's syndrome
Barnes' dilator
Barodense
Baroloid
barometric pressure
Barosperse
Barotrast
barrel-shaped
- cervix, b.
- chest, b.

barrelled
- double b. colostomy

Barrett's esophagus
barrier
- blood-brain b. (BBE)

Bartholin
- anus, B.
- duct, B.
- gland, B.

basal
- cell carcinoma, b.
- cingulum (of teeth), b.
- cistern, b.
- column, b.
- ganglia, b.
- ganglion, b.
- lamina, b.
- metabolic rate, b.
- olfactory bundle of Wallenburg, b.
- plate of placenta, b.
- ridge (of teeth), b .
- sclerosis, b.
- telangiectasia, b.

base
- atelectasis at lung b.
- cerebral peduncle, b. of
- effusion at lung b.
- heart, b. of
- sacrum, b. of
- skull, b. of
- tongue, b. of

baseline
- audiologic testing, b,
- values, b.

basement membrane
bas-fond (a fundus)
basihyoid
basilar
- arachnoiditis, b.
- artery, b.
- crest, b.
- ectasia, b.
- impression, b.
- infiltrate, b.
- invagination, b.
- membrane (of inner ear), b.
- part of occipital bone, b.
- plexus of veins, b.

Additional Entries

basilar *(continued)*
position, b.
rales, b.
sinus, b.
basilaris
cranii, b.
basilateral
basilic
vein, b.
basiocciput
basioccipital
basioglossus
basion
basiotic bone
basis
bundle b.
cordis b.
ossis sacri b.
pedunculi cerebri, b.
prostatae b.
pulmonis b.
basivertebral veins
basket cells
BaSo 4 solution
bas-relief
Bateman equation
bath
acid b.
alkaline b.
antipyretic b.
antiseptic b.
astringent b.
tepid b.
batrachian position
battery
failure, b.
pack rotation, b.
Batho method
Batson's plexus
bat wing formation
bauxite fibrosis
Bayes

Bayes *(continued)*
rule, B.
theorem, B.
BBB (blood brain barrier)
B-cell
B-D lock
BE (barium enema)
beaded
walls, b.
beading of costochondral junction
beam
alignment, b.
collimation, b.
exit point, b.
flattening technique, b.
limiting diaphragm, b.
splitting technique, b.
splitter, b.
shaping blocks, b.
spreading, b.
modification, b.
transport system, b.
data-computerization, b.
size, b.
limiting, b.
data, b.
shielding, b.
monitoring, b.
hardening, b.
energy, b.
penumbra, b.
limiting device, b.
beat
apex b.
atrial premature b.
auricular premature b.
capture b.
ciliary b.
dropped b.
ectopic b.
escaped b.

Additional Entries

beat *(continued)*
forced b.
fusion b.
nodal b.
premature b.
reciprocal b.
skipped b.
ventricular b.
Bechterew
nucleus of B.
pontospinal fasciculus of B.
Beck gastrostomy
Beclere position
becquerel (Bq.)
Becton-Dickinson French catheter scale
bed
air b.
fracture b.
gallbladder b.
Gatch b.
hydrostatic b.
stomach, b. of
water b.
Bell
muscle, B.
nerve, B.
palsy, B.
Bellini
duct, B.
ligament, B.
Benassi position
bench surgery
bending magnet
Benedict gastroscope
benign
febrile convulsion, b.
gastric ulcer, b.
prostatic hypertrophy, b. (BPH)
Bennett fracture
Bentson
guide wire, B.
introducer, B.
bentiromide
benzoate
Berenstein catheter
Bertel position
Bertin
column, B.
ligament, B.
Bertel's position
beryllium (Be)
windowed tube, b.
Best Industries
beta
activity, b.
angle, b.
decay, b.
emission, b.
emitter, b.
emitting nuclide, b.
energy spectrum, b.
hemolytic streptococci, b.
minus particles, b.
particles, b. (electrons)
plus particles, b.
ray, b.
ray applicator, b.
subunit radioimmunoassay, b.
wave, b.
betatron
betazole hydrochloride
Betz
cells, B.
BeV (billion eletron volts) (a/k/a GeV-giga electron volts)
bevel
beveled edge needle
Be window

Additional Entries

bezoar
Bezold abscess
Bi (bismuth)
Bianchi valve
biarticular
biarticulate
biased x-ray tube
biauricular
bibasic
bibeveled
bibulous
bicameral
bicaudate catheter
biceps
    muscle, b.
    tendon, b.
bicipital
    fascia, b.
    groove, b.
    ridges, b.
biconcave
biconvex
bicornuate
    uterus, b.
bicoude' catheter
bicuspid
    aortic valve, b.
    deformity, b.
    teeth, b.
    valve, b.
BIDA (parabutyl derivative)
bidirectional shunt
Biello criteria for V/Q scan
bifurcation
bifid
bifida
    spina b. occulta
bifurcation
    aortic b.
    arterial b.
    Dacron b. prosthesis
Bigelow
    ligament, B. (Y-shaped)
bilateral
    cortical necrosis, b.
    mass effect, b.
    salpingo-oophorectomy, b. (BSO)
Bilbao-Dotter catheter
bile
    capillaries, b.
    cystic b.
    duct, b.
    flow, b.
    gallbladder b.
    leak, b.
    stones, b.
biliary
    atresia, b.
    cirrhosis, b.
    colic, b.
    dyskinesia, b.
    extrahepatic b. obstruction
    imaging, b.
    obstruction, b.
    outflow tract, b.
    radiotracer, b.
    stent, b.
    system, b.
    tract obstruction, b.
    tree, b.
Biligrafin
Biligram
Bilivist
Billroth II anastomosis
Bilopaque
binding energy
binocular length
Binswanger encephalitis
biodistribution
biologic

Additional Entries

biologic *(continued)*
half-life, b. (Tbio)
window, b.
biopsy
aspiration b.
bone marrow b.
brush b.
cold knife conization b.
cone b.
cytological b.
endoscopic b.
excisional b.
incisional b.
needle b.
open lung b.
percutaneous b.
prostate needle b.
punch b.
under x-ray control, b.
wedge b.
wide b.
bioptic gun
biparietal
diameter, b. (BPD)
suture, b.
bipartite
patella, b.
sesamoid, b.
bipedal lymphangiography
bi-phosphor probe
biplane
recording apparatus, b.
sector probe, b.
bipolar cells
Birbeck granules
bird fancier's lung
bird-headed dwarfism
birds' nest lesion
bisacodyl
bismuth (Bi)
alloy, b.
bite block
fixed turban, b.b.
immobilization, b.b.
on a stick, b.b.
bite-wing
Bk (berkelium)
black rubber cork
bladder
atonic b.
autonomous b.
capacity, b.
compression, b.
distended b.
diverticulum of b.
dome of urinary b.
fasiculated b.
filling defect in b.
flap, b.
floor, b.
gall b.
hypertonic b.
hypotonic b.
irritable b.
mucosal pattern, b.
neck contraction, b.
neck obstruction, b.
nervous b.
neurogenic b.
outlet obstruction, b.
paralytic b.
reflex b.
rupture, b.
spastic b.
total b. capacity
trabeculated b.
urinary b.
Blakemore tube
Blalock-Taussig anastomosis
Blalock-Taussig shunt
Blandin glands
blastocyst

Additional Entries

blastopore
bleb
- apical b.
- emphysematous b.

bleeding
- breakthrough b.
- diathesis, b.
- dysfunctional uterine b.
- functional b.
- gastrointestinal b.
- occult b.
- postmenopausal b.
- placentation b.
- tendencies, b.
- time, b.

blind
- biopsy, b.
- ending ureter, b.
- pit, b.
- spot, b.

blindfolded
blind loop (s)
B-line
blink mode
Bloch equation
blocking agent
blighted ovum
block
- anesthesia b.
- arteriovenous b.
- atrioventricular b.
- AV (arteriovenous) b.
- BBB (bundle-branch b.)
- bundle branch b.
- caudal b.
- complete heart b.
- cutter, b.
- epidural b.
- heart b.
- intercostal b.
- intercostal nerve b.
- interventricular heart b.

block *(continued)*
- intraspinal b.
- intraventricular heart b.
- mental b.
- nerve b.
- saddle b.
- second degree heart b.
- spinal b.
- subarachnoid b.
- sympathetic b.
- third degree heart b.
- transsacral b.
- tray, b.

blockage shunt
blocked region
Bloedorn applicator
blood
- brain barrier, b. (BBB)
- chemistry, b.
- containing, b.
- corpuscles, b.
- dyscrasia, b.
- flow, b.
- flow disturbance, b.
- flow measurement, b.
- flow probe, b.
- heparinized b.
- island, b.
- occult b.
- plasma, b.
- platelets, b.
- pool, b.
- sensitized b.
- vessel structural scan, b.
- volume, b.
- volume determination, b.

bloodless
- field, b.
- fold of Treves, b.

Bloom disease
Blount disease

Additional Entries

blow-in fracture
blow-out appearance
blow-out fracture
blue
    brilliant b. dye
    toe syndrome, b.
Blumenbach's plane
blunting
    costophrenic angle, b. of
Blu-Ray printer
blunt tip
blunt tipped catheter
blunting
blurring out
blush of activity
B-mode (brightness modulation)
    dots, B.
    echocardiography, B.
    gray scale ultrasonography, B.
    ultrasound image, B.
board-like rigidity of abdomen
Bocca neck dissection
Bochdalek
    foramen, B.
    gap, B.
Bock equation
body (s)
    accessory b.
    anococcygeal b.
    aortic b.
    carotid b.
    ciliary b.
    coccygeal b.
    cortical accessory b.
    epithelial b.
    foreign b.
    geniculate b.
    Golgi-Mazzoni b.
    Herring b.

body *(continued)*
    hyaline b.
    Luys b.
    malpighian b. of kidney
    mamillary b.
    Nissl's b.
    olivary b.
    penetration, b.
    penis b.
    perineal b.
    pineal b.
    pituitary b.
    polar b.
    quadrigeminal b.
    restiform b.
    retained foreign b.
    scatter, b.
    section radiography b.
    soft tissue foreign b.
    stomach b.
    suprapericardial b.
    surface area, b.
    thyroid b.
    total b. radiation
    trapezoid b.
    ultimobronchial b.
    uterus b.
    vertebral b.
    vitreous b.
    wolffian b.
Bohlet angle
Bohr's
    atom, B.
    model, B.
    theory, B.
bolster
Bolter Hunter method
Boltzmann distribution factor
bolus
bombardment
bone (s)
    accessory b.

Additional Entries

bones (s) *(continued)*
acetabular b.
acromial b.
alar b.
alisphenoid b.
alveolar b.
ankle b.
astragaloid b.
astragaloscaphoid b.
autogenous b. graft
back b.
basal b.
basihyal b.
basilar b.
basioccipital b.
basiotic b.
basisphenoid b.
bone-in-bone appearance
bregmatic b.
calcaneal b.
cancellous b.
capitate b.
carpal b.
cartilage b.
central b.
changes, b.
cheek b.
chevron b.
chips, b.
coccygeal b.
colar b.
compact b.
conduction, b.
coronary b.
cortical b.
costal b.
cranial b.
cribriform b.
cuboid b.
cyst, b.
destruction, b.
ectethmoid b.

bone (s) *(continued)*
endochondral b.
entocuneiform b.
epactal b.
ethmoid b.
exoccipital b.
facial b.
femoral b.
fibular b.
flap, b.
fracture, b.
fragment, b.
frontal b.
hamate b.
haunch b.
homogenous b. graft
humeral b.
hyoid b.
iliac b.
incarial b.
incisive b.
innominate b.
intermediate b.
interparietal b.
intrachondrial b.
ischial b.
island, b.
jugal b.
lacrimal b.
lamellated b.
lentiform b.
lingual b.
lunate b.
malar b.
marrow, b.
marrow aspiration, b.
marrow biopsy, b.
marrow depression, b.
marrow suppression, b.
marrow transplant, b.
mastoid b.
maxillary b.

Additional Entries

bone (s) *(continued)*
- maxilloturbinal b.
- membrane b.
- mesocuneiform b.
- metabolism, b.
- metacarpal b.
- metatarsal b.
- nasal b.
- occipital b.
- odontoid b.
- orbital b.
- orbitosphenoidal b.
- palate b.
- palatine b.
- parietal b.
- pedal b.
- pelvic b.
- periosteal b.
- petrosal b.
- petrous b.
- Pirie's b.
- pisiform b.
- pneumatic b.
- postsphenoidal b.
- postulnar b.
- prefrontal b.
- preinterparietal b.
- premaxillary b.
- presphenoidal b.
- primitive b.
- pterygoid b.
- pubic b.
- pyramidal b.
- radial b.
- radiation, b.
- Riolan's b.
- rudimentary b.
- sacral b.
- scan, b.
- scaphoid b.
- scapular b.
- semilunar b.

bone (s) *(continued)*
- sesamoid b.
- shin b.
- sphenoid b.
- sphenoturbinal b.
- spur, b.
- squamo-occipital b.
- squamous b.
- substitution b.
- supernumerary b.
- suprainterparietal b.
- supraoccipital b.
- suprapharyngeal b.
- suprasternal b.
- survey, b.
- sutural b.
- tarsal b.
- temporal b.
- trapezium b.
- triangular b.
- triquetral b.
- tympanic b.
- ulnar b.
- unciform b.
- uncinate b.
- vesalian b.
- vomer b.
- xiphoid b.
- zygomatic b.

Bonner position

Bonnet capsule

bony
- abnormality, b.
- bridging, b.
- changes, b.
- deposit, b.
- destruction, b.
- dysplasia, b.
- fusion, b.
- island, b.
- landmarks, b.
- lesion, b.

Additional Entries

bony *(continued)*
 osteophyte, b.
 pelvis, b.
 spur, b.
 structures, demineralized b.
 swelling, b.
 thorax, b.
 union, solid b.
boost
 dose, b.
 field, b.
 radiation, b.
 shrinking field technique, b.
border
 cardiac b.
 demarcated b.
 left sternal b.
 right sternal b.
borderline
boron (B)
boronated antibody
Bose hook
Botallo
 duct, B.
 foramen, B.
 ligament, B.
Bouchard's node
Bouchut's tube
bougie a' boule
bound electron
Bovie current
bowel
 adhesions, obstructing b.
 contents, b.
 dilatation, b.
 dilated loops of b.
 disease, functional b.
 disease, inflammatory b.
 distal small b.
 evacuation, b.

bowel *(continued)*
 fluid filled b. loops
 functional b. disease
 gas, superimposed b.
 hyperactive b. sounds
 hypoactive b. sounds
 infarction, b.
 inflammatory b. disease
 irritable b.
 irritable b. syndrome
 loops, b.
 loops, fluid filled b.
 mechanical b. obstruction
 necrosis, b.
 normoactive b. sounds
 obstructing b. adhesions
 obstruction, mechanical b.
 pattern, b.
 prep, b.
 resection, b.
 series, small b.
 sounds, hyperactive b.
 sounds, hypoactive b.
 sounds, normoactive b.
 superimposed b. gas
 syndrome, irritable b.
Bowen's disease
bowing
Bowman's
 capsule, B.
 glands, B.
 membrane, B.
 tube, B.
 type thermistor, B.
box bolus
boxer's fracture
Boyce position
Bozeman's
 catheter, B.
 position, B.

Additional Entries

Bozeman-Fritsch catheter
BPD (biparietal fracture or bronchopulmonary dysplasia)
Bq (becquerel)
Br (bromine)
Braasch bulb catheter
brachial
  arteriography, b.
  artery, b.
  cutaneus nerve, b.
  fascia, b.
  muscle, b.
  node, b.
  plexopathy, b.
  plexus, b.
  veins, b.
brachiocephalic
  arteriography, b.
  artery, b.
  veins, b.
brachiolymphography
brachioradialis muscle
brachium
brachytherapy
Bragg's peak
Bragg-Gray
  cavity theory, B-G
  ionization measurement, B-G
  principle, B-G
braided wire
brain
  activity, electrical b.
  arteries of b.
  blush, b.
  circulation scan, b.
  commissures of b.
  contusion, b.
  cornu of b.
  death, b.
  dura of b.
brain *(continued)*
  hemiatrophy, b.
  imaging, b.
  meninges, b.
  metastases, b. (Mb)
  pathways, b.
  pia of b.
  radiation therapy, whole b.
  scan, b.
  scan, circulation or perfusion study b.
  scan, static image study b.
  sonography, b.
  stem, b.
  stem glioma, b.
  stem infarct, b.
  syndrome, organic b. (OBS)
  veins of b.
  ventricles of b.
  waves, b.
braking (bremsstrahlung) radiation
branch
  block, left bundle b. (LBBB)
  block, right bundle b.(RBBB)
  circumflex b.
branched calculus
branchial
  arches, b.
  cleft cyst, b.
  grooves, b.
Braun hook
brawny
  edema, b.
breast
  architecture, b.
  biopsy, b.

Additional Entries ______________________

breast *(continued)*
  bone, b.
  cystic b.
  engorgement, b.
  lump, palpable b.
  nipple, retraction of b.
  palpable b. lump
  pendulous b.
  ptosis, b.
  retraction of b. nipple
  shadow, b.
  sonogram, b.
  surgical absence of b.
  symmetrical b.
  thickening in the b.
  ultrasound, b.
breathing
  bronchial b.
  continuous positive pressure b.
  CPPB (continuous positive pressure breathing)
  intermittent positive pressure b.
  IPPB (intermittent positive pressure breathing)
  Kussmaul's b.
  labored b.
  shallow b.
  spontaneous b.
bregma
bregmatic fontanelle
bremsstrahlung (braking radiation)
  spectrum, b.
Breuerton view
Brickner position
bridge of nose
bridge of Varolius
bridging osteophyte
bright echo
brightness (B-mode) modulation
brightness level
brilliant blue
Brill-Symmers disease
brim of pelvis
British thermal unit (BTU)
broad
  adhesive band, b.
  bare area, b.
  based, b.
  femoral neck, b.
  ligaments, b.
Broca
  area, B.
  cap, B.
  center, B.
  diagonal band, B.
  gyrus, B.
  limbic lobe of B.
  motor speech area, B.
  parolfactory a., B.
Broden's position
Broder's system
Brodmann's area
Brodel's line
bromine (Br)
Bromsulphalein (BSP)
bronchi
  divisions of b.
  eparterial b.
  hyparterial b.
  intrapulmonary b.
  left b.
  lymphatic capillaries in b.
  right b.
  segmental b.
bronchial
  adenoma, b.
  arteries, b.

Additional Entries ________________________________

bronchial *(continued)*
- arteriography, b.
- asthma, b.
- bifurcation, b.
- brush biopsy, b.
- brushing, b.
- drainage, b.
- fremitus, b.
- mucosa, edema of b.
- nerves, b.
- obstruction, b.
- orifice, b.
- pneumonia, b.
- rales, b.
- remnant, b.
- secretions, thick b.
- spasm, b.
- tree, b.
- washings, b.
- wheezing, b.

bronchiectasis
bronchiole
bronchiolitis obliterans
bronchitis
- acute b.
- acute laryngotracheal b.
- hemorrhagic b.
- membranous b.
- productive b.
- pseudomembranous b.
- staphylococcus b.
- streptococcal b.

bronchoalveolar
- lavage, b.

bronchoalveolitis
bronchoblastomycosis
bronchoblennorrhea
bronchocandidiasis
bronchocavernous
bronchocele
bronchocephalitis
bronchoconstriction
bronchoconstrictor
bronchodilatation
bronchodilator
bronchoesophageal
bronchoesophagology
bronchoesophagoscopy
bronchofiberscope
bronchofibroscopy
bronchogenic
- adenocarcinoma, b.
- carcinoma, b.
- cyst, b.
- oat cell carcinoma, b.

bronchogram
bronchography
- Cope b.

broncholith
broncholithiasis
bronchology
bronchomalacia
bronchomediastinal lymphatic trunks
bronchomotor
bronchomucotropic
bronchomycosis
bronchonocardiosis
bronchopancreatic
bronchopathy
bronchophony
bronchoplasty
bronchoplegia
bronchopleural
bronchopleuropneumonia
bronchopneumonia
bronchopneumonic
bronchopneumonitis
bronchopneumopathy
bronchopulmonary
- aspergillosis, b.
- dysplasia, b. (BPD)
- node (s), b.
- segments, b.

Additional Entries

bronchoradiography
bronchorrhagia
bronchorrhaphy
bronchorrhea
bronchoscopy
    aspiration b.
    fiberoptic b.
bronchosinusitis
bronchospasm
bronchospirochetosis
bronchospirography
bronchospirometer
bronchospirometry
bronchostaxis
bronchostenosis
bronchostomy
bronchotome
bronchotomy
bronchotracheal
bronchotyphoid
bronchovascular
    markings, b.
bronchus (pl. bronchi)
    dexter, b.
    distortion of left main stem b.
    intermedius, b.
    main stem b.
    partial occlusion main b.
    sinister, b.
Broviac catheter
brow-down
    half axial posteroanterior projection, b-d
    hanging head projection, b-d
    position, b-d
    straight posteroanterior projection, b-d
Brown-Roberts-Wells (BRW) CT stereotaxic guide
Brown-Sequard syndrome
brown tumor
brow-up
    cross table lateral projection, b-u
    cross table lateral projection with hanging head, b-u
    frontal anteroposterior projection, b-u
    half axial anteroposterior projection, b-u
    lateral (cross-table) projection, b-u
    position, b-u
Bruch's membrane
bruit
    aneurysmal b.
    carotid b.
    placental b.
    systolic b.
Brunner's
    glands, B.
    hypertrophy, B.
brushing (s)
    tissue, b. of
BRW (Brown-Roberts-Wells) CT stereotaxic guide
Bryant's triangle
BSA (body surface area)
B-scan technique
BSO (buthionine sulphoximine)
BTU (British thermal unit)
bubble
    air b.
    ventriculography, b.
bubbling
    rales, b.
bubbly lung
buccae
buccal
    artery, b.

Additional Entries

buccal *(continued)*
- branches of facial nerve, b.
- cavity, b.
- fat pad, b.
- glands, b.
- mucosa, b.
- nerve, b.
- tube, b.

buccinator
- artery, b.
- muscle, b.
- nerve, b.

buccoaxial
buccoaxiocervical
buccoaxiogingival
buccocervical
buccoclusal
buccoclusion
buccodistal
buccogingival
buccoglossopharyngitis
buccolabial
buccolingual
buccomaxillary
buccomesial
bucconasal membrane
bucco-occlusal
buccopharyngeal
- fascia, b.
- membrane, b.

Buchler afterloading system
Buchler GmbH
Buckbee-Meers resolution plate
bucket
- handle tear of meniscus, b.

buckling
- aorta, b. of
- branchiocephalic vessels, b. of

Buck's fascia
Bucky
- diaphragm, B.
- factor, B.
- film, B.
- oscillating B.
- rays, B.
- table, B.
- tomogram, B.
- vertical, B.
- view, B.

Bucky-Potter grid
Budd-Chiari syndrome
Budin joint
bulb
- aortic b.
- auditory b.
- catheter, b.
- duodenal b.
- duodenal b. and sweep
- eye b.
- gustatory b.
- hair b.
- irritable duodenal b.
- olfactory b.
- posterior cornu, b. of
- scarring of duodenal b.
- spinal b.
- sweep, duodenal b. and
- urethral b.
- vaginal b.
- vestibule, b. of
- vestibulovaginal b.

bulbar palsy
bulbocavernous muscle
bulbourethral glands of Cowper
bulboventricular loop
bulbs of internal jugular vein
bulbus
- cordis, b.
- oculi, b.

Additional Entries

bulbus *(continued)*
olfactorius, b.
urethrae, b.
vestibuli vaginae, b.
bulging
disk, b.
bulk disease
bulky
cervical lesions, b.
site, b.
tumor, b.
bulla ethmoidalis
bullae
bullous
emphysema, b.
bull's eye lesion
bunch of grapes
bundle
aberrant b.
branch block, b.
atrioventricular b.
Bruce's b.
cornucommissural b.
fundamental b.
Kent-His b.
longitudinal medial b.
main b.
medial forebrain b.
Meynert b.
Monakow b.
muscle b.
of His, B.
posterior longitudinal b.
predorsal b.
Schultze b.
sinoatrial b.
solitary b.
thalamomamillary b.
Thorel b.
tubules, b. of
bundle *(continued)*
Turck b.
Wallenburg b.
Vicq d'Azyr b.
Weissmann's b.
bur
cutting b.
drill, b.
hole, b.
Burdach tract
Burnett applicator
Burn's space
bursa (pl. bursae)
omental b.
omentalis b.
pharyngeal b.
prepatellar b.
suprapatellar b.
burst (s)
alpha activity, b. of
fracture, b.
paroxysmal b.
periodic slow b.
butifenin
butionine sulphoximine (BSO)
butterfly
astrocytoma, b.
fracture, b.
needle, b.
pattern, b.
type glioma, b.
buttock
button
distal prostate, b. of
sequestrum, b.
Byford double-ended retractor
bypass
aortocoronary b.
aortoiliac b.

Additional Entries ______

bypass *(continued)*
- aortorenal b.
- arterial b.
- CABG (coronary artery b. graft)
- cardiopulmonary b.
- coronary b.
- coronary artery b.
- femoropopliteal b.
- gastric b.

bypass *(continued)*
- graft, coronary artery b. (CABG)
- intestinal b.
- jejunal b.
- jejunoileal b.
- left heart b.
- partial b.
- pulmonary b.
- right heart b.

Additional Entries

C

C (carbon)
C (coulomb)
Ca (calcium)
CABG (coronary artery by-pass graft)
cachexia
cadmium (Cd)
    chloride, c.
cafe-au-lait spots
CaF2 (calcium fluoride)
Caffey's
    acetabular angle, C.
    disease, C.
cage
    bony rib c.
Cahan's criteria
cake frosting appearance
calamus
    scriptorius, c.
calcaneal
    arteries, c.
    bursa, c.
    nerve, c.
    spur, c.
    sulcus, c.
    tuberosity, c.
calcaneoapophysitis
calcaneoastragaloid
    articulation ligaments, c.
calcaneocavus
calcaneocuboid
calcaneodynia
calcaneofibular
calcaneonavicular
    ligaments, c.
calcaneoplantar
calcaneoscaphoid
calcaneotibial
    ligaments, c.
calcaneovalgocavus
calcaneovalgus
calcaneovarus
calcaneum
calcaneus
calcar
    avis, c.
    femorale, c.
calcarine fissure
calcific
    aortic stenosis, c.
    changes, c.
    density, c.
    deposits, c.
    nodule, c.
    shadows, c.
calcification
    aortic c.
    pineal gland c.
    soft tissue c.
calcified
    aortic valve, c.
    benign granuloma, c.
    blood vessel, c.
    density, c.
    epithelioma, c.
    granuloma, c.
    hematoma, c.
    leiomyoma, c.
    liver lesion, c.
    lymph node, c.
    pineal gland, c.
    plaque, c.
    pleura, c.
    psoas abscess, c.
    pulp, c.
    uterine fibroid, c.
    valve, c.
calcifying hematoma
calcinosis
    intervertebralis, c.

Additional Entries ______________________________

____

____

calcinosis *(continued)*
universalis, c.
calcium (Ca)
balance, c.
chloride Ca 45, c.
chloride Ca 47, c.
ipodate, c.
deposits, c.
oxalate crystals, c.
phosphate, c.
calculus (pl. calculi)
biliary c.
calcium oxalate c.
dental c.
fusible c.
gallbladder c.
lacrimal c.
lucent c.
lung c.
nonopaque c.
opaque c.
prostatic c.
renal c.
salivary c.
staghorn c.
urinary c.
vesical c.
Caldani's ligament
Caldwell position
Caldwell-Luc procedure
Caldwell-Moloy classification
Caldwell position
Caldwell view
calf
bone, c.
caliber
calibration
instrument, c.
source, c.
calibrator
calices (sg. calix)
of kidney, c.
caliectasis
californium (Cf)
neutron brachytherapy, c.
252 radioisotope, c.
caliper,
skinfold c.
calix (pl. calices)
Calleja's islets
callosal
convolution, c.
fissure, c.
callosomarginal
artery, c.
fissure, c.
callosum
corpus, c.
callous
formation, c.
caloric ray
Calori's bursa
Calot's triangle
calvaria
calvarial
thickening, c.
uptake, c.
calvarium
Calve-Perthes disease
calvorimetry
calyceal
cup, c.
cyst, c.
dilatation, c.
diverticulum, c.
stone, c.
syndrome, c.
calyces (sg. calyx)
blunting of c.
pelves c. and ureters
calyx (pl. calyces)
major c.
minor c.

Additional Entries

camera
 Anger c.
 anterior bulbi c.
 oculi c.
 posterior bulbi c.
 vitrea bulbi c.
C-14 aminopyrine
campanula
 halleri, c.
Campbell's
 capsule, C.
 ligament, C.
Camp-Coventry position
Camper's
 angle, C.
 fascia, C.
Camp grid cassette
camptomelic syndrome
 (bending of limbs)
canal (s)
 adductor c.
 Alcock's c.
 alimentary c.
 alveolar c.
 anal c.
 arterial c.
 atrial c.
 atrioventricular c.
 auditory c.
 birth c.
 carotid c.
 central c. of spinal cord
 cervical c.
 cochlear c.
 condylar c.
 condyloid c.
 craniopharyngeaal c.
 crural c.
 dental c.
 ethmoidal c.
 facial c.
 femoral c.

canal (s) *(continued)*
 floor of inguinal c.
 Gartner's c.
 gastric c.
 genital c.
 haversian c.
 Huguier c.
 Hunter's c.
 hyaloid c.
 hypoglossal c.
 incisive c.
 infraorbital c.
 inguinal c.
 lacrimal c.
 mandibular c.
 medullary c.
 nasolacrimal c.
 neural c.
 neurenteric c.
 Nuck c.
 optic c.
 palatine c.
 parturient c.
 pericardioperitoneal c.
 perivascular c.
 Petit's c.
 portal c.
 pterygoid c.
 pterygopalatine c.
 pudendal c.
 pulp c.
 pyloric c.
 ray, c.
 reaming of medullary c.
 root c.
 sacral c.
 Schlemm c.
 semicircular c.
 seminal c.
 spermatic c.
 spinal c.
 spiral c.

Additional Entries ______________________

canal (s) *(continued)*
subsartorial c.
supraciliary c.
supraoptic c.
supraorbital c.
tarsal c.
tensor tympani, c.
tubal c.
umbilical c.
urogenital c.
vaginal c.
vertebral c.
vestibular c.
vidian c.
Volkmann's c.
vomerovaginal c.
zygomaticofacial c.
zygomaticotemporal c.
canaliculi
bone, c. of
dental c.
canaliculus
inferior tympanic c.
innominatus of Arnold c.
mastoid c.
canalis
centralis cochleae, c.
cervicis uteri, c.
reuniens (of Hensen), c.
semicircularis lateralis, c.
semicircularis posterior, c.
semicircularis superior, c.
Canavan's disease
Canavan-van Bogaert-Bertrand disease
cancellous
bone, c.
formation, c.
graft, c.
cancellous *(continued)*
tissue, c.
cancer
in situ, c.
cancericidal
cane
quadripod c.
tripod c.
canescent
canine
eminence, c.
fossa, c.
teeth, c.
cannula
perfusion c.
cannulate
cannulated
activity, c.
biliary tree, c.
femoral artery, c.
cannulation
cannulator
cannulization
canthectomy
canthi (of eyelids) (sg. canthus)
Cantor tube
cap
acrosomal c.
Broca, c. of
duodenal c.
enamel c.
knee c.
skull c.
capacity
bladder c.
diffusing lung c.
FIVC (forced inspiratory vital c.)
forced inspiratory vital c.
forced vital c.
functional vital c.

Additional Entries

capacity *(continued)*
    FVC (forced vital c.)
    FVC (functional vital c.)
    indirect maximum
        breathing c.
    IMBC (indirect maxi-
        mum breathing)
    maximum breathing c.
    residual lung c.
    TIBC (total iron binding
        c.)
    timed vital c.
    total lung c.
    total vital (TV) c.
    total volume c. (TVC)
    tubular excretory c.
    TV (total vital c.)
    TVC (timed vital c.)
    VC (vital c.)
    vital c.
capillaries
    bile c.
    lymphatic c.
capillary
    bed, c.
    drainage, c.
    friability, c.
    hemorrhage, c.
    permeability, c.
    plexus, c.
    sample, c.
    wall, c.
capitate
    bone, c.
capitula
capitular
capitulum
    fibulae, c.
    humeri, c.
    humerus, c. of
    mallei, c.
    stapedis, c.
Caplan's syndrome
capping silhouette
CAPR (combined abdomino-
    perineal resection)
capsula
    articularis, c.
    externa, c.
    extrema, c.
    interna, c.
    lentis, c.
capsular
    adhesions, c.
    artery, c.
capsulation
capsule
    adherent c.
    adrenal c.
    adipose c.
    articular c.
    auditory c.
    bacterial c.
    Bonnet's c.
    Bowman's c.
    cartilage c.
    cerebral c.
    corpora cavernosa of
        penis, fibrous c. of
    Crosby c.
    crystalline c.
    dental c.
    external c.
    fatty c. of kidney
    fibrous c.
    fibrous c. of corpora
        cavernosa of penis
    fibrous c. of kidney
    fibrous c. of testis
    fibrous c. of thyroid
        gland
    Gerota's c.
    Glisson's c.
    glomerular c.

Additional Entries ______________________

capsule *(continued)*
- head, c.
- hepatobiliary c.
- internal c.
- joint c.
- kidney, fatty c. of
- kidney, fibrous c. of
- lens c.
- liver, fibrous c. of
- nasal c.
- optic c.
- perinephric c.
- renal c.
- spleen, fibrous c. of
- suprarenal c.
- synovial c.
- Tenon's c.
- testis, fibrous c. of
- thyroid gland, fibrous c.

capsulectomy

capsulitis
- adhesive c.

caput
- caecum coli, c.
- femoris, c.
- humeri, c.
- medusae, c.
- pancreatis, c.
- tali, c.

carbon (C)
- 11, c.
- C-13 (natural isotope)
- C-14 (radioactive isotope)
- dioxide, c.
- dioxide imaging, c. (15–0 carbon dioxide imaging)
- particles, c.

carboxyhemoglobin

carboxymethylcellulose

carbuncle

carcinoembryonic antigen

carcinoid heart disease

carcinoma-encuirasse

carcinosarcoma

cardiac
- activity, c.
- aneurysm, c.
- arrest, c.
- arrhythmia, c.
- arteriography, c.
- blood pool imaging, c.
- borders, c.
- calcification, c.
- catheter, c.
- catheterization, c.
- compensation, c.
- conduction, c.
- contour, c.
- cycle, c.
- decompensation, c.
- decompression, c.
- defibrillation, c.
- depressant, c.
- dullness, c.
- echogram, c.
- edge, c.
- enzymes, c.
- failure, c.
- flow imaging, c.
- ganglion, c.
- gating, c.
- generator, c.
- glands, c.
- infarction, c.
- insufficiency, c.
- index, mean c. (MCI)
- long axis plane, c.
- massage, c.
- monitor, c.
- murmur, c.
- myxoma, c.
- nerves, c.

Additional Entries ______________________________

cardiac *(continued)*
 notch, c.
 orifice of stomach, c.
 output, c.
 pacemaker, c.
 perfusion, c.
 plexus of nerves, c.
 resuscitation, c.
 sequelae, c.
 shadow, c.
 shock, c.
 short axis plane, c.
 shunt, c.
 silhouette, c.
 sounds, c.
 sphincter, c.
 status, c.
 stimulant, c.
 tamponade, c.
 transaxial emission tomography, c.
 valve leaflets, c.
 variability, c.
cardinal
 ligaments, c.
 symptoms, c.
 veins, c.
Cardio-Conray
cardioesophageal
 junction, c.
cardiogenic
 shock, c.
Cardiografin
cardiogram
 exercise c.
 stress c.
 treadmill c.
cardiograph
cardiographic
cardiography
cardiokymographic
cardiokymography
cardiomalacia
cardiomegaly
 borderline c.
cardiomyopathy
 alcoholic c.
 congestive c.
 infiltrative c.
 peripartum c.
 postpartum c.
 primary c.
 restrictive c.
 secondary c.
cardiopathy
cardiopericarditis
cardioplegia
cardiophrenic angle
cardiopulmonary
 bypass, c.
 resuscitation, c.
cardioscope
cardiospasm
cardiosphygmogram
cardiosphygmograph
cardiotachometer
cardiotachometry
cardiothoracic (CT ratio)
cardiotocography
cardiotocography
cardiotomy
cardiovalvular
cardiovalvulitis
cardiovalvulotome
cardiovalvulotomy
cardiovascular
 accident, c. (CVA)
 arteriosclerotic c. disease (ASCVD)
 atherosclerotic c. disease (ASCVD)
 disease, arteriosclerotic c. (ASCVD)
 disease, atherosclerotic c. (ASCVD)
 renal disease, c.

Additional Entries

cardiovascular *(continued)*
shunt, c.
silhouette, c.
structures, c.
cardioversion
cardioverter
Carey-Coons stent
carina (pl.carinae)
freely movable, c.
sharp and mobile, c.
trachea, c. of
carious
lesion, c.
carmine
indigo c. dye
cariticolinoid
foramen, c.
ligament, c.
C-arm angiographic system
caroticotympanic
artery, c.
nerve, c.
carotid
angiography, c.
arch, c.
arteriogram, c.
arteriography, c.
artery, c.
body, c.
bruit, c.
canal, c.
compression, c.
Doppler, c.
foramen, c.
ganglion, c.
groove, c.
massage, c.
nerve, c.
plexus, c.
pulsation, c.
pulses equal, c.
sheath, c.
sinus, c.

carotid *(continued)*
sinus syndrome, c.
siphon, c.
triangle, c.
carpal
arteries, c.
bones, c.
navicular, c.
necrosis, c.
net-work, c.
tunnel, c.
tunnel decompression, c.
tunnel release, c.
tunnel syndrome, c.
carpocarpal
carpometacarpal
articulations, c.
joints, c.
carpopedal
carpophalangeal
Carpule cartridge
carpus
articulations, c.
curvus, c.
joints, c.
carrier agent
carrier-free specific activity (CFSA)
Carr-Purcell sequence
Carr-Purcell-Meiboom-Gill sequence
Carswell's grapes
cartilage (s)
alar c.
aortic c.
arthrodial c.
articular c.
arytenoid c.
auricular c.
connecting c.
corniculate c.
costal c.
cricoid c.

Additional Entries

cartilage (s) *(continued)*
- cuneiform c.
- epiglottic c.
- epiphyseal c.
- ethmovomerine c.
- floating c.
- hyaline c.
- interosseous c.
- intrathyroid c.
- investing c.
- lacunae c.
- laryngeal c.
- lateral c.
- mandibular c.
- Meckel's c.
- nasal c.
- palpebral c.
- permanent c.
- pinna c.
- Reichert's c.
- Santorini c.
- semilunar c.
- septal c.
- sesamoid c.
- subvomerine c.
- temporary c.
- tracheal c.
- thyroid c.
- triticeal c.
- tympanomandibular c.
- vomeronasal c.
- white fibro c.
- Wrisberg c.
- xiphoid c.

cartilaginification
cartilaginiform
cartilaginoid
cartilaginous
- ring, c.
- ring incised, c.
- septum, c.
- tissue, c.

caruncle
- lacrimal c.
- Morgagni's c.
- morgagnian c.
- sublingual c.
- urethral c.

caruncula lacrimalis
caruncula hymenales
cascade
- electron c.

caseous pneumonia
Casselberry position
Casser's fontanelle
cassette
- holder, c.
- positioned under area of interest, c.

Castaneda (internal-external) drain
Castellani's bronchitis
Castellani's paint
Castleman's disease
CAT (computerized axial tomography)
catheter (listed alphabetically)
catherization
- cardiac c.
- heart c.
- hepatic vein c.
- left cardiac c.
- self c.

catheterize
cathode
- ray, c.
- ray oscilloscope display screen, c.
- ray tube, c. (CRT)

CATT scan (computerized axial transverse tomography)
cauda (pl.caudae)

Additional Entries

cauda *(continued)*
equina, c.
helicis, c.
pancreatis, c.
caudad
caudae
caudal
anesthesia, c.
block, c.
folds, c.
caudalis
caudalward
caudate
lobe, c.
nucleus, c.
process, c.
caudatolenticular
caudatum
caudocephalad
causalgia
cauterization
cauterized
cautery
Bovie c.
button c.
chemical c.
cold c.
electric c.
cavascope
cavern
corpus spongiosum, c's. of
Schnabel's c.
cavernoscope
cavernoscopy
cavernosography
corpus c.
cavernous
arteries, c.
hemangioma, c.
nerves, c.
plexus, c.
cavernous *(continued)*
sinus, c.
sinus venography, c.
space, c.
transformation, c.
cavitated nodule
cavitating
emboli, c.
infection, c.
lesion, c.
cavography
cavosurface
cavovalgus
CBD (common bile duct)
CBF (cerebral blood flow)
CBG (coronary bypass graft)
CBS (chronic brain syndrome)
cc. (cubic centimeter)
CCK (cholecystokinin)
CCT (cranial computed tomography)
Cd (cadmium)
chloride, Cd. (Cd-109)
Ce (cerium)
CEA (carcinoembryonic antigen)
cecal
arteries, c.
fossae, c.
cecectomy
Cecil-Culp urethroplasty
cecocele
cecocentral
cecocolon
cecocolopexy
cecocolostomy
cecofixation
cecoileostomy
cecoplication
cecorrhaphy
cecosigmoidostomy

Additional Entries

cecostomy
cecotomy
cecum
  distal tip of c.
  lymphatic vessels of c.
Celestin tube
celiac
  angiography, c.
  arteriogram, c.
  artery, c.
  axis, c.
  branches of vagus nerve, c.
  ganglion, c.
  plexus, c.
  sprue, c.
cella
cellulae ethmoidales
cellular
  repopulation factor, c.
  swelling, c.
celom (see coelom)
cementoma
centigrade (C)
centigray (cGy)
centimeter (cm)
central
  artery, c.
  axis depth dose, c.
  block, c.
  canal, c.
  canal stenosis, c.
  cells, c.
  disk shaped retinopathy, c.
  fibrous core, c.
  fissure, c.
  gray stratum of cerebral aqueduct, c.
  lesion, c.
  ligament of medulla spinalis, c.
central *(continued)*
  lobe, c.
  necrosis, c.
  nervous system, c.
  ray, c.
  sulcus, c.
  tendinous point of perineum, c.
  tendon of diaphragm, c.
  venous catheter, c.
  venous line, c.
  venous pressure, c.
  zone, c.
cellulose sponge embolic media
centered to table
centigray (cGy.)
centimeter (cm)
central nervous system (CNS)
central processing unit (CPU)
central venous pressure catheter
centriciput
centrifugal
  nerve fibers, c.
centriole
  bodies of ovum, c.
  bodies of spermatozoon, c.
centripetal nerve fibers
centroacinar cells of Langerhans
centrosome
centrum semiovale
cephalic
  folds, c.
  index, c. (CI)
  portion of sympathetic system vein, c.
  presentation, c.

Additional Entries ______________________________

cephalocaudad
  diameter, c.
cephalocaudal
cephalocele
cephalocentesis
cephalohematocele
cephalohematoma
cephaloma
cephalopathy
cephalopelvic
  disproportion, c. (CPD)
cera
  alba, c.
  flava, c.
ceratocricoid ligament
ceratohyal of hyoid bone
cerebellar
  arteries, c.
  fasciculus, c.
  hemangioblastoma, c.
  malformation, c.
  peduncles, c.
  tract of Flechsig, c.
  veins, c.
cerebellomedullary cisterna
cerebellopontine
  angle, c.
cerebellum
  caudal lobe of c.
  caudal peduncle of c.
  cranial lobe of c.
  dorsolateral fissure of c.
  flocculonodular lobe of c.
  gray substance of c.
  herniation of c.
  lobes of c.
  median lobe of c.
  middle peduncle of c.
  narrow middle strip of c.(vermis)
  nucleus dentatus, c.

cerebellum *(continued)*
  peduncles of c.
  posterior lobe of c.
  posterolateral fissure of c.
  primary fissure of c.
  rostral peduncle of c.
  vermis of c.
  white substance of c.
cerebral
  agenesis, c.
  aqueduct, c.
  arteriogram, c.
  artery, c.
  blood flow, c.
  blood flow measurement, c.
  borders of c. hemispheres
  brain flow, c.
  cingulum of c. hemispheres
  cortex electrodes, c.
  edema, c.
  fibers of c. hemispheres
  fissure, c.
  flow scan, c.
  gigantism, c.
  gray substance of c. hemispheres
  gyri, c. hemisphere
  hemispheres, c.
  infarction, c.
  ischemia, c.
  lacunar infarction, c.
  nerve, c.
  peduncle, c. hemisphere
  perfusion, c.
  poles of c. hemisphere
  spinal fluid (CSF) flow scan, c.
  sulci of c. hemisphere

Additional Entries

cerebral *(continued)*
vasculature, c.
veins, c.
vein thrombosis, c.
ventricles, c.
white substance of c. hemisphere
cerebritis
cerebroma
cerebromacular
degeneration, c.
cerebromedullary tube
cerebropathy
cerebrospinal
fasciculus, c.
fibers of internal capsule, c.
fluid, c. (CSF)
fluid imaging, c.
fluid infusion manometry, c.
fluid pleocytosis, c.
nerves, c.
rhinorrhea, c.
spaces, c.
cerebrovascular
accident, c. (CVA)
anterior commissure of c.
cistern of lateral fossa of c.
convolutions of c.
disease, c.
dural covering of c.
flow study, c.
insufficiency, c.
longitudinal fissure of c.
middle commissure of c.
resistance, c.
ventricle of c.
cerium (Ce)
Cerrobend

Cerrobend *(continued)*
block, C.
blocking, C.
cutouts, C.
field, C.
mantle blocks, C.
mask, C.
ceruminous glands
ceruminal
impaction, c.
cervical
adenitis, c.
adenopathy, c.
arch, c.
artery, c.
ascending, c.
biopsy, c.
branch, c.
canal, c.
cancer, c.
curve, reversal of c.
disc syndrome, c.
dysplasia, c.
dystocia, c.
enlargement of medulla spinalis, c.
erosion, c.
esophagus, c.
fascia, c.
ganglia, c.
incompetence, c.
lymph nodes, c.
lymphadenopathy, c.
mobilization, c.
muscles, c.
nerve, c.
nodes, c.
os, c.
pleura, c.
plexus, c.
polyp, c.
radiculopathy, c.

Additional Entries

cervical *(continued)*
rib, c.
smear, c.
spina bifida, c.
spinal block, c.
spine, c.
spine fracture, c.
spondolisthesis, c.
spondylolysis, c.
stenosis, c.
stump, c.
sympathectomy, c.
traction, c.
myelogram, c.
veins, c.
vertebrae, c.
cervicoaxillary
cervicobrachial
cervicolpitis
cervicodorsal
cervicofacial
cervicolabial
cervicolingual
cervico-occipital
cervicoplasty
cervicoscapular
cervicothoracic
cervicovaginitis
cervicovesical
cervix
atrophic c.
conization of c.
effacement of c.
incompetent c.
lip of c.
parous c.
thinning of c.
uteri, c.
cesium (Cs.)
137 c.
applicator, c.
chloride Cs 131, c.

cesium (Cs.) *(continued)*
cylinder, c.
implant, c.
insertion, c.
intracavitary c. therapy
iodide, c. (CsI.)
needle, c.
teletherapy unit, c. (137 Cs)
therapy, c.
tube, c.
CET (coefficient of equivalent thickness)
Cf (californium)
252 Cf radioisotope
CF 20L Olympic colonoscope
CFSA (carrier free specific activity)
11C-glucose
CGR Saturn III accelerator
CGR, AGC Curieton afterloader
CGR Medical Corporation
CGR Opticontact table
cGy. (centigray)
chain
lymphatic c.
ossicular c.
periaortic c.
superior cervical c.
sympathetic c.
chalasia
chamber
anomaly, c.
aqueous c.
calibration, c.
counting c.
diffusion c.
enlargement, c.
hyperbaric c.
ionization c.
polarity, c.

Additional Entries

chamber *(continued)*
- pressures, c.
- pulp c.
- relief c.
- vitreous c.
- voltage, c.

Chamberlain's line
Chamberlain's view
Chamberlain-Towne position
change (s)
- active parenchymal c.
- associated degenerative c.
- cystic c.
- degenerative arthritic c.
- fibrotic c.
- leukoplakic c.
- lytic c.
- minimal calcific c.
- no appreciable c.
- structural c.

channel (s)
- blood c's.
- deep venous c.
- lymph c's.
- perineural c.
- pyloric c.

Chaoul low voltage x-ray tube
characteristic ray
characteristic fluorescent ray
Charcot's arthritis
Charcot-Marie atrophy
Charcot-Marie-Tooth disease
Charnley-Mueller hip prosthesis
Charriere's gauge scale
Chassaignac's tubercle
Chassard-Lapine' maneuver
Chausse projection
Chausse view
Chaussier's line
check
- ligaments, c.

Check-Flo introducer
Chediak-Steinbrinck-Higashi syndrome
cheiloangioscopy
cheilocarcinoma
cheiloscopy
cheilosis
- angular c.

cheilostomatoplasty
cheirobrachialgia
cheiromegaly
cheiroscope
cheirospasm
chelate
chelation
chemical induced hepatitis
chemisorb
chemodectoma
chemosensitization
cherubism
chest
- AP diameter of c.
- barrel c.
- barrel-shaped c.
- excursion, c.
- expansion, c.
- flail c.
- stand, c.
- symmetrical, c.
- wall adhesions, c.
- wall metastases, c.

CHF (congestive heart failure)
Chiari's network (reticulum)
Chiari II type malformation
chiasma
chiasmatic
- cistern, c.
- groove, c.

Chiba fine needle

Additional Entries

Chicago Blue 6B
chicken wing positioning
Chilaiditi's syndrome (interposition of colon)
chimney field
chin depressed toward chest
chin and nose in contact with cassette
chin resting on cassette holder
chip
    bone c.
    fracture, c.
chiropractic films
C3H mammary tumor
chloramine-T
chlorine (Cl)
chlormerodrin Hg 197
chlormerodrin Hg 203
choana (pl.choanae)
choanal
    polyps, c.
cholangioadenoma
cholangiocarcinoma
cholangiogram
    cystic duct c.
    endoscopic c.
    intraoperative c.
    transhepatic c.
    T-tube c.
cholangiography
    intravenous c.
    operative c.
    percutaneous c.
    postoperative c.
    transduodenal c.
cholangiopancreatography
    endoscopic retrograde c. (ERCP)
cholangitis
    sclerosing c.
Cholebrine
cholecyst
cholecystitis
    acute c.
    calculous c.
    chronic c.
    emphysematous c.
    follicular c.
    gaseous c.
    glandularis proliferans, c.
cholecystogram
    intraoperative c.
    oral c.
cholecystography
    four day oral c.
    oral c.
cholecystokinetic
cholecystokinin (CCK)
cholecystolithiasis
cholecystolithotripsy
cholecystopathy
choledochal cyst
choledochogram
choledochoscope
cholelith
cholelithiasis
cholepathia
    spastica, c.
choleretic
cholescintography
    radionuclide test, c.
cholesteatoma
Cholografin
choloscopy
Cholovue
chondroblast
chondroblastoma
chondrocalcinosis
chondrocarcinoma
chondrocranium
chondrodysplasia punctata
chondrodystrophy

Additional Entries

chondrodystrophy *(cont'd)*
familial c.
hereditary deforming c.
hyperplastic
hypoplastic c.
hypoplastic fetal c.
chondroectodermal dysplasia
chondroepitrochlearis muscle
chondroglossus muscle
chondroma
joint c.
sarcomatosum c.
synovial c.
true c.
chondromalacia
chondromatosis
synovial c.
chondromatous
chondromere
chondrometaplasia
tenosynovial c.
chondromucoid
chondromyoma
chondromyxoid fibroma
chondromyxoma
chondromyxosarcoma
chondronecrosis
chondro-osseous
chondro-osteodystrophy
chondropathia
tuberosa, c.
chondropathy
chondroplasia
chondroplast
chondroplastic
chondroplasty
chondroporosis
chondrosarcoma
chondrosarcomatosis
chondrosarcomatous
chondroseptum
chondrosis
chondroskeleton
chondrosome
chondrosteoma
chondrosternal
ligament, c.
chondrosternoplasty
chondrotrophic
chondroxiphoid
ligaments, c.
Chopart's
articulation, C.
fracture, C.
joint, C.
chorda
dorsalis, c.
tympani, c.
chordae tendinae
chordal furrow
choreic
athetoid movements, c.
choreiform
movements, c.
choreoathetoid
choreoathetosis
chorioadenoma
chorioallantoic
chorioamnionitis
chorioangiofibroma
chorioangioma
chorioblastoma
chorioblastosis
choriocarcinoma
choriocele
chorioepithelioma
choriogenesis
chorioid
choriodea
lamina choriocapillaris, c.
chorioma
choriomeningitis
chorion

Additional Entries

chorion *(continued)*
- frondosum, c.
- laeve, c.
- plate, c.
- primitive c.
- shaggy c.

chorionic
- plate, c.
- villi, c.

chorioplacental
chorioretinal
chorioretinitis
chorioretinopathy
choristoblastoma
choristoma
choroid
- artery, c.
- coat of eyeball, c.
- detachment of c.
- plexus, c.
- plexus papilloma, c.

choroidal
- artery, c.
- atrophy, c.
- fissure, c.

choroiditis
- anterior c.
- areolar c.
- central c.
- diffuse c.
- disseminated c.
- Doyne's familial honeycombed c.
- exudative c.
- Forster's c.
- metastatic c.
- senile macular exudative c.
- suppurative c.
- Tay's c.

choroidocyclitis
choroidoiritis
choroidopathy
choroidoretinitis
chromaffin
- cells, c.

chromaffinity
chromaffinoblastoma
chromaffinoma
chromaffinopathy
chromargentaffin
chromate
chromatelopsia
chromatic
chromatid
chromatin
chromatinic
chromatism
chromatize
chromatoblast
chromatogenous
chromatogram
chromatograph
chromatography
chromatoid
chromatology
chromatolysis
chromatopathy
chromatophagus
chromatophil
chromatophilia
chromatophore
chromatophoroma
chromatophoromatosis
chromatophorotropic
chromatoplasm
chromatoptometer
chromatoptometry
chromatosis
chromatoskiameter
chromatosome
chromatotaxis
chromatotropism
chromaturia

Additional Entries

chromesthesia
chromhidrosis
chromic
    acid, c.
    phosphate P 32, c.
chromium (Cr)
    chloride Cr 51
chromocholoscopy
chromocystoscopy
chromogenic
chromometer
chromomycosis
chromoparic
chromopectic
chrompexy
chromophage
chromophil
chromophilic
chromophilous
chromophobe
chromophobia
chromophore
chromophoric
chromophose
chromophototherapy
chromoplasm
chromoplast
chromoptometer
chromoradiometer
chromoretinography
chromorhinorrhea
chromoscope
chromoscopy
chromotherapy
chromotropic
chromourinography
chronaximeter
chronaximetric
chronaximetry
chronic
    active hepatitis, c
    atrophic gastritis, c.
chronic *(continued)*
    back pain, c.
    brain syndrome, c.
    bronchitis, c.
    cystitis, c.
    disease, c.
    dislocation, c.
    granulomatous disease, c.
    heart disease, c.
    hemodialysis, c.
    illness, c.
    obstructive lung disease, c. (COLD)
    obstructive pulmonary disease, c. (COPD)
    process, c.
    stage, c.
    subdural hematoma, c.
    ulcerative colitis, c.
chronograph
chronometry
chronomyometer
chronophotograph
chronoscope
chylangioma
chylaqueous
chyle
chylectasia
chylemia
chylifacient
chylifaction
chyliferous
    vessels, c.
chylocele
chylocyst
chyloderma
chylomediastinum
chylomicrograph
chylopericardium
chyloperitoneum
chylopleura

Additional Entries

chylopneumothorax
chylothorax
chylous
  ascites, c.
  fistula, c.
chyluria
Ci (curie - unit of radioactivity)
CI (cephalic index)
cicatrices
cicatricial
  contraction, c.
  scarring, c.
  tissue, c.
cicatrix
cigarette drain
cilia
ciliariscope
ciliarotomy
ciliary
  arteries, c.
  body, c.
  disc, c.
  ganglion, c.
  glands, c.
  muscle, c.
  nerves, c.
  processes, c.
ciliated
cilioretinal
cilioscleral
ciliospinal
cilium
C15 02 imaging technique
Cimino arteriovenous shunt
cine
  angiography, c.
  camera, c.
  CT scanner, c.
  studies, c.
cineangiocardiography
cineangiography
cine CT scanner
cinedensigraphy
cine-esophagogram
cinefluorography
cinemascopy
cinematic format
cine methods
cinemicrography
cinephlebography
cineradiography
cinerecording
cine study
cine view
cingulate
  fissures, c.
  gyrus, c.
  sulcus, c.
cingulum
  cerebral hemispheres, c. of
C-14 inulin
circle
  diffusion c.
  Haller, c. of
  Willis, c. of
circular
  folds, c.
  microtron, c.
  sinus, c.
  sulcus, c.
circulating
  blood volume, c.
  platelets, c.
circulation
  allantoic c.
  collateral c.
  coronary c.
  fetal c.
  lymph c.
  peripheral c.
  placental c.
  portal c.

Additional Entries

circulation *(continued)*
- pulmonary c.
- sinusoidal c.
- systemic c.
- time, c.
- umbilical c.
- vitelline c.

circulatory
- assist, c.
- collapse, c.
- embarrassment, c.
- overload, c.

circulus
- arteriosus, c.
- vasculosus, c.

circumarticular
circumaxillary
circumbulbar
circumcallosal
circumcorneal
circumcrescent
circumduction
circumference
circumferentia
circumferential
- fibrocartilage, c.
- fracture, c.
- venules, c.

circumflex
- artery, c.
- artery stenosis, c.
- nerve, c.

circumflexus
circumflexed
- branch, c.

circumgemmal
circuminsular
- fissure, c.

circumintestinal
circumlental
circumnuclear
circumocular
circumoral
circumorbital
circumpatellar anastomosis
circumrenal
circumvallate papillae
circumvascular
circumvolute
cirrhosis
- alcoholic c.
- bacterial c.
- biliary c.
- congestive c.
- fatty c.
- Laennec's c.
- metabolic c.
- portal c.
- posthepatic c.
- postnecrotic c.

cirrhotic
- changes, c.
- nodules, c.
- regenerating nodules, c.

cirrus
cistern (s)
- basal c.
- cerebellomedullary c.
- Pecquet, c. of
- Sylvius, c. of
- subarachnoid c's.

cisterna
- ambiens, c.
- basalis, c.
- cerebellomedullaris, c.
- chiasmatica, c.
- chiasmatis, c.
- chyli, c.
- fossae lateralis cerebri, c.
- interpeduncularis, c.
- magna, c.
- venae magnae cerebri, c.

cisternae subarachnoid

Additional Entries

cisternal
  puncture, c.
cisternogram
cisternographic
cisternography
  metrizamide c.
  radionuclide c.
CIS-US 192 Ir hairpin
Civatte's poikiloderma
Civinini's ligament
CKA-3 applicator
CKA-4 circular applicator
CKA-7 circular applicator
Cl (chlorine)
11C-labeled carbon monoxide
clamp
clamped
  aorta cross-c.
Clarke's
  cells, C.
  column, C.
  nucleus, C.
Clark level I
Clark level II
Clark level III
Clark level IV
Clark level V
Clarkson's method
claudication
  intermittent c.
Claudius' cell
claustra
claustral
claustrum
  gutturis, c.
  oris, c.
  virginale, c.
Clave disease
clavicle
clavicula
clavicular
clavicular *(continued)*
  notch of sternum, c.
claviculus
clavipectoral fascia
clay
  colored stool, c.
clean
  catch urine, c.
  voided specimen, c.
cleansing
  breath, deep c.
  enema, c.
clear
  airway, c.
  conjunctivae, c.
  dose-response curve, c.
  liquid diet, c.
  pulmonary fields, c.
  urine effluxing bilaterally, c.
cleavage
  lines, c.
  skin, c.
cleaved cell
cleft
  branchial c.
  face, c.
  lip, c.
  palate, c.
  pudendal, c.
  spinous process, c.
  synaptic c.
  valve leaflet, c.
  vertebral body, c. of
  visceral c.
cleidocostal
cleidocranial
  dysostosis, c.
  dysplasia, c.
click
  ejection c.
  systolic c.

Additional Entries

climacterium
praecox, c.
climatotherapy
clinical diagnostic staging (cTNM)
Clini-Therm Corporation
clinodactyly
clinoid processes
clipping
middle cerebral artery, c. of
clitoris
frenulum of c.
glans of c.
nerves of c.
prepuce of c.
clivus
skull, c. of
sphenoid c.
cloacogenic carcinoma
clonic
convulsion, c.
seizure, c.
tonic seizure, c.(a/k/a clonitonic)
clonogenic cells
clonograph
clonospasm
C-loop
Cloquet
canal, C.
fascia, C.
ganglion, C.
hernia, C.
lymph nodes, C.
closed
angle glaucoma, c.
chest cardiac massage, c.
fracture, c.
incision c. loosely
loop, c.
-loop ventilation system, c.

closed *(continued)*
needle biopsy, c.
reduction of fracture, c.
closing membranes
clot
agonal c.
antemortem c.
blood c.
chicken fat c.
currant jelly c.
laminated c.
marantic c.
passive c.
plastic c.
postmortem c.
clotting
time, c.
clouding
sinuses, c. of
cloudy
fluid, c.
grossly c. fluid
urine, c.
cloverleaf
deformity, c.
skull, c.
clubbing
distal phalanges, c. of
extremities, c. of
clubfoot
clustered polypoid mass
Clysodrast
Cm (curium)
cm. (centimeter)
CMG (cystometrogram)
C-11 monoxide (inhalation)
CNS (central nervous system)
Co (cobalt)
57 Co
48 Co
60 Co
60 Co eye plaque

Additional Entries

Co (cobalt) *(continued)*
60 Co moving strip
60 Co ophthalmic applicator
60 Co single x-ray beam
60 Co teletherapy machine
57 Co bleomycin
137 Co teletherapy machine
coagulability
coagulable
coagulant
coagulate
coagulated
bleeding points clamped and c.
coagulating
Bovie c. current
coagulation
diffuse c.
intravascular c.
disseminated intravascular c.
coagulator
bipolar c.
Bovie c.
coagulogram
coagulopathy
C02 angiography
coarctate
coarctation
abdominal aorta, c. of
aorta, c. of
unusual site of c.
ventricle, c. of
coal worker's pneumoconiosis
coarse
crepitations, c.
folds, c.
rales, c.
rhonchi, c.
coarse *(continued)*
thrill, c.
trabecular pattern, c.
trabeculation, c.
tremor, c.
coarticulation
coat
adventitial c.
buffy c.
corneoscleral c.
sclerotic c.
serous c.
coated
coaxial
catheter, c.
technique, c.
cobalt (Co)
bleomycin (Co-57)
eye plaque (Co-60)
isotope (Co-60)
ophthalmic applicator (Co-60)
teletherapy unit (Co-60)
markers, c.
moving strip, c.
single x-ray beam, c. (Co-60)
cobaltous chloride Co 57
cobaltous chloride Co 60
cobblestone mucosa
Cobb method
Cobra 2 catheter
coccidioidal
coccidioidin
coccidioidomycosis
coccygeal
arteries, c.
body, c.
cornua, c.
gland, c.
nerve, c.
plexus, c.
vertebrae, c.

Additional Entries

coccygeus muscle
coccygodynia
coccyx
cochlea
  aqueduct of c.
  cupula of c.
  lamina spiralis ossea, c.
  modiolus of c.
  scalae of c.
  spiral canal of c.
  vessels of c.
cochlear
  artery, c.
  nerve, c.
  nuclei, c.
  otosclerosis, c.
  root of acoustic nerve, c.
cochleariform process
cochleovestibular
cock-up splint
coded aperture collimator system
Codman's triangle
coefficient
cognitive
  ability, c.
  functioning, c.
cog-tooth of malleus
cogwheel
  rigidity, c.
coherent
  light, c.
  scattering, c.
cohesion
cohesive
Cohnheim's areas
coil
  crossed c.
  Golay c.
  gradient c.
  Helmholtz c.
  receiver c.

coil *(continued)*
  RF (radiofrequency) c.
  shim c.
  solenoid c.
  surface c.
coiled position
coin
  lesion of lung, c.
coincidence
  loss, c.
  peak, c.
cold
  clammy skin, c. and
  cautery, c.
  compress, c.
  knife conization, c.
  lesion, c.
  light, c.
  nodule, c.
  spot, c.
  thyroid nodule, c.
coleocele
coleocystitis
colic
  arteries, c.
  biliary c.
  flexure, c.
  impression, c.
  renal c.
  ureteral c.
  valve, c.
colicky
  pain, c.
coliform
colinephritis
colitis
  acute pseudomembranous c.
  amebic c.
  antibiotic-associated c.
  bacterial c.
  cystica profunda, c.

Additional Entries

colitis *(continued)*
fulminating c.
granulomatous c.
ischemic c.
parasitic c.
pseudomembranous c.
radiation c.
regional c.
segmental c.
transmural c.
ulcerative c.
collagenic fibers
collagenoblast
collagenocyte
collagenogenic
collagenous
collagen vascular disease
collapse
circulatory c.
lung c.
massive c.
periosteal c.
peripheral vascular c.
right lower lobe c.
vertebral c.
collar
bone, c.
brace, c.
cervical c.
incision, c.
collarette
Biet, c. of
collateral
circulation, c.
eminence, c.
fissure, c.
ganglia, c.
ligament, c.
vessels, c.
collateralization
collecting
duct, c.

collecting *(continued)*
system, c.
tubes, c.
tubules, c.
Colles'
fascia, C.
fracture, C.
splint, C.
colliculi
inferior c.
superior c.
colliculus
arytenoid cartilage, c. of
facialis c.
inferior c.
nervi optici c.
superior c.
collimated
collimator
assembly, c.
face, c.
light, c.
rotational c.
collodion
colloid
cyst, c.
goiter, c.
scan, c.
shift, c.
colloidal
198 Au, c.
barium sulfate, c.
gold, c.
32P, c.
collum
anatomicum humeri, c.
distortum, c.
mallei, c.
tali, c.
valgum, c.
coloboma
colohepatopexy

Additional Entries

colon
- abnormality, intrinsic c.
- ascending c.
- conduit, c.
- cut-off sign, c.
- deformity, extrinsic c.
- descending c.
- diverticula of sigmoid c.
- haustra of c.
- haustral markings of c.
- hepatic flexure of c.
- iliac c.
- iliac flexure of c.
- irritable c.
- left c.
- nerves of c.
- pelvic c.
- proximal c.
- resection of c.
- right c.
- sigmoid c.
- spasm of c.
- spastic c.
- splenic flexure of c.
- transverse c.
- tunica mucosa of c.
- tunica muscularis of c.
- tunica serosa of c.
- vessels of c.

colonalgia

colonic
- angiodysplasia
- interposition syndrome, c.
- mucosa, c.
- obstruction, c.
- polyp, c.

colonization
- bacterial c.

colonopathy

colonorrhagia

colonoscope

colonoscopy

colopexotomy

colopexy

colophony

coloplication

coloproctectomy

coloproctitis

coloproctostomy

coloptosis

color-coded image

color Doppler imaging

colorectal

colorectitis

colorectostomy

colorectum

colored
- clay c. stool
- lines of Retzius, c.
- straw c. fluid
- straw c. urine

colorless corpuscles

colorrhaphy

colorrhea

colosigmoidostomy

colostomy
- bag, c.
- closure of c.
- diverting c.
- double-barreled c.
- end-to-side c.
- functioning c.
- Hartmann's c.
- ileotransverse c.
- loop c.
- permanent c.
- sigmoid c.
- sigmoid loop c.
- stoma, c.
- transverse c.
- Wagensteen's c.

colostrum

colotomy

Additional Entries

colovaginal
colovesical
colpectomy
colpocele
colpoceliocentesis
colpoceliotomy
colpocleisis
colpocystitis
colpocystocele
colpocystoplasty
colpocystotomy
colpocystoureterocystotomy
colpocytogram
colpocytology
colpoepisiorrhaphy
colpohyperplasia
colpohysterectomy
colpohysteropexy
colpohysterorrhaphy
colpohysterotomy
colpomicroscope
colpomicroscopic
colpomicroscopy
colpomycosis
colpomyomectomy
colpoperineoplasty
colpoperineorrhaphy
colpopexy
colpoplasty
colpopoiesis
colpopolypus
colpoptosis
colporectopexy
colporrhagia
colporrhaphy
colporrhexis
colposcope
colposcopic
colposcopy
colpospasm
colpostat
colpostenosis
colpostenotomy
colpotherm
colpotomy
colpoureterocystotomy
colpoureterotomy
colpoxerosis
columella
  cochlea, c.
  fornicis, c.
  nasi, c.
columellae
column
  abdominal ring c.
  anal c.
  anterior fauces, c. of
  barium c.
  Bertin, c. of
  cervical Pantopaque c.
  Clarke, c. of
  fornix, c. of
  lumbar Pantopaque c.
  medulla spinalis, c. of
  Pantopaque c.
  rectal c. of Morgagni
  renal c.
  spinal c.
  vagina, c. of
  vertebral c.
columna
  anterior medullae spinalis, c.
  autonomica medullae spinalis, c.
  dorsalis medullae spinalis, c.
  fornicis, c.
  lateralis medullae spinalis, c.
  posterior medullae spinalis, c.
  vertebralis, c.
columnae carneae

Additional Entries

columnar
epithelium, c.
lined esophagus, c.
coma
alcoholic c.
diabetic c.
hepatic c.
hypoglycemic c.
irreversible c.
Kussmaul's c.
metabolic c.
prehepatic c.
comatose
Comberg contact lens
combination duplicator/subtractor
combined
abdominoperineal resection, c. (CAPR)
hemorrhoids, c.
left lateral view, c.
liver-lung imaging, c.
comedocarcinoma
comedogenic
comma-shaped fasciculus
comminuted fracture
commissura laborum anterior
commissura palpebrarum lateralis
commissura palpebrarum medialis
commissural fibers of cerebral hemispheres
commissure (s)
anterior c.
brain c.
corpus callosum, c. of
Gudden c.
habenular c.
hippocampal c.
labia majora, c. of
commissure (s) *(continued)*
medulla spinalis, c. of
middle c.
optic c.
palpebral c.
posterior c.
supraoptic c.
commissurorrhaphy
aortic c.
mitral c.
pulmonary c.
tricuspid c.
commissurotomy
committed stem cell (CSC)
common
atrium, c.
atrioventricular valve, c.
bile duct, c.
carotid artery, c.
dental germ, c.
duct exploration, c.
duct stone, c.
femoral artery, c.
hepatic tube, c.
iliac artery, c.
iliac lymph nodes, c.
iliac vein, c.
integument, c.
interosseous artery, c.
ligament, c.
peroneal nerve, c.
communicating
artery, c.
bursa, c.
hydrocephalus, c.
compact tissue
comparison
film, c.
view, c.
compartment
anterior tibial c.
medial c. of knee

Additional Entries ______________________

compartment *(continued)*
syndrome, c.
compartmentalization
compatible
compensated
cardiac status, c.
compensating filter
compensatory
atrophy, c.
emphysema, c.
hypertrophy, c.
competence
complete
abortion, c.
absence of pericardium, c.
amputation, c.
atrioventricular canal, c.
block, c.
bowel obstruction, c.
breech position, c.
clinical remission, c.
emptying of bladder, c.
heart block, c.
hemostasis, c.
left bundle branch block, c. (LBBB)
right bundle branch block, c.(RBBB)
complex
anomalous c.
antigen-antibody c.
atrial c.
auricular c.
echo, c.
factor IX c.
Golgi c.
immune c.
major histocompatability c.
mutliple spike c.
QRS c.

complex *(continued)*
RS c.
sonic liver mass, c.
symptom c.
ventricular c.
whole-body counting method, c.
complicated field block
complicated plaque
complication shunt
component
anterior c.
anxiety c.
articular c.
brain wave c.
variable c.
composite
graft, c.
compound
comminuted fracture, c.
dislocation, c.
fracture, c.
ganglion, c.
joint, c.
nevus, c.
compress
cold c.
dry c.
hot moist c.
compression
bandage, c.
bulky c. dressing
carotid c.
cerebral c.
cord c.
deformity c.
digital c.
dressing, c.
external c.
extrinsic c.
fracture of spine, c.
soft tissue c. injury

Additional Entries ______________________

compression *(continued)*
- median nerve c.
- nerve root c.
- spinal cord c.
- type deformity, c.
- umbilical cord c.

compressor naris muscle
compromised host
Compton
- effect, C.
- electrode, C.
- interactions, C.
- pre-detector scatter, C.
- process, C.
- scatter, C.
- -scattered photons, C.

computation of beams
computed
- axial tomography, c. (CAT) scan
- reconstruction, c.
- transmission tomography, c.

computer-enhanced nuclear scan
computerized
- tomography, c. (CT)
- transverse axial tomography, c. (CTAT)

concatenate
concatenation
concave
- mirror, c.
- socket, c.

concavity
- spine with scoliosis, c. of

concavoconcave
concavoconvex
concealed
- hemorrhage, c.

concentric
- atrophy, c.

concentric *(continued)*
- constriction, c.
- cylinder, c.
- hypertrophy, c.
- lesion, c.

concept
conception
- products of c.

concha
- auricula, c. of
- nasal c.
- nasalis inferior, c.

conchae
conchal crest
conchiform
conchoscope
conchotome
conchotomy
concussion
- abdominal c.
- brain c.
- cerebral c.

condensing osteitis
conductance
conduction
- aberrant c.
- abnormality, c.
- air c.
- anomalous c.
- bone c.
- cardiac c.
- deafness, nerve c.
- defect, c.
- delayed c.
- disturbance, c.
- intraventricular c. defect
- myocardial c. defect
- studies, c.
- system, catrioventricular c.
- velocity, motor nerve c.
- ventricular c.

Additional Entries

conductive heating
condylar
    joint, c.
condyle
    femoral c.
    mandible, c. of
    medial c.
    occipital c.
    tibial c.
condyloid
    articulation, c.
    canal, c.
    foramen, c.
    fossa, c.
    process of mandible, c.
cone
    biopsy, c.
    bipolars of retina, c.
    projection, c.
    retinal c.
    shaped orbit, c.
coned
    down view, c.
    lateral view, c.
    left lateral view, c.
    projection
configuration
confluence
    nodules, c. of
    sinuses, c. of
confluent
    rash, c.
    shadows, c.
congenital
    absence, c.
    anomaly, c.
    atresia, c.
    cleft palate, c.
    cyst, c.
    defect, c.
    disease, c.
    dislocation, c.
congenital *(continued)*
    fistula, c.
    heart disease, c.
    hernia, c.
    hip dislocation, c.
    immunity, c.
    lesion, c.
    lung hernia, c.
    malformation, c.
    myocarditis, c.
    megacolon, c.
    polycystic kidney, c.
    syphilis, c.
congested
congestion
    active c.
    bronchial c.
    chronic passive c.
    interstitial c.
    nasal c.
    pulmonary c.
    upper respiratory c.
    vascular c.
    venous c.
congestive
    failure, c.
    glaucoma, c.
    heart failure, c. (CHF)
conglomerate
congruence angle
conical catheter
conical papillae
conization
    cold knife c.
    cervical c.
    electrocautery c.
conjoined
    tendon, c.
conjugate
    diagonal c.
    diameter of pelvic inlet, c.

Additional Entries

conjugate *(continued)*
  diameter of pelvis, c.
  eye movements, c.
  gaze, c.
  measurements, c.
conjunctiva
  bulbar portion of c.
  caruncle lacrimalis c.
  fornix c.
  lacus lacrimalis c.
  palpebral portion of c.
  plica semilunaris c.
connecting fibrocartilage
connective
  tissue, c.
    areolar c.t.
    fibrous c.t.
    loose c.t.
    tubing, c.
connector
Conn's syndrome
conoid
  ligament, c.
  tubercle, c.
Conradi's line
Conray-30
Conray-43
Conray-325
Conray-400
consciousness
  altered state of c.
  clouding of c.
  impaired c.
  lapses of c.
  loss of c.
  threshold of c.
  transient loss of c.
consistency
  doughy c.
  nodular c.
  uniform c.
constant potential
constricted
  blood vessels, c.
  pupils, c.
constricting
  lesion, c.
constriction
  apical c.
  concentric c.
  deformity, c.
constrictive
  pericarditis, c.
  ring, c.
constrictor
  pharyngis, c.
  urethrae muscles, c.
contact
  jelly, c.
  paste, c.
content
  abdominal c.
  bowel c.
contiguous
continence
  fecal c.
  urinary c.
continuous
  drainage, c.
  echo Doppler, c.
  irrigation, c.
  lesion, c.
  monitoring, c.
  positive pressure airway, c.
  positive pressure breathing (CPPB), c.
  remission, c.
  wave argon laser, c.
  wave (CW) ultrasound, c.
Contour Fabricators, Inc.
contra-angle
contra-aperture

Additional Entries

contracted
bladder, c.
cecum, c.
pooling, c.
contraction
active c.
anodal c.
atrial c.
Braxton Hicks c.
Dupuytren's c.
nodal premature c.
PAC (premature atrial) c.
paroxysmal c.
premature atrial c.
premature auricular c.
right ventricular c.
supraventricular premature c.
tertiary c.
contracture
abduction c.
adduction c.
bladder neck c.
Dupuytren's c.
flexion c.
vesical neck c.
Volkmann's c.
contralateral
chain, c.
node, c.
contrast
agent warmer, c.
barium enema, air-c.
border, c.
column, c.
double c. visualization
enema, c.
echocardiography, c.
enhancing mass, c.
esophagoscopy, c.
gastrointestinal study, c.
contrast *(continued)*
filled vessels, c.
laryngography-pharyngography, c.
material, c.
media, c.
soaked tampon, c.
study, c.
visualization, double c.
contrecoup fracture
control
biopsy under x-ray c.
bladder c.
infectious diseae c.
measures, c.
pneumatic tourniquet c.
contused lung
contusion (s)
cerebral c.
lung c.
conus
arteriosus, c.
distraction, c.
elasticus, c.
medullaris, c.
conventional generator
convergent ray
converging
hole, c.
collimator, c.
convex
lens, c.
surface, c.
convexity
lens, c. of
spine with scoliosis, c. of
convoluted
tubes of kidney, c.
tubules, c.
convolution
callosal c.
frontal c.

Additional Entries ______________________

convolution *(continued)*
 occipitotemporal c.
 parietal c.
convolutional
 atrophy, c.
 markings, c.
Cook JB2 catheter
Coolidge vacuum tube
cooling curve
Cooper's ligament
COPD (chronic obstructive pulmonary disease)
Cope
 bronchography, C.
 cutting needle, C.
 loop catheter, C.
 needle, C.
 nephrostomy tube, C.
 outfit needle, C.
copious
 bleeding, c.
 drainage, c.
 lavage of wound, c.
 mucoid material, c.
co-planer set-up
copper seeds
copper (Cu)
copper-7 (IUD) intrauterine device
copula
cor
 pulmonale, c.
 triatriatum, c.
coracoacromial
 ligament, c.
coracobrachialis muscle
coracoclavicular
 fascia, c.
 ligament, c.
coracohumeral
 ligament, c.
coracoid
coracoid *(continued)*
 notch, c.
 process of scapula, c.
 tuberosity, c.
coracoiditis
coracoradialis
coracoulnaris
60 Co radioisotope
coralliform
cord
 compression, c.
 decompression, spinal c.
 gangliated c.
 genital c.
 false vocal c.
 heel c. lengthening
 palpable venous c.
 spermatic c.
 spinal c.
 spinal c. decompression
 stripping, vocal c.
 structures, c.
 true vocal c.
 umbilical c.
 vocal c.
 vocal c. nodule
 vocal c. stripping
cordal
cordate
cordectomy
cordiform
Cordis
 Injector I, C.
 Injector II, C.
 lymphography injector, C.
corditis
core
coreoplasty
Cormed infusion pump
cornea
 abrasion of c.

Additional Entries

corneal
corpuscles, c.
endothelium, c.
epithelium, c.
spaces, c.
transplant, c.
trauma indicator, c.
tube, c.
Cornelia de Lange's syndrome
corneoscleral
cornified pearls
cornu
Ammonis, c.
anterius medullae spinalis, c.
coccyx, c.
cutaneum, c.
ethmoid c.
posterius medullae spinalis, c.
cornua
coccyx, c. of
hyoid bone, c. of
lateral ventricles, c. of
majora, c.
minora, c.
sacrum, c. of
thyroid cartilage, c. of
cornual
portion of uterus, c.
cornuate
cornucommissural
corona
glandis, c.
radiata, c.
Zinn's c.
coronal
arc, c.
image, c.
plane, c.
projection, c.
coronal *(continued)*
section, c.
sulcus, c.
suture, c.
view, c.
coronary
angiogram, c.
arteries, c.
arteriogram, c.
arteriography, selective c.
arteriosclerosis, c.
artery byass graft, c. (CABG)
artery occlusive disease, c.
atherosclerosis, c.
blood flow, c.
bypass procedure, c.
cineangiography, c.
circulation, c.
embolism, c.
insufficiency, c.
ligament, c.
loop catheter, c.
occlusion, c.
plexus, c.
sinus, c.
sinus anomaly, c.
sinus ostium, c.
stomach, c. of
sulcus of heart, c.
thrombosis, c.
vein of stomach, c.
veins of heart, c.
coronoid
fossa, c.
process, c.
corpora
arantii, c.
atretica, c.
bigemina, c.

Additional Entries ______________________________

____

____

cor pulmonale
corpus
callosum, c.
callosum lipoma, c.
cavernosography, c.
cavernosum, c.
ciliare, c.
femoris, c.
fibulae, c.
geniculatum laterale, c.
geniculatum mediale, c.
Highmori, c.
humeri, c.
incudis, c.
luteum, c.
luteum cyst, c.
luteum, hemorrhagic, c.
maxillae, c.
ossis hyoidei, c.
oss. ilii, c.
ossis ischii, c.
ossis pubis, c.
penis, c.
radii, c.
spongiosum, c.
sterni, c.
striatum, c.
tali, c.
tibiae, c.
ulnae, c.
uteri, c.
vertebrae, c.
vitreum, c.
corpuscles
blood c.
genital c.
Golgi c.
Grandry c.
granular c.
Hassall c.
corpuscles *(continued)*
Herbst c.
Mazzoni c.
Meissner c.
pacinian c.
renal c.
Ruffini c.
Wagner c.
correlation
clinical c.
time, c.
corrosive scarring
cortex (pl. cortices)
cerebellum, c. of
cerebral c.
cerebrum, c. of
kidney, c. of
lymph nodes, c. of
renal c.
sensory c.
suprarenal c.
Corti's
ganglion, C.
membrane, C.
cortiadrenal
cortical
arches, c.
atrophy, c.
bone, c.
bone graft, c.
calcification, c.
deafness, c.
defect, c.
desmoid, c.
echogenicity, c.
fracture, c.
function, c.
glomeruli, c.
graft, c.
hyperplasia, c.

Additional Entries ___

cortical *(continued)*
necrosis, c.
lesions, c.
opacification, c.
sulci, c.
thickness, c.
thinning, s.
cortices
corticifugal
corticipetal
corticoadrenal
corticoafferent
corticoautonomic
corticobulbar
tract, c.
corticocerebral
corticodiencephalic
corticoefferent
corticofugal
corticomedullary junction
corticomesencephalic
corticopenducular
corticospinal
tract, c.
corticosteroid
corticosuprarenaloma
corticothalamic
corticotropin
repository, c.
zinc hydroxide, c.
cosmesis
cosmic ray
costa
costae
costal
angle, c.
arch, c.
bone, c.
cartilage, c.
element, c.

costal *(continued)*
groove, c.
margin, c.
pleura, c.
process, c.
tuberosity, c.
costocentral
articulation, c.
costocervical
trunk, c.
costochondral
junction, c.
costocoracoid
ligament, c.
membrane, c.
costocoracoideus muscle
costomediastinal sinus
costophrenic (CP) angle
blunting of c. a.
costopleural
costopneumopexy
costoscapula
costoscapularis
costosternal
angle, c.
articulations, c.
costosuperior
costotransverse
articulations, c.
ligament, c.
costovertebral
angle, c. (CVA)
costoxiphoid
ligament, c.
C02 suture
cotton wool spots
cotyloid
cavity, c.
ligament, c.
coude' catheter

Additional Entries ______

coulomb (C)
coulombic forces
Coumadin
Councill
  catheter, C.
  nephrostomy, C.
counter pulsation
count ratio (C2/C1) method
coupling
  gel, c.
  spin, c.
Courvoisier
  gallbladder, C.
Coutard's x-ray irradiation method
cover plate
Cowper's
  glands, C.
  ligaments, C.
coxa valga hip deformity
coxa vara hip deformity
coxal articulation
Coyle's position
CP (costophrenic) angle
CPD (cephalopelvic disproportion)
cpm (cycles per minute)
cps (cycles per second)
CPU (central processing unit)
Cr (chromium)
crackling
  fine c. rales
cradle
cranial
  activity, c.
  arachnoid, c.
  bones, c.
  dura mater, c.
  fossa, c.
cranial *(continued)*
  pia mater, c.
  sympathetics, c.
  vault, c.
cranioacromial
cranioaural
craniobuccal
craniocaudad
  view, c.
craniocaudal
craniocerebral
cranioclast
craniofacial
  appliance, c.
  dystocia, c.
craniograph
craniography
craniometaphyseal dysplasia
craniometer
craniopharyngeal
  spasm, c.
craniopharyngeus
craniopharyngioma
craniophore
cranioplasty
craniopuncture
craniosclerosis
cranioscopy
craniospinal
craniostenosis
craniosynostosis
craniotomy
craniotonoscopy
craniotopography
cranium
  bifidum occultum, c.
crater
  active ulcer c.
51 Cr chromium
  51 Cr labeling

Additional Entries

CRE (cumulative radiation effect)
crease
 inframammary c.
 nasolabial c.
creeping thyroiditis
cremaster
cremasteric
 artery, c.
 fascia, c.
 muscle, c.
crescentic mass
crescents of Gianuzzi
crescendo murmur
crest (s)
 ampullary c.
 basilar c.
 conchal c.
 ethmoidal c.
 frontal c.
 iliac c.
 incisor c.
 infratemporal c.
 infundibuloventricular c.
 internal occipital c.
 intertrochanteric c.
 lacrimal c.
 maxillary c.
 nasal c.
 neural c.
 obturator c.
 occipital c.
 palatine c.
 pubic c.
 right atrial c.
 sphenoidal c.
 supinator c.
 supramastoid c.
 tibial c.
 trochanteric c.
crests (s) *(continued)*
 of tubercles, c.
 urethral c.
 vestibular c.
cretinism
cribriform
 fascia, c.
 plate of ethmoid, c.
cricoarytenoideus
 lateralis muscle, c.
 posterior muscle, c.
cricoarytenoid
 ligament, c.
 muscles, c.
cricoid
 cartilage, c.
cricopharyngeal
cricothyroid
 artery, c.
 ligament, c.
 membrane, c.
 muscle, c.
cricotracheal
 ligament, c.
 space, c.
cri-du-chat syndrome
crimping tool
Crisp and Gosevek weighted retractor
crista
 acustica, c.
 ampullaris, c.
 anterior fibulae, c.
 colli costae, c.
 falciformis, c.
 galli, c.
 temporalis, c.
 vestibuli, c.
CRL (crown rump length)
Crohn's disease

Additional Entries

Cronkhite-Canada syndrome
Crookes' vacuum tube
cross
    anteroposterior recumbent position, c.
    clamping of aorta, c.
    sectional echocardiography, c.
    sectional projection, c.
    sectional views, c.
    table lateral decubitus view, c.
    table lateral simulator film, c.
    table lateral view, c.
    table oblique view, c.
crossed
    coil design, c.
    commissural fibers, c.
    filling, c.
    grid, c.
    pyramidal tract, c.
    renal ectopia, c.
crosshairs alignment
crosshatched areas
crosshatching
crossing
    arteriovenous (AV) c.
    needles, c.
crossover pattern
cross-sectional echocardiography
cross-sectional view
cross-table lateral view
Crouzon syndrome
crown
    resorption, c.
    rump length, c.(CRL)
    rump measurement, c.
    tooth, c. of
crowning
    infant's head, c. of
CRT (cathode ray tube)
crucial
    anastamosis, c.
    ligament, c.
cruciate
    crural ligament, c.
    eminence of occipital bone, c.
    incision, c.
    ligament, c.
    ligament of atlas, c.
    ligaments of knee, c.
cruciform
crura
    diaphragm, c. of
    fornix, c. of
    penis, c. of
    stapes, c. of
    subcutaneous inguinal ring, c. of
crural
    arch, c.
    fascia, c.
    ligament, c.
    nerve, c.
    septum, c.
    sheath, c.
crureus muscle
crus
    fornicis, c.
crush injury
crusta
    cerebral peduncle, c. of
Cruveilhier
    atrophy, C.
    glenoid ligaments of C.
    fascia, C.
crux (pl. cruces)

Additional Entries ______________________

crux (pl. cruces) *(continued)*
heart, c. of the
cryesthesia
crymodynia
cryoanalgesia
cryocardioplegia
cryocautery
cryoextraction
cryohypophysectomy
cryometer
cryopathy
cryoprobe
cryoprotective
cryoscope
cryosectional anatomy
cryostat
cryosurgery
cryothalmectomy
cryotherapy
cryotolerant
crypt (s)
Luschka's c.
Lieberkuhn, c. of
cryptic
cryptitis
cryptodeterminant
cryptoempyema
cryptoglioma
cryptoleukemia
cryptolith
cryptomenorrhea
cryptophthalmia
cryptophthalmos
cryptopodia
cryptopyic
cryptoradiometer
cryptorchidectomy
cryptorchidism
cryptorrhea
crystal

crystal *(continued)*
configuration, c.
face, c.
scatter, c.
shape, c.
scintillation detector, c.
crystalline lens
cortical substance of c. l.
nucleus of c.l.
Cs (cesium)
137 Cs. isotope, c.
needle, c.
tube, c.
CSC (committed stem cell)
CSF (cerebrospinal fluid)
C-shaped border
C-shaped configuration
CsI (cesium iodide)
137 Cs isotope
needle, 137 Cs
teletherapy unit, 137 Cs
tube, 137 Cs
CT (computerized tomography) scan
cine CT scan
directed biopsy, CT
enhanced CT scan
guided biopsy, CT
metrizamide enhanced CT
millisecond CT scan
number display, CT
scout image, CT
CTAT (computerized transverse axial tomography)
C15–02 technique
cTNM (clinical diagnostic staging)
CT x-ray tube
Cu (copper)

Additional Entries

Cuatico needle
cubic centimeter (cc.)
cubic millimeter (cu.mm.)
cubicle
cubital
  tunnel syndrome, c.
  vein, c.
cubitocarpal
cubitoradial
cubitus
cuboid
  bone, c.
cuboideonavicular articulation
cuff
  pneumatic c.
  vaginal c.
cuffing
cul-de-sac
  conjunctival c.
  Douglas c.
  free fluid in c.
  posterior c. of vagina
  uterine c.
  vaginal c.
culdocentesis
culdoscope
culdoscopy
culdotomy
culmen (pl. culmina)
  cerebelli, c.
cumbersome motions
cu. mm. (cubic millimeter)
cumulative radiation effect (CRE)
cuneate
  nucleus, c.
  tubercle, c.
cuneatus
cuneiform

cuneiform *(continued)*
  bone, c.
  cartilages, c.
  ligament, c.
  tubercle, c.
cuneocuboid
  articulation, c.
  joint, c.
cuneonavicular
cuneoscaphoid
cuneus
cuniculi
cup
  acetabular c.
  arthroplasty c.
  calyceal c.
  optic c.
cupped
cupping
  disc, c. of
  nerve, c. of
  optic c.
cupric acetate Cu 64
cupula
  cochlea, c. of
  pleura, c. of
cupulae
cupulogram
cupulolithiasis
cupulometry
curative
  resection, c.
curet
curettage
  cervical c.
  diagnostic c.
  dilatation and c.
  dull c.
  endocervical c.
  endometrial c.

Additional Entries ____________________

curettage *(continued)*
fractional c.
sharp c.
suction c.
vacuum c.
curie (Ci-unit of radioactivity)
curiegram
curie-hour
curietherapy
Curietron afterloading system
curioscopy
curium (Cm)
Curling's ulcer
current
curricula
curriculum
Curry intravascular retriever set
curvature
antrum, c. of
cervical c.
flattening of normal lumbar c.
greater c.
lesser c.
stomach, c. of
curve
stripping technique, c.
curved
biopsy forceps, c.
forceps, c.
laryngeal cannula, c.
needle, c.
curves of vertebral column
curvilinear
calcifications, c.
echogenic structure, c.
incision, c.
cushingoid
cushingoid *(continued)*
facies, c.
Cushing's
disease, C.
syndrome, C.
cushion (s)
auditory tube, c. of
endocardial c.
epiglottis, c. of
type ventricular septal defect, c.
cusp (s)
aortic c.
bicuspid valve c.
semilunar c.
tricuspid valve c.
cuspid
cuspidate
cuspides (sg.cuspis)
cuspis (pl.cuspides)
custom-made blocks
cut across tumor
cutaneous
cervical nerve, c.
external nerve, c.
internal nerve, c.
lesser internal nerve, c.
middle nerve, c.
nerves, c.
cutdown
arterial c.
venous c.
cuticle
root sheath, c. of
cuticula
dentis, c.
cuticulae
cuticulum
cutis (the skin)
laxa, c.

Additional Entries

cutis (the skin) *(continued)*
plate, c.
cutoff
cutting teeth
Cuvier
canal, C.
duct, C.
CVA (cerebrovascular accident)
CVD (cardiovascular disease)
CVP (central venous pressure) line
CW (continuous wave)
Doppler, CW
ultrasound, CW
cyanocobalamin Co 57
cyanocobalamin Co 60
cyanosis
clubbing and edema, c.
extremities, c. of
nailbeds, c. of
cyanotic
cyclectomy
cycle duration
cyclic
cyclocryotherapy
cyclodiathermy
cycloduction
cycloelectrolysis
cyclogram
cyclomastopathy
cyclophorometer
cyclophosphamide cystitis
cycloplegia
cycloplegic
cycloscope
cyclospasm
cyclostat
cyclotherapy
cyclothyme
cyclothymic
cyclotomy
cyclotron
radiation, c.
Cydex
cylinder
cast, c.
cylindrical
plug, c.
cylindrocellular
cylindroid
cylindroma
cylindromatous
cylindrosarcoma
cymba conchae
cymbiform
cynanthropy
cyogenic
cyotrophy
cyrtography
cyrtometer
cyst
adenocarcinoma, c.
apical c.
aspiration, c.
Baker c.
Bartholin duct c.
blue-dome c.
bronchial c.
bronchogenic c.
chocolate c.
corpus luteum c.
dermoid c.
embryonal c.
enteric c.
follicular c.
formation c.
functional ovarian c.
gastroenteric c.
hemorrhagic c.

Additional Entries

cyst *(continued)*
inclusion c.
lutein c.
meibomian c.
morgagnian c.
multiloculated c.
multilocular c.
nabothian c.
neurenteric c.
ovarian c.
paranephric c.
parapelvic c.
parovarian c.
peripelvic c.
pilonidal c.
pyelogenic c.
retention c.
sebaceous c.
simple c.
synovial c.
theca-luteum c.
tubo-ovarian c.
cystadenocarcinoma
cystadenoma
mucinous c.
serous c.
cystadenosarcoma
cystic
adenoma, c.
adenomatoid malformation, c.
artery, c.
astrocytoma, c.
breast, c.
cervicitis, c.
changes, c.
chronic c. cervicitis
disease of lung, c.
duct, c.
duct cholangiogram, c.

cystic *(continued)*
fibrosis, c.
hygroma, c.
medial necrosis, c.
neoplasm, c.
odontoma, c.
ovarian mass, c.
tumor, benign c.
vein, c.
cystica
cystitis c.
pyelitis, c.
ureteritis, c.
cysticolithectomy
cysticolithotripsy
cysticorrhaphy
cysticotomy
cystine
cystis
fellea, c.
cystitis
chronic c.
cystica, c.
glandularis, c.
hemorrhagic c.
interstitial c.
irradiation c.
cystitome
cystitomy
cystlike malformation
cystoblast
cystocarcinoma
cystocele
cystocolostomy
cystodiaphanoscopy
cystoduodenostomy
cystodynia
cystoelytroplasty
cystoenterocele
cystoepiplocele

Additional Entries

cystoepithelioma
cystofibroma
cystogastrostomy
Cystografin
cystogram
excretory c.
postvoiding c.
retrograde c.
voiding c.
cystography
air c.
double contrast c.
cystojejunostomy
Roux-en-Y c.
Cystokon
cystolith
cystolithiasis
cystolithic
cystoma
cystomatitis
cystomatous
cystometer
cystometrogram (CMG)
cystometry
cystomorphous
cystomyoma
cystomyxoadenoma
cystomyxoma
cystonephrosis
cystoparalysis
cystopexy
cystophotography
cystoplasty
cystoplegia
cystoproctitis
cystoprostatectomy
cystoproctostomy
cystopyelitis
cystopyelography
cystopyelonephritis
cystoradiography
cystorrhaphy
cystorrhea
cystosarcoma
cystosclerosis
cystoscope
cystoscopy
biopsy, c. and
fulguration, c. and
cystospasm
cystostaxis
cystostomy
cystotomy
cystourethritis
cystourethrocele
cystourethrogram
voiding c. (VCUG)
cystourethrography
chain c.
cystourethroscope
cytochrome oxidase enzyme system
cytocidal agent
cytocidal effect
cytoclasis
cytodiagnosis
cytodifferentiation
cytogenic
analysis, c.
cytogenous
cytology
ABC (aspiration biopsy c.)
aspiration biopsy c.
exfoliative c.
cytoma
cytomegalic inclusion disease
Cytomel
cytometer
cytometry

Additional Entries

cytonecrosis
cytopathic
cytopenia
cytophagous
cytophotometer
cytophotometric
cytophotometry
cytophylactic
cytophylaxis
cytoplasmically
cytosine arabinoside
cytoskeletal
cytoskeleton
cystostome
cytotherapy
cytotoxic
Czermak's spaces

Additional Entries

D

D (dose in cGy)
dacrycystalgia
dacryoadenalgia
dacryoadenitis
dacryoblennorrhea
dacryocanaliculitis
dacryocyst
dacryocystalgia
dacryocystectasia
dacryocystis
dacryocystitis
    acute d.
    chronic d.
    phlegmonous d.
    syphilitic d.
    trachomatous d.
    tuberculous d.
dacryocystitome
dacryocystoblennorrhea
dacryocystocele
dacryocystography
dacryocystoptosis
dacryocystorhinostenosis
dacryocystorhinostomy
dacryocystorhinotomy
dacryocystostenosis
dacryocystostomy
dacryocystosyringotomy
dacryocystome
dacryocystotomy
dacryogenic
dacryohelcosis
dacryohemorrhea
dacryolith
dacryolithiasis
dacryoma
dacryon
dacryopyorrhea
dacryopyosis
dacryorhinocystotomy
dacryorrhea
dacryoscintigraphy
dacryosinusitis
dacryosolenitis
dacryostenosis
dacryosyrinx
dactyledema
dactylogram
dactylography
dactylogryposis
dactylolysis
dactylomegaly
dactylophasia
dactyloscopy
dactylospasm
dactylosymphysis
Dalkon shield
Dalrymple's sign
Dandy-Walker
    cyst
    syndrome
dartos
    muscle, d.
    reflex, d.
    tunic, d.
dasymeter
Darwin, auricular tubercle of
daughter nuclide
decibel (db)
dead
    brain d.
    end, d.
    space, d.
    time, d.
De Bakey Type 1, Type 2, Type 3
debris
    amorphous d.
    cell d.
    cholesteatoma d.

Additional Entries ______________________

____

____

debris *(continued)*
desquamating d.
necrotic d.
debulking
decacurie
decagram
decalcification
decalcify
decaliter
decameter
decannulation
decay
characteristics, d.
constant, d.
deceleration
decentering
decerbellation
decerebrate
posturing, d.
rigidity, d.
decerebration
decerebrize
decidua
basalis, d.
capsularis, d.
menstrual d.
parietalis, d.
placentalis, d.
stratus compactum of d.
stratum spongiousum of d.
unaltered or boundary layer of d.
vera d.
decidual
cast, d.
cells, d.
retention of d. fragment
tissue, d.
deciduate
deciduoma
deciduous
deciduous *(continued)*
placenta, d.
teeth, d.
tissue, d.
decigram
deciliter (dl.)
decimeter
decompensation
abdominal d.
cardiac d.
carpal tunnel d.
cerebral d.
heart d.
median lobe d.
nerve d.
thoracic outlet d.
decompression
abdominal d.
cardial d.
carpal tunnel d.
cerebral d.
heart d.
median nerve d.
orbit, d. of
pericardial d.
spinal cord d.
thoracic outlet d.
deconvolution analysis
decortication
arterial d.
lung, d. of
renal d.
decreased nodal activity
decrescendo
murmur, d.
decubitus
care, d.
film, d.
position, d.
projection, d.
ulcer, d.
view, d.

Additional Entries

deep
abdominal ring, d.
artery of penis, d.
auricular artery, d.
cerebral veins, d.
cervical artery, d.
crural arch, d.
epigastric artery, d.
epigastric artery, d.
epigastric vein, d.
fascia, d.
femoral artery, d.
iliac circumflex artery, d.
iliac vein, d.
lingual artery, d.
muscle invasion, d.
muscles of back, d.
palmar arch, d.
peroneal nerve, d.
petrosal nerve, d.
plantar artery, d.
seated tumor, d.
stomal invasion, d.
suctioning, d.
sylvian vein, d.
temporal arteries, d.
temporal nerves, d.
transverse fascia of leg, d.
ulcer, c.
venous channel, d.
venous thrombosis, d.
defatted
defect
aortic septal d.
atrioseptal d.
birth d.
bony d.
congenital d.
extradural d.
extrinsic d.

defect *(continued)*
filling d.
interatrial septal d.
interventricular septal d.
intrinsic d.
lucent d.
mucosal d.
myocardial conduction d.
neurological d.
polypoid filling d.
segmental d.
visual field d.
deferent
duct, d.
defibrillation
atrial d.
electrical d.
ventricular d.
deficit
focal neurological d.
pulse d.
sensory d.
visual field d.
deformans
arteritis d.
arthrosis d.
endarteritis d.
osteitis d.
osteochondritis d.
spondylitis d.
deformity
Arnold-Chiari d.
bony d.
cloverleaf d.
compression d.
congenital d.
constriction d.
coxa vara d.
funnel d.
gibbous d.

Additional Entries ______________________________

____

____

deformity *(continued)*
gross d.
hallux valgus d.
inversion d.
Madelung's d.
metatarsus primus varus d.
pectus excavatum d.
pigeon breast d.
scar d.
silver-fork d.
skeletal d.
Sprengel's d.
swan-neck d.
trigger finger d.
valgus d.
varus d.
degeneration
ascending d.
congenital macular d.
cystic d.
ascending d.
disciform macular d.
fatty d.
fibrous d.
gray d.
hepatolenticular d.
macular d.
myxomatous d.
progressive lenticular d.
retinal d.
secondary d.f
spinal cord d.
spongy d. of central nervous system
Wallerian d.
degenerative
arthritis, d.
atrophy, d.
bone changes, d.
bone disease, d.
degenerative *(continued)*
cells, d.
changes, d.
disc calcification, d.
disease, d.
joint disease, d. (DJD)
spurring, d.
tic, d.
De George syndrome
deglutition
mechanism, d.
dehydrocholate sodium
Deiters'
cells, D.
nucleus, D.
Dejerine-Klumpke paralysis
Dejerine-Landouzy dystrophy
Dejerine-Lichtheim phenomenon
Dejerine-Sottas atrophy
delayed
complication, d.
conduction, d.
dentition, d.
emptying, d.
healing, d.
image, d.
suture fusion, d.
transfer flap, d.
union of fracture, d.
Delclos
applicator, D.
vaginal cylinder, D.
delineation of target volume
delivery
abdominal d.
breech d.
cesarean d.
forceps d.
full term, normal d.

Additional Entries ______________________

delivery *(continued)*
normal spontaneous d. (NSD)
spontaneous vaginal d.
DeLouche afterloading system
delta
activity, d.
bursts of d. activity
gap, d.
ray, d.
deltoid
ligament, d.
muscle, d.
tuberosity, d.
deltoideus muscle
DEM (diethyl maleate)
demeure catheter
demilunes of Heidenhain
demineralization
bony structures, d. of
demodulator
Demour's membrane
demyelinating disease
dendrite
dendrons
Denonvilliers'
aponeurosis, D.
fascia, D.
dens
axis, d.
scrotinus, d.
view, d. (of cervical spine)
dense
adhesions, d.
capillary blush, d.
enhancing, d.
nodule, d.
densimeter
densitometer
densitometry
density
calcified d.
ill-defined d.
increased d.
linear increase d.
nodular d.
pulmonary d.
radiolucent d.
radiopaque d.
soft tissue d.
spin d.
densography
dental
appliance, d.
artery, d.
canaliculi, d.
disclosing agent, d.
formulae, d.
furrow, d.
interproximal survey, d.
lamina, d.
nerve, d.
occlusal, d.
panoramic, d.
periapical, d.
pulp, d.
sac, d.
dentate
fissure, d.
gyrus, d.
ligament, d.
line, d.
nuclei, d.
suture, d.
dentes
canini, d.
decidui, d.
incisivi, d.
molares, d.
permanentes, d.
dentibuccal
dentigerous follicular cyst

Additional Entries

dentilabial
dentilingual
dentimeter
dentin
    bridge, d.
    intertubular d.
    secondary d.
dentinal
    canaliculi, d.
    fibers, d.
    matrix, d.
    sheath of Neumann, d.
    tubules, d.
dentinogenesis imperfecta
dentition
    deciduous d.
    delayed d.
    permanent d.
    precocious d.
    predeciduous d.
    primary d.
    retarded d.
    secondary d.
    transitional d.
dentoalveolar
dentoalveolitis
dentofacial
Denuce's ligament
denucleated
denudation
deossification
deoxyribonucleic acid (DNA)
Depage position
depopulation
dephase
depot
    fat d.
depression
    bone marrow d.
    congenital chondrosternal d.
    involutional d.

depression *(continued)*
    nasal bone d.
    involutional d.
    pacchionian d.
    postpartum d.
    reactive d.
    respiratory d.
depressomotor
depth
    dose, d.
    ionization, d.
    penetration, d. of
de Quervain's
    disease, d.
    thyroiditis, d.
derangement
    internal d. of knee
dermabrader
dermabrasion
dermad
dermal
    backflow, d.
    reactivity indicator, d.
    sinus, d.
dermatitis
    actinic d.
    ammonia d.
    herpetiformis d.
    radiation d.
    seborrheic d.
    stasis d.
    weeping d.
dermatoarthritis
dermatoautoplasty
dermatocele
dermatochalasis
dermatoconjunctivitis
dermatodysplasia
dermatofibroma
dermatofibrosarcoma
    protuberans, d.
dermatofibrosis

Additional Entries ________________

dermatograph
dermatographism
dermatoheteroplasty
dermatoid
dermatologic
dermatolysis
dermatome
    air-driven d.
dermatomegaly
dermatomere
dermatomycosis
dermatomyoma
dermatomyositis
dermato-ophthalmitis
dermatopathic
    lesion, d.
dermatopathology
dermatopathy
dermatophilosis
dermatophylaxis
dermatoplasty
dermatorrhagia
dermatorrhexis
dermatosclerosis
dermatosis
dermatosome
dermatoparaxis
dermatotherapy
dermic
    coat of hair follicle, d.
dermis
dermitis
dermograph
dermohygrometer
dermoid
    cyst of ovary, d.
dermoidectomy
dermolipoma
dermolysin
dermometer
dermomyotome
dermopathy
dermovascular
DES (diethylstilbestrol)
Descemet's membrane
descemetocele
descending
    aorta, d.
    colon, d.
    comma-shaped fasciculus, d.
    coronary artery, d.
    limb of Henle's loop, d.
    oblique muscle, d.
    palatine artery, d.
    process of lacrimal bone, d.
    ramus of hypoglossal nerve, d.
    ramus of ischium, d.
    ramus of os pubis, d.
    thoracic aorta, d.
DESC.FNC (descending facial nerve canal)
Deschamps needle
Desilets-Hoffman introducer
Desjardins' point
desmepithelium
desmethylmisonidazole (DMM)
desmid
desmocranium
desmography
desmohemoblast
desmoid
    tumor, d.
desmoma
desmoneoplasm
desmopathy
desmopexia
desmoplasia
desmoplastic
    fibroma, d.
desmopyknosis

Additional Entries

desmorrhexis
desmosome
desmotomy
desorption
desquamated
  cells, d.
  epithelium, d.
desquamation
destruction
  area of bone, d.
destructive
  phase, d.
detachable mini-silicone balloon
detached
  loose body, d.
  retina, d.
detachment
  medial meniscus, d. of
  retinal d.
  vitreous d.
detector
  array, d.
  efficiency, d.
  head of gamma scintillation camera, d.
  source geometry, d.
  surface, d.
  system, d.
deterioration
  macular d. of retina
dethyroidism
dethyroidize
detonation
detorsion
detrusor
  function, d.
  muscle, d.
  sphincter dyssynergia, d.
  urinae muscle, d.
deuterium
  oxide, d.
deuteron
deuteropathy
developmental
  arest, d.
  defect, d.
deviation
  abnormal left axis d.
  axis d.
  from normal, d.
  nasoseptal d.
  tongue d.
  tracheal d.
  ulnar d.
  ureters, d. of
device
  intrauterine d.
  IUD (intrauterine)
  metallic long screw fixation d.
  plate and screw fixation d.
dexter
dexterity
dextrad
dextral
dextrality
dextraural
dextrocardia
dextrocardiogram
dextrocerebral
dextroclination
dextrocular
dextrocularity
dextroduction
dextrogastria
dextrogram
dextrogyration
dextromanual
dextropedal
dextroposition
dextrorotatory
dextrosinistral

Additional Entries

diabetes insipidus
diabetic
    acidosis, d.
    cataract, d.
    coma, d.
    gangrene, d.
    ketoacidosis, d.
    neuritis, d.
    retinopathy, d.
diagnosis
    differential d.
    histological d.
    pathological d.
    presumptive d.
    provisional d.
    tissue d.
diagnostic
    curettage, d.
    laparoscopy, d.
    x-ray tube, d.
diagonal band of Broca
dialysis
    chromic ambulatory peritoneal (CAPD) d.
    chronic maintenance d.
    kidney d.
    maintenance d.
    peritoneal d.
    solution, d.
diamagnetic shift
diametaphyseal
diametaphysis
diameter
    anteroposterior (AP) d.
    bispinous d.
    cephalocaudal d.
    chest d.
    conjugate d.
    cranial d.
    extracanthic d.
    intercanthic d.
    pelvic d.
diameter *(continued)*
    pelvic inlet, d. of
    pupil, d. of
    transverse d. of heart
diamond-shaped dose distribution
diapedesis
diphanometry
diaphanoscope
diaphanoscopy
diaphoretic
diaphragm
    Akerlund spiral type d.
    Bucky d.
    Bucky-Potter d.
    dome of d.
    elevation of d.
    excursion of d.
    free air under d.
    leaves of d.
    level of d.
    lymphatic vessels of d.
    muscles of d.
    optic d.
    pelvic d.
    rupture of d.
    urogenital d.
    vaginal d.
diaphragma
    sellae, d.
diaphragmatic
    elevation, d.
    hernia, d.
    lymph nodes, d.
    pleura, d.
diaphragmatocele
diaphyseal
    sclerosis, d.
diaphyses
diaphysial
diaphysis
diaphysitis

Additional Entries

diaplacental
diaplasis
diaplastic
diapophysis
diapositive mask
diarthrodial
diarthroses
diarthrosis
diarticular
diaschisis
diascope
diascopy
diastalsis
diastaltic
diastasis
    recti abdominis, d.
diastatic
diastematocrania
diastematomyelia
diastolic
    blood pressure, d.
    blow, d.
    decrescendo murmur, d.
    gallop, d.
    gradient, d.
    murmur, d.
    pressure, d.
    thrill, d.
    volume, d.
diathermy
diatrizoate
    meglumine, d.
    sodium, d.
    sodium I 125, d.
    sodium I 131, d.
diatrizoic acid
dicephaly
diechoscope
dielectric
    heating, d.
    liquids, d.
diencephalon
diethylene triamine pentaacetic acid (DTPA) renal scan
diethyl maleate (DEM)
diethylstilbestrol (DES)
diffraction waves
diffuse
    atrophy, d.
    idiopathic skeletal hyperostosis, d. (DISH)
    infiltration, d.
    infiltrative process, d.
    intra-abdominal activity, d.
    nodular process, d.
    osteoporosis, d.
    peritonitis, d.
    pulmonary calcification, d.
    spasm, d.
    toxic goiter, d.
    type, d.
    pulmonary parenchymal disease, d.
    spasm, d.
diffused light
diffusely eroded
diffusion
    chamber, d.
    double d.
    gel, d.
digastric
    fossa, d.
    muscle, d.
    nerve, d.
    triangle, d.
digestion
    artificial d.
    gastric d.
    gastrointestinal d.
    intestinal d.
    organs of d.

Additional Entries ____________

digestion *(continued)*
- pancreatic d.
- peptic d.
- primary d.
- salivary d.

digit (s)
- articulations of d.
- joints of d.
- supernumerary d.

digital
- angiography, d.
- arteries, d.
- arteries of foot, d.
- arteries of hand, d.
- block anesthesia, d.
- compression, d.
- computed tomography, d.
- dilatation, d.
- epididymis, d. fossa of
- examination, d.
- femur, d. fossa of
- fluorography, d.
- fluoroscopic system, d.
- imaging, d.
- lateral plantar, d. nerve of
- magnetic resonance, d.
- median d. nerve
- musculocutaneous d. nerve
- nerve, d.
- radial d. nerve
- radiography, d.
- ray, d.
- subtraction angiography (DSA), d.
- ulnar d. nerve
- vascular imaging (DVI), d.
- vein, d.

digitalis

digitalis *(continued)*
- effect, d.
- toxicity, d.

digitalization

Digitron DVI/DSA computer

digitoplantar

digitus

dihydroxycholecalciferol

diiodotyrosine

dilatable tube

dilatation
- aneurysmal d.
- calyceal d.
- cervical d.
- collecting system, d.
- curettage, d. and
- digital d.
- effacement and d.
- esophageal d.
- urethral d.

dilated
- annulus, d.
- blood vessels, d.
- cervix, d.
- heart, d.
- loops of bowel, d.
- ventricle, d.
- ventricular chambers, d.

dilating balloon catheter

dilution factor

dimension

dimethylnitrosamine

dimethylsuccinic acid

dimercaptosuccinic acid (DMSA) renal scan

diminished
- breath sounds, d.
- reflexes, d.

diminution

Dimmer's keratitis

dimple

dimpling

Additional Entries

dimpling *(continued)*
skin d.
Diodrast
diohippuric acid I 125
diohippuric acid I 131
Dionosil
diopsimeter
diopter
dioptometer
dioptometry
dioptoscopy
diotyrosine I 125
diotyrosine I 131
DIP (distal interphalangeal) joint
diphenylhydantoin
diphenylhydramine hydrochloride
diphtheria toxin for Schick test
diplogram
diploic
space widening, d.
vein, d.
diploid
diplopia
binocular d.
heteronymous d.
homonymous d.
monocular d.
paradoxical d.
torsional d.
vertical d.
diplopiometer
diploscope
dipolar interaction
dipole
dipyramidole
direct
auscultation, d.
blue 1, d.
blue 53, d.

direct *(continued)*
catheterization, d.
cell kill, d.
cerebellar fasciculus, d.
extension, d.
invasion, d.
laryngoscopy, d.
needle puncture, d.
puncture, d. (DP)
ray, d.
retroperitoneal pneumography, d.
tract of Flechsig, d.
pyramidal tract, d.
x-ray method, d.
discernible radiolucent metal cement interface
discharge tube
discission
cataract d.
cervix uteri d.
lens, d. of
pleura, d. of
posterior d.
discission needle
discography
discoid
atelectasis, d.
lupus erythematosus, d.
meniscus, d.
discopathy
traumatic d.
discordant
discrete
lesion, d.
mass, d.
nodule, d.
discus
articularis, d.
disease
Acosta's d.
active parenchymal d.

Additional Entries ______

disease *(continued)*
active pulmonary d.
acute cardiovascular d.
acute infectious d.
acute respiratory d.
Adams-Stokes d.
Addison's d.
Albers-Schonberg d.
allogeneic d.
Almeida's d.
Alper's d.
alpha-chain d.
Alzheimer's d.
Apert-Crouzon d.
Aran-Duchenne d.
arterial occlusive d.
arteriosclerotic cardio-
vascular d.
Ayerza's d.
Bamberger-Marie d.
Banti's d.
Barlow's d.
Barraquer's d.
Basedow's d.
Bayle's d.
Bazin's d.
Bekhterev's d.
Behcet's d.
Berger's d.
Bernhardt's d.
Besnier-Boeck d.
Best's d.
Bielschowsky-Jansky d.
Biermer's d.
Blocq's d.
Bloodgood's d.
Blount's d.
Boeck's d.
Bornholm d.
Bowen's d.
Breda's d.
Bright's d.

disease *(continued)*
Brill's d.
Brill-Symmers d.
Brill-Zinsser d.
Buerger-Grutz d.
Busse-Buschke d.
Caffey's d.
caisson d.
California d.
Calve-Perthes d.
Camurati-Engelmann d.
Canavan's d.
cardiovascular renal d.
cat-scratch d.
celiac d.
Chagras-Cruz d.
Charcot-Marie-Tooth d.
Christian-Weber d.
Christmas d.
chronic granulomatous
d.
chronic obstructive pul-
monary d. (COPD)
chronic renal d.
Coats' d.
collagen d.
collagen vascular d.
communicable d.
complicating d.
Concato's d.
congenital d.
congenital heart d.
contagious d.
Cori's d.
coronary heart d.
Cowden's d.
coxsackievirus A. d.
Creutzfeldt-Jakob d.
Crigler-Najjar d.
Crohn's d.
Crouzon's d.
Cruveilhier's d.

Additional Entries

disease *(continued)*
Cushing's d.
cystine d.
cystic d.
cytomegalic inclusion d.
Darier's d.
Darling's d.
deficiency d.
degenerative disc d.
degenerative joint d.
Dejerine-Sottas d.
demyelinating d.
de Quervain's d.
Dercum's d.
Devic's d.
discogenic d.
diverticular d.
Duchenne's d.
Duchenne-Aran d.
Duhring's d.
Dukes' d.
Duplay's d.
Durand-Nicolas-Favre d.
Ebstein's d.
Economo's d.
Engelmann's d.
Erb's d.
Erb-Goldflam d.
Eulenburg's d.
extrapyramidal d.
Fabry's d.
Fahr-Volhard d.
familial d.
Fanconi's disease
Farber's d.
Feer's d.
fibrocystic d.
fifth d.
focal d.
Forbes' d.
Fordyce's d.
Fothergill's d.

disease *(continued)*
fourth d.
Fox-Fordyce d.
Frei's d.
Freiberg's d.
Friedlander's d.
Friedreich's d.
functional d.
functional bowel d.
Gamna's d.
Garre's d.
Gaucher's d.
Gee-Herter-Heubner d.
Gee-Thaysen d.
Gierke's d.
Gilbert's d.
Gilles de la Tourette's d.
Glanzmann's d.
Glisson's d.
glycogen storage d.
Goldflam's d.
Goldflam-Erb d.
graft-versus-host d.
Graves' d.
Greenfield's d.
Gull's d.
Gunther's d.
H d.
Hailey-Hailey d.
Hamman's d.
Hand's d.
hand-foot-and-mouth d.
Hand-Schuller-Christian d.
Hanot's d.
Hansen's d.
Hartnup's d.
Hashimoto's d.
heavy-chain d.
Heerfordt's d.
Heine-Medin d.
hemoglobin d.

Additional Entries ______________________

disease *(continued)*
hemolytic d.
Hers' d.
Heubner-Herter d.
hip-joint d.
Hippel's d.
Hippel-Lindau d.
Hirschsprung's d.
His-Werner d.
Hodgkin's d.
Hodgson's d.
hookworm d.
Hutchinson-Gilford d.
hyaline membrane d.
hydatid d.
hypertensive cardiovascular d.
Iceland d.
immune-compl,ex d.
infectious d.
inflammatory bowel d.
intercurrent d.
iron-storage d.
ischemic heart d.
Jensen's d.
Kawasaki d.
Kienbock's d.
kinky hair d.
Klippel's d.
Kohler's bone d.
Krabbe's d.
Kufs' d.
Kugelberg-Welander d.
Kummell's d.
Kussmaul's d.
Lafora's d.
Legg-Calve-Waldenstrom d.
legionnaires' d.
Leiner's d.
Leriche's d.
Letterer-Siwe d.

disease *(continued)*
Libman-Sacks d.
Lignac-Fanconi d.
Lindau's d.
Lindau-von Hippel d.
Little's d.
Lobstein's d.
Lowe's d.
Lutz-Splendore-Almeida d.
Madelung's d.
Majocchi's d.
maple bark d.
Marchiafava-Micheli d.
Marie's d.
Marie-Bamberger d.
Marie-Strumpell d.
Marie-Tooth d.
mast cell d.
Mediterranean d.
medullary cystic d.
Menetrier's d.
Meniere's d.
Merzbacher-Pelizaeus d.
Meyer's d
Mikulicz's d.
Milroy's d.
Minamata d.
Mitchell's d.
mixed connective tissue d.
Mobius' d.
Mondor's d.
Morquio-Ulrich d.
Morton's d.
Morvan's d.
mosaic d.
motor neuron d.
Nicholas-Favre d.
Niemann-Pick d.
Norrie's d.
occlusive vascular d.

Additional Entries

disease *(continued)*
Ollier's d.
Oppenheim's d.
organic brain d.
Ormond's d.
Osgood-Schlatter d.
Osler's d.
Osler-Vaquez d.
Owren's d.
Paget's d.
Parkinson's d.
Parrot's d.
Pel-Ebstein d.
Pelizaeus-Merzbacher d.
Pellegrini-Stieda d.
peptic ulcer d.
periodontal d.
peripheral vascular d.
Perthes' d.
Peyronie's d.
Pfeiffer's d.
Pick's d.
pink d.
polycystic d.
polycystic kidney d.
polycystic d. of ovary
Pompe's d.
Poncet's d.
Pott's d.
pulseless d.
Quincke's d.
Raynaud's d.
Recklinghausen's d.
Rendu-Osler-Weber d.
rheumatic heart d.
rheumatoid d.
Riggs' d.
Ritter's d.
Roger's d.
Rokitansky's d.
Sandhoff's d.
San Joaquin Valley d.

disease *(continued)*
Schamberg's d.
Scheuermann's d.
Schilder's d.
Schimmelbusch's d.
Schlatter-Osgood d.
Schonlein's d.
Schonlein-Henoch d.
Schuller's d.
Schuller-Christian d.
secondary d.
self-limited d.
serum d.
severe combined immunodeficiency d.
sickle cell d.
Simmonds' d.
sixth d.
Smith-Strang d.
Spielmeyer-Vogt d.
Stanton's d.
Still's d.
Stokes-Adams d.
storage d.
Strumpell-Leichtenstern d.
Strumpell-Marie d.
Sturge-Weber d.
Stuttgart d.
Sudeck's d.
Sutton's d.
Swift's d.
Tangier d.
Teschen d.
Thomsen's d.
thyrocardiac d.
thyrotoxic heart d.
trophoblastic d.
usual childhood d.
valvular heart d.
Vaquez's d.
venereal d.

Additional Entries ______________________

____

____

disease *(continued)*
  Vincent's d.
  Vogt-Spielmeyer d.
  Volkmann's d.
  von Hippel's d.
  von Jaksch's d.
  Willebrand's d.
  Waldenstrom's d.
  wasting d.
  Weber-Christian d.
  Weil's d.
  Werlhof's d.
  Wernicke's d.
  Westphal-Strumpell d.
  Whipple's d.
  white muscle d.
  Whitmore's d.
  Wilson's d.
  Winckel's d.
  Wolman's d.
DISH (diffuse idiopathic skeletal hyperostosis)
DISIDA (diisopropylacetanilide iminodiacetic acid/disofenin)
disintegrate
disk (disc)
  bulge, d.
  cervical d. syndrome
  choking of d.
  cupping of d.
  degenerative d. disease
  extruded d.
  herniated d.
  herniated intervertebral d.
  interpubic d.
  interspace, d.
  intervertebral d.
  lumbar d.
  lumbosacral d.
  margin, d.

disk (disc) *(continued)*
  Merkel tactile d.
  optic d.
  protrusion, d.
  ruptured d.
  sharp d.
  space, d.
  space narrowing, d.
  syndrome, cervical d.
  well-outlined d.
disintegration
diskiform
diskitis
diskogram
diskography
dislocation
dismemberment
disofenin
displaced labrum
displacement
  activity, d.
  fracture fragments, d. of
display zoom
disporous
disposition
disproportion
  cephalopelvic d.
dissecans
  osteochondritis d.
  osteochondrosis d.
dissect
dissecting
  aneurysm, d.
dissection
  and snare tonsillectomy, d.
  aortic d.
  blunt d.
  blunt and sharp d.
  finger d.
  sharp d.
  subperiosteal d.

Additional Entries ______________________

disseminated
    carcinoma, d.
    intravascular coagulation (DIC), d.
    melanoma, d.
dissimilate
dissimilation
dissipation
dissociation
    arteriovenous d.
    atrioventricular d.
    auriculoventricular d.
dissonance
distad
distal
    convoluted tubule, d.
    interphalangeal (DIP) joint, d.
    phalanges, clubbing of d.
    phalanx, d.
    small bowel, d.
distant site
distended
    abdomen, d.
    bladder, d.
    neck veins, d.
distention
    abdominal d.
    gaseous d.
    jugular vein d.
distichiasis
distobuccal
distobocco-occlusal
distobuccopulpal
distocervical
distoclination
distoclusion
distogingival
distolabial
distolabioincisal
distolingual
distolinguoincisal
distolinguo-occlusal
distolinguopulpal
disto-occlusal
disto-occlusion
distopulpal
distopulpolabial
distopulpolingual
distortion
distoversion
distress
    adult respiratory d. syndrome (ARDS)
    emotional d.
    epigastric d.
    fetal d.
    respiratory d.
    respiratory d. syndrome (RDS)
distribution
    Boltzmann d.
    gaussian d.
    inhomogeneous tracer d.
    nerve d.
    uniform d.
disuse
    atrophy, d.
diurese

diuresis
    tubular d.
diuretic renography
divergent ray
diverging
    collimator, d.
    hole, d.
diverticula (sg. diverticulum)
diverticular
diverticularization
diverticulectomy
diverticulitis
diverticulogram
diverticulopexy

Additional Entries

diverticulosis
diverticulum (pl.diverticula)
 bladder d.
 false d.
 Graser's d.
 Heister's d.
 intestinal d.
 intramural d.
 Kirchner's d.
 Meckel's d.
 Nuck's d.
 pharyngoesophageal d.
 pressure d.
 pulsion d.
 Rokitansky's d.
 scattered d.
 sigmoid colon d.
 traction d.
 Zenker's d.
diverting
 colostomy, d.
division (s)
 bronchi, d. of
 cells, d. of
dkg. (decagram)
dkl. (decaliter)
dkm. (decagram)
dl. (deciliter)
DLE (discoid lupus erythematosus)
Dmax (maximum dose)
DMM (desmethylmisonidazole)
DMSA (dimercaptosuccinic acid) renal scan
Dobbhoff tube
dog-ear effect
dog's ear sign
dog-leg technique
Dohle's disease
dolichocephalic
dolichocephaly
dolichomorphic
dolichopellic
dolichosigmoid
Dollinger's tendinous ring
dolorimeter
dolorimetry
dome
 blue d. cyst
 bladder, d. of
 diaphragm, d. of
 urinary bladder, d. of
domed cylinder
dominant
 circumflex coronary artery, d.
 left coronary artery, d.
 right coronary artery, d.
Donder's glaucoma
donor
 bone graft d.
 site, d.
Donovan bodies
Doppler
 carotid D.
 color D.
 continuous-echo D.
 effect, D.
 evaluation D.
 imaging, D.
 pulsed-wave (PW) D.
 shift, D.
 ultrasonography, D.
 ultrasound, D.
Doplette monitor
Dorno's ray
dorsa
dorsad
dorsal
 aortae, d.
 artery of penis, d.

Additional Entries

dorsal *(continued)*
- aspect, d.
- carpal artery, d.
- cutaneous nerves, d.
- elevated position, d.
- fissure of medulla oblongata, d.
- flap, d.
- indentation, d.
- interossei muscles, d.
- interosseous artery, d.
- interosseous nerve, d.
- lamina, d.
- lithotomy position, d. (dorsolithotomy)
- mesogastrium, d.
- metacarpal arteries, d.
- metacarpal veins, d.
- nasal artery, d.
- nerve, d.
- peripheral band, d.
- position, d.
- pulmonary nerves, d.
- recumbent position, d.
- reflex, d.
- rigid position, d.
- scapular nerves, d.
- slit, d.
- spinal artery, d.
- spine, d.
- surface, d.
- veins, d.
- venous arch, d.
- vertebrae, d.
- vestibular nucleus, d.

dorsiduct
dorsiflexion
dorsipalmar oblique view
dorsiplantar view
dorsispinal
dorsoanterior
dorsocephalad
dorsointercostaal
dorsolateral
dorsolithotomy
dorsolumbar
dorsomedian
- fissure of medulla oblongata, d.

dorsomesial
dorsonasal
dorsonuchal
dorsoposterior
dorsoradial
dorsosacral position
dorsoscapular
dorsoventrad
dorsoventral
dorsum
- ilii, d.
- linguae, d.
- nasi, d.
- scapulae, d.
- sellae, d.
- of tongue, d.

dose
- calculation, d.
- calibrator, d.
- correction algorithms, d.
- distribution, d.
- equivalent, d.
- increments, d.
- perturbation, d.
- profile half-width, d.
- reciprocity, d.
- reduction factor (DRF), d.
- survival curve, d.

dosimeter
dosimetric calculations
dosimetrist
dosimetry

Additional Entries ________________

dosimetry *(continued)*
film, d.
Dos Santos needle
dot brightnesses
Dotter intravascular retriever set
Dotter-Judkins technique
double
annihilation escape peak, d.
aortic arch, d.
armed mattress suture, d.
barreled colostomy, d.
contrast arthrogram, d.
contrast barium enema, d.
contrast media, d.
contrast study, d.
contrast visualization, d.
current catheter, d.
decidual sac, d.
dose technique, d.
emulsion film, d.
exposure technique, d.
footling presentation, d.
gutter guide, d.
inlet right ventricle, d.
lumen balloon catheter, d.
lumen balloon sheath catheter, d.
lumen tube, d.
outlet right ventricle, d.
peak bolus, d.
photon imaging, d.
photon scanner, d.
plane implant, d.
renal pelvis, d.
step gait, d.
uterus, d.
vision, d.
doubling time (DT)
doubly
bleeders d. clamped and ligated
doughnut
plane, d.
doughy
consistency, d.
Douglas'
cry, D.
cul-de-sac, D.
pouch, D.
Down syndrome
downsloping depression
doxorubicin
Doyere's eminence
DP (direct puncture or dorsipalmar)
dr. (dram)
drainage
bag, d.
capillary d.
catheter d.
continuous suction d.
incision and d. (I&D)
postural d.
system, d.
tidal d.
tube d.
underwater seal d.
dram (dr.)
draining lymph nodes
Dressler disease
Drew-Smythe catheter
DRF (dose reduction factor)
Drinker respirator
drip infusion nephrotomography
dromedary hump
dromograph
dromotropism
drop

Additional Entries

drop *(continued)*
- foot d.
- wrist d.

dropped
- periodic d. beat

drowned lung
drug-induced gastric erosions
drum
- ear d.

drusen
Druy stent
DSA (digital subtraction angiography)
DT (doubling time)
DTPA (99mTc-diethylene-triamine penta-acetic acid)
- aerosol lung imaging, DTPA

dual
- contrast, d.
- electron beam field, d.
- energy unit, d.
- foil system, d.
- photon absorptiometry, d.

Duchenne-Aran muscular atrophy
Duchenne-Erb paralysis
Duchenne-Landouzy dystrophy
duct (s)
- aberrant d.
- accessory pancreatic d.
- acoustic d.
- adipose d.
- alimentary d.
- allantoic d.
- alveolar d.
- archinephric d.
- arterial d.
- Bartholin's d.
- Bellini's d.

duct (s) *(continued)*
- Bernard's d.
- bile, common, d.
- bile, interlobular, d.
- biliary d.
- biliferous d.
- Blasius' d.
- Bochdalek's d.
- branchial d.
- bulbourethral glands, d. of
- canalicular d.
- cell carcinoma, infiltrated d.
- cervical d.
- choledochous d.
- chyliferous d.
- cloacal d.
- cochlear d.
- common bile d.
- common hepatic d.
- Coschwitz' d.
- cowperian d.
- craniopharyngeal d.
- Cuvier, d. of
- cystic d.
- cystic d. cholangiogram
- deferent d.
- dilatation of bile d.
- efferent d.
- ejaculatory d.
- endolymphatic d.
- exploration of common d.
- excretory d.
- frontonasal d.
- galactophorous d.
- gall d.
- Gartner's d.
- gasserian d.
- genital d.
- gutteral d.

Additional Entries ______________________

duct (s) *(continued)*
- Haller's aberrant d.
- Hensen's d.
- hepatic d.
- hepaticopancreatic d.
- hepatocystic d.
- hypophyseal d.
- incisive d.
- incisor d.
- injection, d.
- intercalated d.
- interlobular d.
- lacrimal d.
- lacrimonasal d.
- lactiferous d.
- Leydig's d.
- lingual d.
- Luschka's d.
- lymphatic d.
- mammary d.
- mammillary d.
- mesonephric d.
- metanephric d.
- milk d.
- mullerian d.
- nasal d.
- nasofrontal d.
- nasolacrimal d.
- nasopharyngeal d.
- nephric d.
- of Arantius d.
- of Botallo d.
- of bulbourethral gland, exretory, d.
- of Cuvier, d.
- of epididymis, d.
- of epoophoron, d.
- of epoophoron, longitudinal, d.
- of gallbladder, d.
- of His, d.
- of Muller, d.

duct (s) *(continued)*
- of Pecquet, d.
- of prostate gland, d.
- of Rivinus, d.
- of Santorini, d.
- of seminal vesicle, d.
- of seminal vesicle, excretory, d.
- of Steno, d.
- of testis, exretory, d.
- of Vater, d.
- of Wirsung, d.
- of Wolff, d.
- omphalomesenteric d.
- ovarian d.
- pancreatic d.
- pancreatic accessory d.
- pancreatic minor d.
- papillary d.
- paramesonephric d.
- paraurethral d.
- parotid d.
- perilymphatic d.
- primordial d.
- pronephric d.
- prostatic d.
- Rathke's d.
- Reichel's cloacal d.
- renal d.
- Rokitansky-Aschoff d.
- sacculoutricular d.
- salivary d.
- Schuller's d.
- secretory d.
- semicircular d.
- seminal d.
- Skene's d.
- spermatic d.
- sphincter muscle of bile d.
- Stensen's d.
- sublingual d.

Additional Entries

duct (s) *(continued)*
submandibular d.
submaxillary d.
suderiferous d.
sweat d.
tear d.
testicular d.
thoracic d.
thyroglossal d.
thyrolingual d.
umbilical d.
urogenital d.,
utriculosaccular d.
vitelline d.
vitellointestinal d.
Walther's d.
Wharton's d.
wolffian d.
ductal
cell carcinoma, infiltrating d.
dilatation, d.
ectasia, d.
hyperplasia, d.
papilloma, d.
pattern, d.
ductular
ductule
ductus
aberrans, d.
aberrans halleri, d.
Arantii, d.
arteriosus, d.
arteriosus, patent d.
arteriosus, reversed d.
biliferi, d.
choledochus, d.
cochlearis, d.
cowperi, d.
cuvieri, d.
cysticus, d.
deferens, d.

ductus *(continued)*
ejaculatorius, d.
endolymphaticus, d.
epididymidis, d.
epoophori longitudinalis, d.
excretorius glandulae bulbourethrales, d.
excretorius vesiculae seminalis, d.
glandulae bulbourethralis, d.
hepaticus communis, d.
hepaticus dexter, d.
hepaticus sinister, d.
incisivus, d.
interlobulares, d.
lacrimales, d.
lactiferi, d.
lingualis, d.
lobi caudati dexter, d.
lobi caudati sinister, d.
lymphaticus dexter, d.
mesonephricus, d.
Muelleri, d.
nasolacrimalis, d.
pancreaticus, d.
pancreaticus accessorius, d.
paramesonephricus, d.
paraurethrales, d.
parotideus, d.
perilymphatici, d.
prostatici, d.
reuniens, d.
semicirculares, d.
semicircularis anterior, d.
semicircularis lateralis, d.
semicircularis posterior, d.

Additional Entries ____________________

ductus *(continued)*
semicircularis superior, d.
spermaticus, d.
sublingualis major, d.
sublinguales minores, d.
submandibularis, d.
submaxillaris (Wharton), d.
sudoriferus, d.
thoracicus, d.
thoracicus dexter, d.
thyroglossus, d.
utriculosaccularis, d.
venosus, d.
Wolffi, d.
Duddell's membrane
Duhot's line
Duhring's disease
Duhrssen's incision
Dukes' classification
Dukes' disease
dullness
percussion, d. to
shifting d.
dumbbell
needle, d.
tumor, d.
dummy
ribbons, d.
seeds, d.
source, d.
wire, d.
dumping
syndrome, d.
Duncan's
folds, D.
position, D.
duodenal
atresia, d.
bulb and sweep, d.
cap, d.

duodenal *(continued)*
C-loop, d.
deformity, d.
fossae, d.
glands, d.
papilla, d.
scarring, d.
stump, d.
sweep, d.
ulcer, d.
duodenectomy
duodenitis
duodenocholangeitis
duodenocholecystostomy
duodenocholedochotomy
duodenocolic
duodenocystostomy
duodenoduodenostomy
duodenoenterostomy
duodenogastric reflux
duodenogram
duodenography
hypotonic d.
duodenohepatic
duodenoileostomy
duodenojejunal
flexure, d.
fold, d.
fossa, d.
duodenojejunostomy
duodenolysis
duodenopancreatectomy
duodenopyloric
constriction, d.
duodenorrhaphy
duodenoscope
duodenoscopy
duodenostomy
duodenotomy
duodenum
prompt spill into d.
second portion of d.

Additional Entries

duodenum *(continued)*
suspensatory ligament of d.
Duografin
duplex system
duplication
collecting system, d. of
kidney, d. of
Du Pont Cronex
duplicator subtractor, D.P.C.
printer, D.P.C.
subtraction film, D.P.C.
duplex ultrasound
duplicator
Dupre's disease
Dupuytren's
contracture, D.
dura
dural
ectasia, d.
membrane, d.
plate, d.
puncture, d.
sinus, d.
sac, d.
vascular supply, d.
dura mater
arteries of d.m.
brain, d.m. of
cranial d.m.
endosteal layer, d.m. of
meningeal layer, d.m. of
nerves, d.m. of
processes, d.m.
spinal cord, d.m. of
veins, d.m. of
venous sinuses, d.m. of
Durand's disease
Durand-Nicolas-Favre disease
duraplasty
Durck's nodes
Duret's lesion
Durham's tube
Duroziez' disease
Dutton's disease
Duverney's foramen
DVI (digital vascular imaging)
DVT (deep venous thrombosis)
dwarfism
achondroplastic d.
bird-headed d.
Dy (dysprosium)
dye
brilliant green d.
indigo carmine d.
radiopaque d.
residual d.
Dynamax 88 digital subtraction angiography x-ray tube
dynamic
flow study, d.
range, d.
rays, d.
dynamograph
dynamometer
dynamopathic
dynamoscope
dynamoscopy
dysarthria
dysarthric
dysarthrosis
dysautonomia
dyscephaly
dysequilibrium
dysfunctional
labor, d.
uterine bleeding, d.
dysgenopathy
dysgerminoma

Additional Entries

dysglandular
dyskinesia
    biliary d.

dyskinetic
    aneurysm, d.
    contraction, d.
    motion, d.
dysmenorrhea
    congestive d.
    essential d.
    inflammatory d.
    membranous d.
    obstructive d.
    primary d.
    secondary d.
    spasmodic d.
dysmyelinating disease
dysostosis
    cleidocranial d.
    craniofacial d.
    mandibulofacial d.
    metaphyseal d.
    multiplex d.
    orodigitofacial d.
dyspepsia
dyspeptic
dysperistalsis
dysphagia
dysphasia
dysplasia
    bronchopulmonary d.
    cervical d.
    diaphyseal d.
    epiphyseal d.
    epiphysealis hemimelica, d.
    focal d.
dysplasia *(continued)*
    mammary d.
    metaphyseal d.
    thymic d.
dyspnea
dyspneic
dysprosium (Dy)
dysrhythmia
dyssymmetry
dyssynergia
    detrusor-sphincter d.
dyssystole
dysthymia
dysthymiac
dysthyroid
dysthyroidism
dystocia
    fetal d.
dystonia
dystrophia
dystrophic
    calcification, d.
dystrophy
    Becker's muscular d.
    Duchenne's muscular d.
    Landouzy-Dejerine d.
    Leyden-Moebius d.
    limb-girdle muscular d.
    myotonic d.
    ocular muscle d.
    progressive muscular d.
    pseudohypertrophic muscular d.
    Salzmann's nodular corneal d.
dysuria
dysuric

Additional Entries

E

- Eagle-Barrett syndrome
- ear
  - canal, external e.
  - cauliflower e.
  - cavity, middle e.
  - external e.
  - internal e.
  - middle e.
  - outer e.
  - semicircular canals of e.
  - tympanic cavity of e.
  - vestibule of e.
- eardrum
  - injection of e.
  - retraction of e.
  - ruptured e.
- early
  - abortion, e.
  - changes, e.
  - collection, e.
  - diastolic murmur, e.
  - osteoarthritis, e.
  - satiety, e.
  - scleroderma, e.
  - venous drainage, e.
- Eastman Kodak
- easy
  - bruisability, e.
  - friability, e.
- Eaton-Lambert syndrome
- Eberstaller medial frontal sulcus
- Eberth's lines
- Ebner's fibrils
- Ebstein's
  - angle, E.
  - anomaly, E.
  - lesion, E.
- eburnation
- eburnitis
- EC (electron capture)
- ECAT (emission computer assited tomography)
- ecaudate
- ECC (electrocorticogram)
- eccentric
  - hypertrophy, e.
  - lesion, e.
- ecchondroma
- ecchymoma
- ecchymosis
- ecchymotic
- eccrine glands
- ECG (electrocardiogram)
- echinococcal cyst
- echo
  - amphoric e.
  - pattern, e.
  - metallic e.
  - planar imaging, e.
  - texture, e.
  - time, e.
- ECHO (echocardiography)
- echocardiogram
  - sector scan e.
  - two-dimensional (2–D) e.
- echocardiography
- echodense
- echoencephalogram
- echoencephalography
- echoencephalography
- echogenic
  - area, e.
  - foci, e.
  - material, e.
- echogenicity
- echogram
  - pelvic e.

Additional Entries ____________________

echography
echoic
echolucent
halo, e.
rim, e.
echopathy
echophonocardiography
echophony
echophotony
echopraxia
echorenography
echo
bright e.
spin, e.
strength, e.
time, e. (TE)
weak e.
Eck's fistula
Ecker's fissure
Ecker's fluid
eclampsia
puerperal e.
uremic e.
eclamptic
toxemia, e.
eclipse
ECOG performance status
Economo's encephalitis
ectasia
mammary duct, e. of
ectatic
ecterograph
ectethmoid
ectocardia
ectocervical
ectocervix
ectocolon
ectocolostomy
ectocondyle
ectocuneiform
ectocytic
ectoderm
ectodermal
dysplasia, e.
plate, e.
ectodermoidal
ectodermosis
ectogenous
ectoglobular
ectogony
ectolysis
ectomere
ectomesoblast
ectomorph
ectonuclear
ectoperitoneal
ectoperitonitis
ectopia
ectopic
activity, ventricular e.
beats, ventricular e.
calcification, e.
eruption, e.
fetal heart, e.
gastric mucosa, e.
insertion, e.
kidney, e.
ossification, e.
pacemaker, e.
pancreas, e.
pregnancy, e.
thyroid, e.
ureter, e.
ventricular activity, e.
ventricular beats, e.
ectoplasm
ectoplast
ectoscopy
ectostosis
ectotoxemia
ectrodactyly
ectrometacarpia
ectrometatarsia
ectrophalangia

Additional Entries

ectropion
ectrosis
ectrosyndactyly
eczema
contact e.
herpeticum e.
eczematization
eczematogenic
eczematoid
eczematous
eddy current
Edebohl's position (a/k/a Simon's position)
edema
angioneurotic e.
brain e.
brawny e.
cardiac e.
dependent e.
interstitial e.
nerve root e.
pedal e.
peripheral e.
pitting e.
pretibial e.
presacral e.
pulmonary e.
Quincke's e.
vasogenic e.
edematous
edentulous
Eder-Puestow metal olive dilator
edge
enhancement, e.
fimbriated e.
gradient, e.
liver e.
palpable liver e.
smooth liver e.
wound e.
eddy current
Edinger-Westphal nucleus
EDR (effective direct radiation)
edrophonium chloride
Edsall's disease
EDTA (ethylenediamine tetra-acetic acid)
EEG (electroencephalogram)
efface
effacement
additive e.
cervix, e. of
dilatation, e. and
effect
digitalis e.
Doppler e.
mass e.
sedative e.
side e.
Somogyi e.
therapeutic e.
traumatic e.
effective half-life
efferent
arteriolar dilatation, e.
arteriole, e.
artery, e.
duct, e.
glomerular artery, e.
loop, e.
nerve, e.
neuron, e.
vessels, e.
view, e.
efficacy
efflorescence
efflorescent
effluent
effluxing
ureteral orifices e. clear urine
effort

Additional Entries ______________________________

effort *(continued)*
  inspiratory e.
effusion
  bloody e.
  cardiac e.
  hemorrhagic e.
  joint e.
  knee joint, e. of
  malignant e.
  pericardial e.
  pleural e.
EG (esophagogastric) junction
Egan's technique
egersimeter
EGG (electrogastrogram)
eggshell calcification
eggshell-like
egobronchophony
EHBD (extrahepatic biliary duct)
Ehlers-Danlos syndrome
Ehrenritter's ganglion
EIA (electroimmunoassay)
Eichhorst's atrophy
Eichstedt's disease
E.I. du Pont De Nemours & Company
eighth nerve
eikonometer
Einhorn esophageal dilator
Eisenmenger
  anomaly, E.
  complex, E.
  syndrome, E.
ejaculator urinae muscle
ejaculatory ducts
ejection
  click, systolic e.
  fraction, e.
  murmur, e.
EKG (electrocardiogram)
elastic
  arteries, e.
  fibers, e.
  fibrocartilage, e.
  laminae of cornea, e.
  membrane of larynx, c.
elapsed timer
elasticity
elastofibroma
Elastoplast
elbow
  joint, e.
  tennis e.
elbowed catheter
Eldebohls' position (a/k/a Simon's position)
Eldorado 8 cobalt unit
electrical
  charge, e.
  discharge, e.
  energy, e.
  forces, e.
  stimulation response, e.
Electrical Musical Industries scan
electroacupuncture
electroanalgesia
electroaugmentation
electrobioscopy
electrocardiogram (ECG)
  borderline e.
  exercise e.
  gracing, e.
  serial e.
  stress e.
  treadmill e.
  12 lead e.
electrocardiograph
electrocardiography
electrocardiophonogram
electrocardiophonograph
electrocardioscopy

Additional Entries

Electro-Catheter Corporation
electrocautery
  Bovie e.
  unit, e.
electroincision
electrocochleograph
electrocochleography
electrocorticogram
electrocorticography
electrocystography
electrocystoscope
electrode
  active e.
  bipolar e.
  Bugbee e.
  calomel e.
  depolarizing e.
  disk-type surface e.
  exciting e.
  hydrogen e.
  internal e.
  impregnated e.
  indifferent e.
  internal e.
  nasopharyngeal e.
  negative e.
  pacemaker e.
  point e.
  positive e.
  ring-type surface e.
  silent e.
  therapeutic e.
  wire break, e.
electrodermal
electrodermatome
electrodesiccation
electrodiagnosis
electrodiagnostics
electroencephalogram (EEG)
  isoelectric e.
  normal waking e.
  sleep e.
electroencephalograph
electroencephalography
electroencephaloscope
electroexcision
electrofluoroscopy
electrogastroenterostomy
electrogastrogram
electrogastrograph
electrogastrography
electrogram
  His bundle e.
electrography
electrohysterogram
electrohysterography
electroimmunodiffusion
electrokinetic
electrokymogram
electrokymograph
electrokymography
electrolysis
electromagnetic
  decay, e.
  irradiation, e.
  radiation, e.
  spectrum, e.
  vibrations, e.
electromechanical injector
electrometer
electrometrogram
electromigratory
electromyogram (EMG)
electromyograph
electromyography
electron
  arc therapy, e.
  beam, e.
  beam dosimetry, e.
  beam flatness, e.
  beam symmetry, e.
  boost, e.
  capture, e.
  density, e.

Additional Entries ______

electron *(continued)*
energy, e.
field asymmetry, e.
gun, e.
linear accelerator, e.
microscopy, e.
spin, e.
stream, e.
volt, e. (eV)
electronegativity
electroneurography (ENG)
electroneurolysis
electroneuromyography
electronic
equilibrium, e.
linear accelerator, e.
subtraction, e.
summation device, e.
electronystagmogram (ENG)
electronystagmograph
electronystagmography
electro-oculogram
electro-oculography
electro-olfactogram
electro-osmosis
electroparacentesis
electrophoresis
electrophoretic
pattern, e.
electrophoretogram
electrophotometer
electroplexy
electroradiometer
electroresection
electroretinogram
electroretinograph
electroretinography
electroscission
electroscope
electrosection
electrospectogram
electrospectrography
electrospinogram
electrostatic
charge, e.
unit, e.
electrostenolysis
electrostethograph
electrostimulation
electrostriatogram
electrosurgery
electroureterogram
electroureterography
Elema-Schonander Mimer II
head unit, E.S.M. II
rotating chair, E.S.M. II
lymphography injector, E.S.M. II (Siemens-Elema AB)
eleoma
eleometer
eleoplast
elephantiasis
elevated
bladder flap, e.
diaphragm, e.
flap, e.
elevator
periosteal e.
eleventh nerve
Elliot's position
ellipsoid
approximation, e.
joint, e.
elliptic elongation
Ellis
compensator filter system, E.
filter, E.
formula, E.
line, E.
Ellis-Garland line
Ellis van Creveld syndrome
Eloesser flap

Additional Entries

elongation
aorta, e. of
correction, e.
Elschnig's bodies
Elscint Excel 905 scanner
Elsner's asthma
emaciated
Emax (maximum energy)
embarrassment
circulatory e.
respiratory e.
embolectomy
emboli
embolic
phenomena, e.
phenomenon, e.
occlusion, e.
origin, e.
thrombosis, e.
emboliform
embolism
air e.
cerebral e.
coronary e.
fat e.
inflective e.
miliary e.
paradoxical e.
pulmonary e.
embolization
embolus
fat e.
saddle e.
embryoblast
embryograph
embryography
embryoid
embryoma
embryonal
carcinoma, e.
cell, e.
cell carcinoma, e.

embryonal *(continued)*
cyst, e.
nephroma, e.
sarcoma, e.
embryonic
neural tube, e.
omphalomesenteric duct, e.
embryoniform
embryonization
embryopathy
rubella, e.
embryoscope
embryotome
embryotomy
embryotrophy
emesis
basis, e.
gravidarum, e.
EMG (electromyogram)
EMI scan (Electrical Musical Industries scan)
eminence
arcuate e.
articular e.
canine e.
cruciate e.
frontal e.
hypothenar e.
iliopectineal e.
iliopubic e.
intercondyloid e.
malar e.
medial e.
parietal e.
pyramidal e.
thenar e.
eminentia
arcuata, e.
articularis, e.
ossis temporalis, e.
pyramidalis, e.

Additional Entries ______________________

emissary
- vein, e.
- vessel, e.

emission
- CT scan, e.
- computer assisted tomography, e. (ECAT)
- computed tomography (ECT) scan, e.
- radiation, e. of

emitted radiation
Emmert-Gellhorn pessary
emotiomuscular
emotiovascular
emphysema
- atrophic e.
- bullous e.
- centrilobar e.
- hypoplastic e.
- interlobar e.
- interstitial e.
- intestinal e.
- lobar e.
- mediastinal e.
- obstructive e.
- of conjunctiva, e.
- pulmonary e.
- splanchnic vasculature e.
- subcutaneous e.
- surgical e.
- Swyer-James e.
- vesicular e.

emphysematous
- bleb, e.
- infection, e.
- pyelonephritis, e.

empty gestational sac
empty sella syndrome
empty vaginal cylinder
empyema
- interlobar e.
- loculated e.

empyemic
empyesis
empyocele
emulsion film
enamel cells
- droplet e.c.
- epithelium, e.c. of
- fibers of e.c.
- organs, e. c. of
- teeth, e.c. of

enanthema
enanthematous
enanthrope
enarthritis
enarthrosis
en bloc
- dissection, e. b.

encanthis
encapsulated
- abscess, e.
- collection, e.
- empyema, e.
- sessile implants, e.
- tumor, e.

encase
encasement of cardiac electrode
encephalalgia
encephalasthenia
encephalatrophy
encephalemia
encephalic
encephalitic
encephalitis
- acute disseminated e.
- herpes e.
- lead e.
- postinfection e.
- postvaccinal e.

encephalization
encephalo-arteriography
encephalocele

Additional Entries

encephaloclastic
encephalocoele
encephalocystocele
encephalodialysis
encephalodysplasia
encephalogram
encephalography
encephaloid
encephaloma
encephalomalacia
encephalometer
encephalomyelitis
  acute disseminated e.
  benign myalgic e.
  granulomatous e.
  postinfectious e.
  postvaccinal e.
encephalomyelocele
encephalomyeloneuropathy
encephalomyelopathy
encephalomyeloradiculitis
encephalomyeloradiculo-
 neuritis
encephalomyeloradiculopathy
encephalomyocarditis
encephalon
encephalonarcosis
encephalopathy
  biliary e.
  bilirubin e.
  hepatic e.
  hypernatremic e.
  lead e.
  myoclonic e.
  portal-system
  Wernicke's e.
encephalopuncture
encephalopyosis
encephaloradiculitis
encephalorrhagia
encephalosclerosis
encephaloscope
encephaloscopy
encephalosepsis
encephalosis
encephalospinal
encephalothlipsis
encephalotome
encephalotomy
enchondroma
enchondromatosis
enchondromatous
enchondrosarcoma
enchondrosis
enchylema
enchyma
enclave
enclitic
encranial
encranius
encyesis
encyopyelitis
encysted effusion
endangiitis
endaortic
endarterectomize
endarterectomy
endarterial
endarteritis
  deformans, e.
  obliterans, e.
  prolifcrans, e.
endarterium
endarteropathy
end-artery
endaural
end-body
end-bulbs of Krause
end-feet
end-diastolic gated blood
 pool image
endoabdominal
endoaneurysmorrhaphy
endoappendicitis

Additional Entries

endoauscultation
endobronchial
endobronchitis
endocardial
    cushion, e.
    cushion defect, e.
    fibroelastosis, e.
endocardiopathy
endocarditis
    atypical verrucous e.
    bacterial e.
    Loffler's e.
    mural e.
    mycotic e.
    nonbacterial thrombotic e.
    nonbacterial verrucous e.
    prosthetic valve e.
    rheumatic e.
    rickettsial e.
    vegetative e.
endocardium
endocavitary irradiation
endoceliac
endocellular
endocervical
    canal, e.
    curettage, e.
    polypectomy, e.
endocervicitis
endocervix
endochondral
endochorion
endochrome
endocolitis
endoconidiotoxicosis
endocranial
endocraniosis
endocranium
endocrine glands
endocrinopathy
endocurietherapy
endocrinotherapy
endocyclic
endocyst
endocystitis
endocyte
endodiascope
endodiascopy
endoenteritis
endogastric
endogastritis
endogenous
endoglobular
Endografin
endolabyrinthitis
endolaryngeal
    mold, e.
endolarynx
endolymph
endolymphatic
endomastoiditis
endometria
endometrial
    curettage, e.
    echo, e.
    hyperplasia, e.
    implant, e.
    polyp, e.
    tissue, e.
endometrioid
endometrioma
endometriosis
endometriotic
endometritis
endometrium
    early secretory e.
    proliferative e.
endometry
endomitosis
endomitotic
endomyocarditis
endomysium

Additional Entries

endonasal
endoneural
endoneuritis
endoneurium
endoneurolysis
endonuclear
endonuclease
endonucleolus
endoparasite
endopelvic
    fascia, e.
endoperiarteritis
endopericardial
endopericarditis
endoperimyocarditis
endoperineuritis
endoperitoneal
endoperitonitis
endophasia
endophlebitis
endophthalmitis
endophytic
endoplasm
endoplast
endopolyploid
endopolyploidy
endopredator
endoradiography
end-organs
endoreduplication
endosalpingitis
endosalpingoma
endosalpingosis
endosalpinx
endoscope
endoscopic
    cholangiogram, e.
    retrograde cholangiopancreatography (ERCP), e.
endoscopy
endosecretory
endosepsis
endoskeleton
endosmosis
endosmotic
endosporium
endosteal
    layer, e.
    portions of cortex, e.
endosteitis
endosteoma
endostethoscope
endosteum
endostoma
endosymbiont
endosymbiosis
endothelia
endothelial
endothelialization
endotheliitis
endothelioblastoma
endotheliocyte
endotheliocytosis
endothelioid
endotheliolysin
endothelioma
endotheliomatosis
endotheliomyoma
endotheliosarcoma
endothelium
endothyropexy
endotoxic
endotoxicosis
endotoxin
endotracheal
    tube (ET), e.
endotracheitis
endotrachelitis
endourethral
endouterine
endovaccination
endovasculitis
end-plates of Kuhne

Additional Entries

end-systolic gated blood pool image
enema
  air contrast barium e.
  analeptic e.
  barium e.
  contrast e.
  double contrast e.
  Fleet e.
  full-column barium e.
  retention e.
  soapsuds e.
energy
  content, d.
  dependence, e.
  resolution, e.
  window, e.
en face view
ENG (electronystagmography or electroneurography)
Engel-Lysholm maneuver
Engelmann's diease
Engelmann's disk
English position (a/k/a lateral recumbent position)
Engman's disease
engorged
engorgement
  breast e.
  neck veins, e. of
  pulmonary vessels, e. of
  vascular e.
  venous e.
enhanced CAT scan
enhancement
  dense e.
  ring e.
enhancing
  nodule, e.
  lesion, e.
enlarged nodes
enlargement
enlargement *(continued)*
  heart, e. of
enlarging defect
ENI (elective inguinal node irradiation)
enophthalmos
enostosis
en plaque
ensiform
  appendix, e.
  process, e.
entad
ental
entasia
entepicondyle
enteradenitis
enteral
enterectasis
enteric
  coated, e.
  cyst, e.
enteritis
  pseudomembranous e.
  regional e.
  terminal e.
enteroanastomosis
enterobiasis
enterobiliary
enterocele
enterocentesis
enterocholecystostomy
enterocholecystotomy
enterocleisis
enteroclysis
enterocoele
enterocolectomy
enterocolitis
  antibiotic-associated e.
  hemorrhagic e.
  necrotizing e.
  pseudomembranous e.
enterocolostomy

Additional Entries

enterocutaneous
enterocyst
enterocystocele
enterocystoma
enterodynia
enteroenterostomy
enteroepiplocele
enterogastric
    reflux, e.
enterogenous
enteroglucagon
enterogram
enterograph
enterography
enterohepatitis
enterohepatocele
enterohepatopexy
enterohydrocele
enterointestinal
enterokinase
enterokinetic
enterokinin
enterolith
enterolithiasis
enterolysis
enteromegaly
enteromere
enteromerocele
enteromycosis
enteromyiasis
enteroneuritis
enteronitis
enteroparesis
enteropathogen
enteropathogenesis
enteropathogenic
enteropathy
    gluten e.
enteropexy
enteroplasty
enteroplegia
enteroptosis
enteroptotic
enterorenal
enterorrhagia
enterrhaphy
enterorrhexis
enteroscope
enterosepsis
enterosite
enterosorption
enterospasm
enterostaxis
enterostenosis
enterostomal
enterostomy
enterotome
enterotomy
enterotoxemia
enterotoxigenic
enterotoxin
enterotropic
enterovaginal
enterovenous
enterovesical
enteroviral
enterovirus
entity
entoblast
entocele
entochondrostosis
entochoroidea
entocone
entoconid
entocornea
entocuneiform
entoderm
entodermal
entoectad
entome
entomere
entomion
entomology
entophthalmia

Additional Entries

entoplasm
entoplastic
entoptic
entoptoscope
entoptoscopy
entoretina
entosthoblast
entotympanic
entropion
entropy
enucleate
enucleation
    cyst, e. of
    eyeball, e.
enuresis
envelope
    glass e.
EOG (electro-olfactogram)
EOM (extraocular movement)
EOMI (extraocular muscles intact)
eosinophil
    corpuscles, e.
eosinophilia
eosinophilic
    gastroenteritis, e.
    granuloma, e.
epactal bones
eparterial
    branch, e.
epencephalon
Ependorf angiocatheter
ependyma
ependymal
    cells, e.
    cyst, e.
    enhancement, e.
    layer, e.
ependymitis
ependymoblast
ependymoblastoma
ependymocyte
ependymoma
ependymopathy
epibulbar
epicanthal
epicanthus
epicarcinogen
epicardia
epicardiectomy
epicardiolysis
epicardium
epicentral
epicoele
epicoeloma
epicondyle
epicondylitis
epicondylus
epicoracoid
epicorneascleritis
epicostal
epicranial
    aponeurosis, e.
epicranium
epicrisis
epicystitis
epicystotomy
epicyte
epidemiography
epidermal
    inclusion cyst, e.
epidermatitis
epidermatoplasty
epidermic
    coat, e.
epidermicula
epidermidalization
epidemis
epidermitis
epidermoid
    cyst, e. degeneration
    inclusion cyst, e.
epidermoidoma

Additional Entries ____________________

____

____

epidermolysis
epidermolytic
epidermophytosis
epidermopoiesis
epidermotropic
epididymal
epididymectomy
epididymis
appendix of e.
testis, e.
epididymitis
epididymodeferentectomy
epididymodeferential
epididymography
epididymotomy
epididymovasectomy
epididymovasotomy
epidural
abscess, e.
anesthesia, e.
extravasation, e.
hematoma, e.
hemorrhage, e.
space, e.
epidurography
epiesophageal
epigastric
epigastrium
epigastrius
epigastrocele
epiglottidectomy
epiglottiditis
epiglottis
cushion of e.
tubercle of e.
epilation
epimandibular
epimenorrhagia
epimenorrhea
epimocroscope
epinephritis
epinephroma
epineural
epineurium
epiotic
center of temporal bone, e.
epiphyseal
activity, e.
cartilage, e.
coxa vara, e.
fracture, e.
growth plate, e.
lines, e.
epiphyses
epiphysis
fibular e.
tibial e.
epiphysiodesis
epiphysioid
epiphysiolysis
epiphysiometer
epiphysiopathy
epiphysis
epiphysitis
epiphytic
epipleural
epiplocele
epiploectomy
epiploenterocele
epiploic
foramen, e.
epiplomerocele
epiplomphalocele
epiploplasty
epiplosarcomphalocele
epiploscheocele
epipyramis
episclera
episcleral
tissue, e.
episcleritis
epispinal
episplenitis

Additional Entries

epistasis
epistatic
epistaxis
episternal
episternum
epistropheus
epitarsus
epithalamus
commissure of e.
habenular nuclei of e.
pituitary body of e.
epithelia
epithelial
epithelialization
epithelialized
crater, e.
healed niche, e.
scar, e.
epitheliitis
epithelioblastoma
epithelioceptor
epitheliochorial
epitheliogenic
epithelioglandular
epithelioid
epitheliolysis
epitheliolytic
epithelioma
epitheliomatosis
epitheliomatous
epitheliomuscular
epitheliosis
epitheliotropic
epithelium
ciliated e.
columnar e.
enamel e.
germinal e.
glandular c.
laminated e.
seminiferous e.
squamous e.
epithelium *(continued)*
stratified of cornea e.
transitional e.
epitrochlear
epitrochleo-anconaeus muscle
epituberculosis
epiturbinate
EPITYMP (epitympanum)
epitympanic
recess, e.
Epstein's disease
epulis
equation
Bloch e.
Fick e.
Stewart-Hamilton e.
equator
lens, e. of
equilateral
equilibration
equilibrator
equilibrium
equinovarus
equinus
equipotential
equipotentiality
equivalence
equivalent
equivocal
E.R.Squibb & Sons
eradicate microscopic disease
Erb-Charcot disease
Erb-Duchenne paralysis
Erb-Goldflam disease
ERCP (endoscopic retrograde cholangiopancreatography)
erect
lateral projection, e.
position, e.
posterioanterior projection, e.

Additional Entries

erect *(continued)*
  view, e.
ERG (electgroretinogram)
ergodynamograph
ergoesthesiography
ergogram
ergograph
ergometer
Erich arch bar
eroded lamina dura
erosion
  cervical e.
  gastric mucosal e.
  superficial e.
erosive
  osteoarthritis, e.
erotogenic
erratic
eruption
  Kaposi's varicelliform e.
erysipelas
erysiphake
erythema
  nodosum, e.
erythematosus
  lupus e.
erythroblastosis
  fetalis, e.
  neonatorum, e.
erythrochromia
erythroclasis
erythroclastic
erythrocyanosis
erythrocyte
  achromic e.
  basophilic e.
  hypochromic e.
  normochromic e.
  orthochromic e.
  polychromic e.
  sedimentation rate, e. (ESR)
erythrocyte *(continued)*
  target e.
erythrodermic disease
erythroid
  cells, e.
  precursors, e.
erythrokeratodermia
erythrokinetic
erythroleukemia
erythrometer
erythropathy
erythropenia
erythropoiesis
erythropoietic marrow
erythrosine sodium
escape
  beats, e.
  nodal e.
  vagal e.
  ventricular e.
escargot curve
eschar
escharotic
Esmarch bandage
esogastritis
esophagalgia
esophageal
  arteries, e.
  atresia, e.
  axis, e.
  bougienage, e.
  dilatation, e.
  diverticulum, e.
  dysmotility, e.
  glands, e.
  hiatus, e.
  manometry, e.
  motility, e.
  nerves, e.
  perforation, e.
  plexus, e.
  stricture, e.

Additional Entries

esophageal *(continued)*
tumor, e.
varices, e.
web, e.
esophagectasia
esophagitis
reflux, e.
esophagobronchial
esophagocardiomyotomy
esophagocele
esophagogastric (EG) junction
esophagogastroscopy
esophagogastrostomy
esophagogram
esophagography
esophagojejunogastrostomosis
esophagojejunoplasty
esophagojejunostomy
esophagolaryngectomy
esophagology
esophagomalacia
esophagometer
esophagomycosis
esophagomyotomy
esophagopharynx
esophagoplasty
esophagoplication
esophagoptosis
esophagorespiratory
esophagoscope
flexible e.
rigid e.
esophagoscopy
esophagospasm
esophagostenosis
esophagostoma
esophagostomiasis
esophagostomy
esophagotome
esophagotomy
esophagotome
esophagotomy
esophagotracheal
esophagus
abdominal e.
Barrett's e.
cervical e.
lymphatic vessels of e.
nerves of e.
thoracic e.
tunica mucosa of e.
esophoria
esotropia
Esser's graft
established
airway, e.
esthesia
esthesic
ethesioblast
esthesiometer
esthesioneuroblastoma
ET (endotracheal) tube
etherometer
ethiodized oil
Ethiodol
ethiofos
ethmoid
air cells, e.
antrum, e.
bone, e.
perpendicular plate of e.
sinus, e.
uncinate process of e.
vertical plate of e.
ethmoidal
arteries, e.
canals, e.
cells, e.
notch, e.
process, e.
sinuses, e.
sine, e.

Additional Entries

ethmoidectomy
ethmoiditis
ethmoidotomy
ethmolacrimal
ethmomaxillary
ethmonasal
ethmopalatal
ethmosphenoid
ethmoturbinal
ethmovomerine
    cartilage, e.
ethmography
ethylenediaminetetra-acetic acid (EDTA)
ethylene glycol
ethylene hydroxydiphosphonate
etidronate
etifenin
Eu (europium)
eudiometer
eukaryon
eukaryosis
Eulenburg's disease
eumenorrhea
eumetria
eumorphism
euoxic
eupancreatism
eupepsia
eupeptic
euplastic
euploid
europium (Eu)
eustachian
    tube, e.
    valve, e.
eusystole
eusystolic
euthyroid
eutonic
eutopic
eutrophia
eV (electron volt)
Evac-Q-Kwik
evacuated
    blood clots, e.
    tissue, e.
    tube, e.
evacuation
    dilatation and e.
evacuator
evagination
evaluation shunt
evanescent
Evans
    blue, E.
    classification, E.
    Type 1 fracture, E.
    Type 2 fracture, E.
eventration
    diaphragm, e. of
eversion
evisceration
    eyeball, e. of
evoked
    auditory response (AER), e.
    sensory resonse (SER), e.
    visual resonse (VER), e.
Ewald tube
Ewing's
    sarcoma, E.
    tumor, E.
exacerbation
exanthema
exanthemata
exanthematous
exarteritis
exarticulation
excavation
    optic disk, e. of
    rectouterine e.

Additional Entries ______________________

____

____

excavation *(continued)*
- retrovesical e.
- vesicouterine e.

exchange
- coupling e.
- forces, e.
- narrowing e.
- respiratory e.
- sheath set, e.
- transfusion, e.

excise
excision
excisional
- wedge biopsy, e.

excitation voltage
excrescence
- fleshy e.

excrescent
excreta
excrete
excretin
excretion
- biliary e.
- contrast material, e. of
- dye, e. of
- urinary e.

excretory
- cystogram, e.
- duct, e.
- pyelogram, e.
- system, e.
- urogram, e.
- urography, e.

excursion
- chest e.
- diaphragm, e. of
- free and equal e.
- respiratory e.

excursive
exencephaly
exenteration
- orbital contents, e. of

exenteration *(continued)*
- total pelvic e.

exercise gated-wall motion study
exfoliation
exfoliative
- cytology, e.
- gastritis,, e.

exit
- dose, e.
- foramina, e.
- foraminal stenosis, e.
- -to-entrance dose penetration, e.

exocardial
exocyclic
exodeviation
exogastric
exogastrula
exometer
exopathy
exophoria
exophthalmic
exophthalmogenic
exophthalmometer
exophthalmometric
exophthalmometry
exophthalmos
exophytic
- lesion,e.
- mass, e.
- tumor, e.

exoplasm
exoskeleton
exosmosis
exosplenopexy
exostosis
exothermic
exothymopexy
exotropia
exotropic
expanded cervix

Additional Entries

expansile lytic lesion
expansion
    chest e.
    lung e.
expectoration
    bloody e.
    cough and e.
expiration
    forced e.
    prolonged e.
expiratory
    flow, e.
    grunting, e.
    trapping of air, e.
    wheezing, e.
explosive
    diarrhea, e.
    stool, e.
exponential function
exposure rate constant
expulsion
    contraction, e.
expulsive
exsanguinate
exsorption
exstrophy
    bladder, e. of
    cloaca, e. of
extended-field irradiation
extensometer
extension
    tear drop e.
exterior
    skull, e.
external
    arcuate ligament, e.
    auditory canal, e.
    auditory meatus, e.
    calcaneal artery, e.
    calcaneo-astragaloid ligament, e.
    canthus, e.

external *(continued)*
    circumflex artery, e.
    cutaneous nerve, e.
    beam, e.
    beam irradiation, e.
    cuff pressure, e.
    geniculate, e.
    iliac artery, e.
    inguinal ring, e.
    intercostal muscles, e.
    jugular vein, e.
    lateral ligament, e.
    ligament of malleus, e.
    magnetic field, e.
    malleolar artery, e.
    mammary artery, e.
    oblique artery, e.
    organs, e.
    plantar artery, e.
    plantar nerve, e.
    popliteal nerve, e.
    pterygoid muscle, e.
    pterygoid nerve e.
    pudic artery, e.
    respiratory nerve of Belli, e.
    saphenous vein, e.
    semilunar fibrocartilage, e.
    spermatic artery, e.
    spermatic fascia, e.
    spermatic nerve, e.
    sphincter ani muscle, e.
    topography, e.
externalize
extorsion
extra-adrenal
extra-articular
extra-axial
    collection, e.
    lesion, e.
    tumor, e.

Additional Entries

extrabronchial
extrabuccal
extrabulbar
extracapsular
extracardial
extracarpal
extracellular
extracerebral
extraconal lesion
extracorporeal
    dissection, e.
extracorticospinal
extracranial
extract
    pituitary e.
    thyroid e.
extraction
    breech e.
    flap e.
    foreign body, e. of
    intracapsular cataract e.
    magnetic e.
    serial e.
    vacuum e.
extradural
    anesthesia, e.
    compression, e.
    defect, e.
    hematoma, e.
    hemorrhage, e.
    lymphatics, e.
    mass, e.
extraepiphyseal
extragenital
extrahepatic
    biliary duct, e. (EHBD)
extraligamentous
extraluminal gas collection
extralymphatic metastases
extramalleolus
extramarginal
extramastoiditis
extramedullary
    hemopoiesis, h.
extrameningeal
extramural
    extension, e.
extranasation
extraneous
extranodal extension
extranuclear
extraocular
extraoculogram
extraosseous
    localization, e.
    soft tissue, e.
extraparenchymal
extrapelvic
extrapericardial
extraperineal
extraperiosteal
extraperitoneal
extraplacental
extraplantar
extrapleural
    disease, e.
    mass, e.
    sign, e.
extrapolation
extraprostatic
extrapulmonary
    site, e.
extrapyramidal
    symptoms, e.
    system, e.
extrarenal calyx
extraskeletal
extraspinal
    veins, e.
extrasystole
    atrial e.
    atrioventricular e.
    infranodal e.
    interpolated e.

Additional Entries

extrasystole *(continued)*
nodal e.
retrograde e.
ventricular e.
extrathecal
extratracheal
extraureteral
extravasation
extravascular
extraventricular
extraversion
extremitas acromialis
extremity
extrinsic
allergic alveolitis, e.
colon deformity, e.
compression, e.
defect, e.
muscles, e.
pressure, e.
extrophy
extrude
extruded
disc fragment, e.
extruded *(continued)*
lumbar disc, e.
extubate
extubation
exudate
bloody e.
mucopurulent e.
watery e.
exudation
exudative
exumbilication
ex vacuo
eye
bulb of e.
Klieg e.
pink e.
eyeball
eyebrow
eyed probe
eyelid
canthus of e.
muscles of e.
ptosis of e.
tarsi of e.

Additional Entries

F

F (fluorine)
F (farad)
Fab (fragment antigen binding)
fabella
fabellae
face
  shield, f.
facet
  artifact, f.
  arthropathy, f.
  articular f.
  hypertrophy, f.
  joint, f.
facial
  artery, f.
  bones, f.
  canal hiatus, f.
  lymph nodes, f.
  nerve, f.
  nevus, f.
  plethora, f.
  vein, f.
facing film holder
faciobrachial
faciocephalgia
faciocervical
faciolingual
facioplasty
facioplegia
facioscapulohumeral
factitial hyperthyroidism
Fahr's disease
fail safe
failed external version
failure
  acute respirtory f.
  cardiac f.
  chronic renal f.
  congestive heart f.

failure *(continued)*
  hepatic f.
  left ventricular heart f.
  pacemaker f.
  renal f.
  respiratory f.
  right-sided heart f.
falciform
  body, f.
  ligament, f.
falcine region
falling load
fallopian
  aqueduct, f.
  arch, f.
  artery, f.
  ligament, f.
  tube, f.
fallout
Fallot
  tetralogy of F.
false
  aneurysm, f.
  color scale, f.
  cord, f.
  labor, f.
  ligaments, f.
  -negative, f.
  negative myelography, f.
  -positive, f.
  pregnancy, f.
  vocal cord, f.
false ligaments
  bladder, f.l. of
  pelvis, f.l. of
  ribs, f.l. of
  vocal cords, f.l. of
falx
  aponeurotica, f.
  cerebelli, f. of

Additional Entries ______________________

____

____

falx *(continued)*
- cerebri, f.
- inguinalis, f.

fan
- beam, f.
- needle technique, f.
- shaped appearance, f.

Fanconi syndrome
Farber disease
farmer's lung
fascia
- abdominal f.
- anal f.
- ankle f.
- antebrachial f.
- arm f.
- axillary f.
- bicipital f.
- brachial f.
- brachii f.
- buccopharyngeal f.
- Buck's f.
- bulbar f.
- bulbi f.
- Camper's f.
- cervical f.
- clavipectoral f.
- Colles' f.
- colli f.
- coracoclavicular f.
- coracoclavicularis f.
- cremasteric f.
- cribriform of thigh f.
- cribrosa f.
- cruris f.
- dartos f.
- deep f.
- deltoid f.
- diaphragmatic f.
- dorsal f.
- external oblique f.
- external spermatic f.

fascia *(continued)*
- Gerota's f.
- iliac f.
- innomata f.
- intercolumnar f.
- intercosal f.
- intercrural f.
- internal spermatic f.
- investing f. of neck
- lata, f.
- leg, f.
- lumbar f.
- lumbodorsal f.
- masseteric f.
- middle spermatic f.
- of abdomen, f.
- obturator f.
- orbital f.
- palmar f.
- palpebral f.
- paraspinous f.
- parotideomasseteric f.
- pectoral f.
- pelvic f.
- penile f.
- perineal f.
- perinephric f.
- perivesical f.
- pharyngobasilar f.
- phrenicopleural f.
- piriformis f.
- plantar f.
- popliteal f.
- pretracheal f.
- prevertebral f.
- psoas f.
- pubocervical f.
- pubovesicocervical f.
- rectovaginal f.
- rectovesical f.
- rectus f.
- renalis f.

Additional Entries ______________________

fascia *(continued)*
retropectoral f.
Scarpa's f.
Sibson's f.
subvesical f.
spermatic external f.
subscapular f.
subscapularis f.
superficial f.
supraspinata f.
supraspinatous f.
temporal f.
Tenon's f.
thigh f.
thoracic region f.
transversalis f.
transverse f.
triangular f.
underlying f.
upper extremity f.
urogenital diaphragm f.
vertebral f.
vesicovaginal f.
fasciagram
fasciagraphy
fascial
flap, f.
graft, f.
layer, f.
plane, f.
sheath, f.
fasciaplasty
fascicle
fascicular
fasciculated
fasciola
cinerea, f.
fasciolae
fast
growing, f.
imaging, f.
neutron, f.

fast *(continued)*
screen cassette, f.
fat
absorption, f.
brown f.
containing area, f.
deposition, f.
embolism, f.
embolus, f.
filled region, f.
graft, f.
infiltration, f.
layer, f.
line, f.
necrosis, f.
pad, f.
plane, f.
subcutaneous f.
total body f.
fatty
capsule of kidney, f.
component, f.
degeneration of heart, f.
fauces
arches of f.
isthmus of f.
muscles of f.
pillars of f.
faucial arch
Fc (fragment crystallizable)
FDP (frontodextra posterior)
FDT (frontodextra transversa)
Fe (iron) Fe 52; Fe 59)
feathering of border
fecal
impaction, f.
incontinence, f.
material, f.
retained f. material
vomiting, f.
fecalith

Additional Entries

feces
retained f.
scybalous f.
feeder vessel
feeding
gavage f.
tube, f.
Fell tube
Felty syndrome
femora
femoral
aortic flush catheter, f.
arteriography, f.
artery, f.
bone, f.
canal, f.
circumflex arteries, f.
condyle, f.
cortices, f.
cutaneous nerve, f.
epiphysis, f.
fossa, f.
head, f.
hernia, f.
muscle, f.
neck, f.
nerve, f.
ring, f.
septum, f.
shaft, f.
sheath, f.
triangle, f.
vein, f.
visceral renal curve catheter, f.
femorocele
femoroiliac
femorotibial
femur
diaphysis (shaft) of f.
length of f.
fenestra
fenestra *(continued)*
cochleae, f.
ovalis, f.
rotunda, f.
vestibuli, f.
fenestrae
fenestral otosclerosis
fenestrate
fenestrated
compression plate, f.
fenestration
Fereol's nodes
fermium (fm)
Ferrein's
canal, F.
tubes, F.
ferric
chloride Fe 59, f.
ion, f.
ferromagnetic
implant, f.
relaxation, f.
ferrous
citrate Fe 59, f.
sulfate Fe 59, f.
ferrule
fetal
age, f.
asphyxia, f.
bradycardia, f.
circulation, f.
death, f.
distress, f.
heart detected, f.
heart monitor, f.
heart motion, absent f.
heart tones (FHT), f.
lobulation, f.
lung maturity, f.
membranes, f.
pole, f.
fetography

Additional Entries

fetometry
fetoplacental
fetoscope
fetoscopy
fetus
    foramen ovale in f.
    macerated f.
FFD (focus-film distance)
18F-fluorodeoxyglucose
fiber
    A f.
    alpha f.
    alveolar f.
    apical f.
    arcuate f.
    B f.
    basilar f.
    beta f.
    C f.
    collagenous f.
    dentinal f.
    depressor f.
    dietary f.
    elastic f.
    extrafusal f.
    Gerdy's f.
    Gottstein f.
    gray f.
    intercrural f.
    intrafusal f.
    medullated f.
    motor f.
    Muller's f.
    muscle f.
    myelinated f.
    nerve f.
    olfactory projection f.
    olivo-cerebellar f.
    osteogenic f.
    postganglionic f.
    precollagenous f.
    preganglionic f.
fiber *(continued)*
    pressor f.
    projection f.
    Purkinje, f. of
    radicular f.
    reticular f.
    Sharpey's f.
    spindle f.
    sudomotor f.
    sustentacular of Muller f.
    tactile discrimination, f. of
    taste, f.
    Tomes' f.
    touch f.
    unmyelinated f.
    vasomotor f.
    white f.
    zonular f.
fiberoptic
    endoscopy, f.
    scope, f.
fibers
    muscles split in line of f.
fibercolonoscope
fibergastroscope
fiberoptic
    flexible system, f.
    light source, f.
fiberscope
fibrae
    annulares, f.
    pontis profundae, f.
    propriae, f.
fibrillation
    atrial f.
    auricular f.
    paroxysmal atrial f.
    ventricular f.
fibrin body
fibrinolytic agent

Additional Entries

fibrinogen I 125
fibrinoscopy
fibrinogenous
    exudate, f.
fibroadenoma
fibroadenosis
fibroangioma
fibroareolar
fibroatrophy
fibroblast
fibroblastic
fibroblastoma
fibrocalcific
fibrocartilage
    circumferential f.
    connecting f.
    interarticular f.
    intervertebral f.
    semilunar f.
    stratiform f.
    yellow f.
    white f.
fibrocartilaginous
    lamina, f.
fibrochondritis
fibrochondroma
fibrocollagenous
fibrocyst
fibrocystic
    cystoma, f.
    disease, f.
    residual, f.
fibrocystoma
fibrodysplasia (myositis) ossificans progressiva
fibroelastic
fibroelastosis
fibroenchondroma
fibroepithelioma
fibrofatty tissue
fibrofibrous
fibroid

fibroid *(continued)*
    calcified uterine f.
    intramural f.
    palpable f.
    serosal f.
    uterine f.
    uterus, f.
fibroma
    cystic f.
    ossifying f. of bone
    uterine v.
fibromatoid
fibromatosis
    gingival f.
    palmar f.
    plantar f.
fibromatous
fibromuscular
    dysplasia, f.
    hyperplasia, f.
    plaque, f.
fibromyoma
fibromyositis
fibromyxosarcoma
fibropapilloma
fibroplasia
    intimal f.
    medial f.
    subadventitial f.
fibropurulent
fibrosarcoma
fibrosclerosis
fibrosis
    congenital hepatic f.
    cystic f.
    diffuse interstitial pulmonary f.
    endomyocardial f.
    idiopathic pulmonary f.
    interstitial f
    mediastinal f.
    perihilar f.

Additional Entries

fibrosis *(continued)*
periureteric f.
pulmonary f.
fibrous
capsule of Glisson, f.
cortical defect, f.
dysplasia, f.
histiocytoma, f.
rings of heart, f.
septa, f.
sheaths of flexor tendons, f.
sheaths of fingers, f.
sheaths of toes, f.
tunic of eyeball, f.
tunic of kidney, f.
union, f.
fibrovascular
fibroxanthoma
fibroxanthomatous cell proliferation
fibula
nutrient artery of f.
fibular
artery, f.
bone, f.
epiphysis, f.
muscle, f.
nerve, f.
notch, f.
shaft, f.
vein, f.
Fick
bacillus, F.
equation, F.
position, F.
principle, F.
FID (free induction decay)
field
block anesthesia, f.
bloodless f.
defect, visual f.
field *(continued)*
defining shield, f.
dry f.
edge, f.
flatness, f.
gradient, f.
higher f.
lower f.
lung f.
midlung f.
operative f.
probe coupling, f.
shaping, f.
size, f.
sterile f.
symmetry, f.
verification, f.
view, f.
vision, f. of
visual f. defect
weightings, f.
Fielding's membrane
fifth
metacarpal bone, f.
metatarsal bone, f.
nerve, f.
filament
ammeter, f.
circuit, f.
filiform
follower, f. and
papillae of tongue, f.
-tipped catheter, f.
filling
defect, f.
film
AP f.
Bucky f.
comparison f.
contrast, f.
cross-table lateral f.
density, f.

Additional Entries

film *(continued)*
  expiratory f.
  flat plate f.
  gamma, f.
  imaging, f.
  late f.
  lateral f.
  lateral decubitus f.
  limited f.
  localization f.
  low-contrast f.
  oblique f.
  overhead f.
  PA f.
  plain f.
  portable f.
  post evacuation f.
  post reduction f.
  post void f.
  preliminary f.
  processing technique, f.
  prone f.
  scout f.
  screen unit, f.
  sequential f.
  serial f.
  spot f.
  stress f.
  subtraction f.
  supine f.
  translateral f.
  upright f.
  x-ray f.
filament
filum
  terminale, f.
fimbria
  ovarian f.
fimbriae
  uterine tube, f. of
fimbriated
  end, f.
fimbriation
fimbriocele
fine
  detail radiography, f.
  needle, f.
  -needle biopsy, f.
  -needle aspiration (FNA), f.
  -needle aspiration biopsy (FNAB), f.
  -needle transhepatic cholangiography (FNTHC), f.
fine needle biopsy
finger-like white matter edema
Finney's pyloroplasty
Finsen
  light, F.
  rays, F.
Firma AB Kifa
first
  cuneiform bone, f.
  dorsal metacarpal artery, f.
  dorsal metacarpal bone, f.
  dorsal metatarsal artery, f.
  dorsal metatarsal bone, f.
  echelon, f.
  interspace vessels, f.
  order subtraction, f.
  pass imaging, f.
  pass radionuclide angiocardiography, f.
  pass radionuclide angiography, f.
  pass-through, f.
  pass view, f.
  transit curve, f.

Additional Entries

Fischgold's
- bimastoid line, F.
- digastric line, F.

fission
- fragment, f.
- production, f.
- reaction, f.

fissionable nuclei

fissura
- antitragohelicina, f.
- calcarina, f.
- cerebri lateralis , f.
- cerebri longitudinalis, f.
- collateralis, f.
- hippocampi, f.
- parietoccipitalis, f.
- petrotympanica, f.
- prima cerebelli, f.
- secunda cerebelli, f.

fissure (s)
- abdominal f.
- abdoccippital f.
- Ammon's f.
- amygdaline f.
- anal f.
- angular f.
- antitragohelicine f.
- ape f.
- basilar f.
- basisylvian f.
- branchial f.
- Broca's f.
- Burdach's f.
- calcarine f.
- callosal f.
- callosomarginal f.
- central f.
- cerebral f.
- choroid f.
- collateral f.
- corneal f.
- craniofacial f.

fissure (s) *(continued)*
- Ecker's f.
- enamel f.
- entorbital f.
- ethmoid f.
- glaserian f.
- great f.
- great horizontal f.
- Helne's f.
- hippocampal f.
- horizontal f.
- inferofrontal f.
- intercerebral f.
- interparietal f.
- intratonsillar f.
- lacrimal f.
- longitudinal f.
- mandibular f.
- maxillary f.
- median f.
- oblique f.
- occipital f.
- occipitosphenoidal f.
- oral f.
- orbital f.
- palpebral f.
- Pansch's f.
- paracentral f.
- parietooccipital f.
- parietosphenoid f.
- paroccipital f.
- petrobasilar f.
- petromastoid f.
- petrooccipital f.
- petrosal f.
- petrosphenoidal f.
- petrosquamosal f.
- petrosquamous f.
- petrotympanic f.
- portal f.
- postcentral f.
- posterolateral f.

Additional Entries

fissure (s) *(continued)*
precentral f.
precuneal f.
prepyramidal f.
presylvian f.
primary f.
pterygoid f.
pterygomaxillary f.
pterygopalatine f.
pterygotympanic f.
pudendal f.
retrocuticular f.
Rolando, f. of
sagittal f.
Santorini's f.
Schwalbe's f.
secondary f.
sign, f.
sphenoidal f.
sphenomaxillary f.
sphenooccipital f.
sphenopetrosal f.
squamotympanic f.
subfrontal f.
subsylvian f.
subtemporal f.
superfrontal f.
supertemporal f.
sylvian f.
Sylvius, f. of
tentorial f.
transtemporal f.
transverse f.
transverse occipital f.
tympanic f.
tympanomastoid f.
tympanosquamous f.
umbilical f.
zygal f.
zygomaticosphenoid f.
fissure sign of congestive heart failure
fistula
ureterocolic f.
ureteroenteric f.
vesicovaginal f.
vesicocolic f.
fistulae
fistulogram
fixation
complement test, f.
device, f.
internal f.
latex f.
muscle, f.
open reduction and internal f.
skeletal, f.
test, f. complement
fixed
cone, f.
perfusion defect, f.
shield, f.
Fixster device
fL (femtoliter)
18 F labeled fluorodeoxyglucose
flaccid
hemiplegia, f.
paralysis, f.
Flack's node
flail
chest, f.
joint, f.
valve, f.
flange
with a keel, f.
flanging tool
flank
pain, f.
stripe, f.
flap
bone f.
delayed transfer f.

Additional Entries

flap *(continued)*
- double pedicle f.
- island f.
- localized advancement f.
- myocutaneous f.
- necrosis, f.
- pedicle f.
- skin f.
- sliding f.
- tear of meniscus, f.
- tube f.
- tunnel f.
- viable f.
- V-Y f.
- Z f.

flare
- phenomenon, f.
- reactions, f.
- response, f.

flat
- abdomen, f.
- circular lesion, f.
- electroencephalogram, f.
- foot, f.
- jugular veins, f.
- pelvic contour, f.
- plate, f.

flattened
- effect, f.

flattening
- filter, f.
- nasolabial fold, f. of
- normal lumbar curvature, f. of
- rib margin, f. of
- T wave f.

flavum

Flechsig
- area, F.
- cerebellar tract of F.
- oval area of F.

Fleet's enema

Fleischmann's hygroma

Fleischner lines

Flemming center

Fletcher applicator 111

Fletcher colpostat

Fletcher-Suit (FS)
- applicator, FS
- ovoid, FS
- tandem, FS

flex

flexible
- endoscopy, f.
- fiberoptic system, f.
- guide wire, f.
- spring wire tip, f.

fleximeter

flexion
- contracture, f.
- crease, f.
- extension projections, f.
- maneuver, f.
- palmar f.
- passive f.
- plantar f.
- semiupright weightbeaaring spot film, f.
- tear drop, f.

flexor knot of Henry

Flexsteel ribbon retractor

flexural area

flexure
- caudal f.
- cephalic f.
- cervical f.
- colic f.
- cranial f.
- dorsal f.
- duodenojejunal f.
- hepatic f.
- lumbar f.
- mesencephalic f.
- nuchal f.

Additional Entries

flexure *(continued)*
pontine f.
sacral f.
sigmoid f.
splenic f.
ventral cephalic f.
flickering light
flip angle
floatation mattress
float coil
floater
stringy vitreous f.
floating
kidney, f.
rib, f.
floccular
fissure, f.
flocculus
flood
fields, f.
source, f.
floor
anterior cranial fossa, f. of
bladder, f. of
fourth ventricle, f. of
inguinal canal, f. of
mouth, f. of
pelvic f.
plate of medulla spinalis, f.
flora
intestinal f.
mixed common f.
oral f.
flow
antegrade blood f.
cerebral brain f.
current, f. of
directed catheter, f.
directed detachable miniature balloon catheter, f.

flow *(continued)*
Doppler flow meter
energy, f. of
forced expiratory f.
forced inspiratory f.
gradient, f.
imaging, f.
instrument, f.
laminar air f.
maximal expiratory f.
maximum terminal f.
meter, Doppler f.
peak expiratory f.
peak inspiratory f.
physiologic f.
rates, f.
related enhancement, f.
related intensity reduction, f.
scan, f.
studies, f.
tract, f.
FLP (left frontoposterior)
FLT (left frontotransverse)
fluid
air f. level
allantoic f.
amniotic f.
ascitic f.
aspirated f.
balance, f.
blood-tinged f.
cerebrospinal f.
cloudy f.
collection, f.
dialysis f.
Douglas, f. in pouch of
extracellular f.
filled gallbladder, f.
filled urinary bladder, f.
fluid interface, f.
fluid level, f.

Additional Entries

fluid *(continued)*
- free f.
- hyperalimentation f.
- interstitial f.
- intestinal f.
- intracellular f.
- intravascular f.
- intravenous f.
- labyrinthine f.
- level, f.
- loculated f.
- Muller's f.
- overload, f.
- purulent f.
- retention, f.
- Scarpa's f.
- seminal f.
- serosanguinous f.
- serous f.
- signals, f.
- straw-colored f.
- synovial f.
- turbid f.
- volume f.
- xanthochromic f.

fluoresce

fluorescein
- angiography, f.
- isocyanate, f.
- sodium, f.

fluorescence
- secondary f.

fluorescent
- antibody staining, f.
- imaging, f.
- rays, f.
- screen, f.
- source, f.
- staining, f.
- treponemal antibody, f.

fluorine 18F

fluorodeoxyglucose

fluorography

fluorometer

fluorometry

fluoronephelometer

fluorophotometry

fluororoentgenography

fluoroscope

fluoroscopic
- control, f.
- view, f.

fluoroscopy

flush
- angiogram, f.
- malar f.
- method, f.

flutter
- atrial f.
- auricular f.
- diaphragmatic f.
- fibrillation, f.
- heart f.
- mediastinal f.
- ventricular f.

flux
- bilious f.

fluxion

Fm (fermium)

FN (facial nerve)

FNA (fine-needle aspiration)

FNAB (fine-needle aspiration biopsy)

FNTHC (fine needle transhepatic cholangiography)

foaming agent

foam pad

focal
- abnormality, f.
- atrophy, f.
- consolidation, f.
- defect, f.
- gigantism, f.
- hyperactivity, f.

Additional Entries

focal *(continued)*
hyperemia, f.
lambdoid defect, f.
lesion, f.
lung disease, f.
mass, f.
nodular hyperplasia, f.
osteolysis, f.
seizure, f.
skin disease, f.
spot, f. (FS)
spot blurring, f.
spot size, f.
stenosis, f.
vault lucency, f.
vault sclerosis, f.
foci
infection, f. of
focimeter
focus
film distance, f.
Ghon f.
infection, f. of
focused
grid, f.
transducer, f.
focusing cup
Fogarty embolectomy catheter
fold (s)
alar f.
amniotic f.
axillary f.
aryepiglottic f.
buttocks, f. of
caudal f.
cecal f.
cephalic f.
ciliary f.
circular f.
conjunctival f.
costocolic f.

fold (s) *(continued)*
crescenteric f.
Douglas' f.
duodenojejunal f.
duodenomesocolic f.
epicanthal f.
epigastric f.
false vocal f.
fimbriated f.
gastric f.
gastric rugal f.
gastropancreatic f.
genital f.
glossoepiglottic f.
gluteal f.
horizonatal f. of rectum
ileocecal f.
inframammary f.
infrapatellar f.
labioscrotal f.
lacrimal f.
longitudinal f.
malleolar f.
medullary f.
mesonephric f.
mucobuccal f.
mucosal f.
mucous f.
nail f.
nasolabial f.
neural f.
rectouterine f.
rectovesical f.
rugal f.
sacrogenital f.
salpingopalatine f.
salpingopharyngeal f.
semilunar f.
semilunar f. of colon
semilunar f. of conjunctiva
serosal f.

Additional Entries

fold (s) *(continued)*
spiral f.
thickened f.
transverse f.
Treves f.
umbilical f.
ureteric f.
urogenital f.
uterovesical f.
uterus f.
ventricular f. of larynx
vestigial f. of Marshall
vocal f.
Foley
balloon, F.
catheter, F.
Folius' muscle
follicle
agminated f.
graafian f.
hair f.
intestinal f.
Lieberkuhn's f.
lingual f.
lymph f.
malpighian f.
Montgomery f.
nabothian f.
ovarian f.
sebaceous f.
solitary f.
thyroid f.
vesicular f.
follicular cyst
folliculitis
folliculoma
folliculosis
folliculus
Fonar Corporation
Fonar QED Beta 3000 MRI gantry
fontactoscope
Fontana's
markings, F.
spaces, F.
fontanelle/fontanel
anterior f.
anterolateral f.
frontal f.
mastoid f.
occipital f.
posterior f.
posterolateral f.
quadrangular f.
sagittal f.
sphenoid f.
triangular f.
foot
arches of f.
fascia of f.
muscles of f.
phalanges of f.
platform, f.
rest, f.
footling
breech presentation, f.
double f.
foramen
aortic f.
apical f.
auditory f.
Bochdalek f.
caroticocinoid f.
cecal f.
cecum, f.
condyloid f.
cotyloid f.
emissary spenoidal f.
epiploic f.
epiploicum f.
esophageal f.
ethmoidal f.
great f.
Huschke f.

Additional Entries

foramen *(continued)*
incisive f.
infraorbital f.
interventricular f.
intervertebral f.
jugular f.
Key and Retzius, f. of
lacerum f.
Luschka f.
Magendie f.
magnum f.
mandibular f.
mastoid f.
medullary f.
mental f.
Monro, f. of
nutrient f.
obturator f.
optic f.
ovale, f.
palatine f.
parietal f.
postglenoid f.
pterygopalatine f.
pterygospinous f.
quadrate f.
rotundum f.
sacral f.
Scarpa's f.
sciatic f.
singulare f.
sphenoidal emissary f.
sphenopalatine f.
spinosum, f.
squamosal f.
Stenson f.
sternal f.
stylomasoid f.
supraorbital f.
supratrochlear f.
temporomalar f.
thebesian f.

foramen *(continued)*
thyroid f.
transversarium f.
transverse f.
vena caval f.
venarum minimarum f.
vertebral f.
vertebroarterial f.
Vesalii f.
Weitbreht's f.
Winslow, f. of
zygomatic f.
zygomaticofacial f.
zygomatico-orbital f.
zygomaticotemporal f.

foramina
intervertebral f.

foraminal
space, f.

foraminotomy

forced
beat, f.
expiration, f.
expiratory flow, f. (FEF)
forced expiratory spirogram, f. (FES)
feeding, f.
inspiratory flow, f. (FIF)
inversion, f.
respiration, f.
tremor, f.
vital capacity, v. (FVC)

forearm
fascia of f.
muscles of f.

forebrain

forefinger

forefoot

foregut
duplication, f.

forehead

foreign body

Additional Entries

foreign body *(continued)*
 localization, f.b.
 needle localization, f.b.
 soft tissue f.b.
Forel's
 commissure, F.
foreskin
 hooded f.
form
 filamentous f.
 granulocyte, band f.
 nonfilamented f.
 segmented f.
 stab f.
 wave f.
Formad's kidney
formation
 abscess f.
 bat-wing f.
 callus f.
 excessive callus f.
 reaction, f.
 reticular f.
 scar tissue, f.
 shunt, f.
formulator
fornix (pl. fornices)
 anterior f.
 based conjunctival flap, f.
 brain, f. of
 body of brain, f.
 cerebri of brain, f. of
 cerebrum, f. of
 columns of brain, f. of
 conjunctivae inferior, f.
 conjunctivae superior, f.
 crura of brain, f. or
 pharyngis, f.
 pharynx, f. of
 posterior f.
 sacci lacrimalis, f.

fornix *(continued)*
 vaginae, f.
 vaginal f.
Forestier disease
Forssell's sinus
forwardscatter factor
fossa (pl. fossae)
 acetabular f.
 adipose f.
 antecubital f.
 articular f.
 canine f.
 cecal f.
 cerebellar f.
 cerebral f.
 cochlearis f.
 condyloid f.
 coronoid f.
 cranial f.
 cubital f.
 digastric f.
 digital f.
 duodenal f.
 duodenojejunal f.
 epigastric f.
 ethmoid f.
 ductus venosus, f. for
 gallbladder, f. for
 glenoid f.
 hyaloid f.
 hypophyseal f.
 ileocecal f.
 iliac f.
 incisive f.
 incudia f.
 inferior vena cava f.
 infraclavicular f.
 infraspinatous f.
 infratemporal f.
 intercondyloid f.
 interpeduncular f.
 intrabulbar f.

Additional Entries

fossa (pl. fossae) *(continued)*
ischiorectal f.
ischiorectalis f.
Jobert's f.
jugular f.
lacrimal f.
liver f.
mandibular f.
mastoid f.
nasal f.
navicular f.
navicularis, f.
occipital f.
olecranon f.
olfactory f.
oral f.
ovalis of fascia lata, f.
ovalis femoris, f.
ovalis of heart, f.
ovarian f.
pararectal f.
paravesical f.
patellar f.
pericecal f.
peritoneal f.
pharyngeal f.
piriform f.
pituitary f.
popliteal f.
posterior f.
prostatic f.
pterygoid f.
pterygopalatine f.
radial f.
renal f.
retrocecal f.
retroperitoneal f.
retroureteric f.
rhomboid f.
rhomboidea f.
Rosenmuller, f.
sagittal f.

fossa (pl. fossae) *(continued)*
scaphoid f.
skull, f. of
sphenomaxillary f.
subarcuate f.
sublingual f.
submandibular f.
subnasal f.
subpyramidal f.
subscapular f.
subsigmoid f.
supinator f.
supraclavicular f.
supraspinatous f.
supraspinous f.
supratonsillar f.
sylvian f.
temporal f.
terminalis f.
tibiofemoral f.
tonsillar f.
triangular f.
trochanteric f.
trochlear f.
urachal f.
vermian f.
vesicae felleae f.
vestibular f.
Waldeyer's f.
zygomatic f.

Foster frame
Foster Kennedy syndrome
fountain decussation of Meynert
fourchette
four day oral cholecystography
four-field
pelvic box technique, f.
plan, f.
setup, f.
quadrant involvement, f.

Additional Entries

four-field *(continued)*
technique, f.
x-ray beam dosimetry, f.
Fourier
analysis, F.
imaging, F.
phase, F.
transform algorithm, F.
four-in-hand necktie
fourth
metacarpal bone, f.
metatarsal bone, f.
nerve, f.
ventricle, f.
four-view study
four-winged catheter
Fowler's position
Fr (francium)
fraction
ejection f.
fractional
biopsy, f.
curettage, f.
emission, f.
fractionated brachytherapy
fractography
fracture
avulsion f.
Barton's f.
basal neck f.
Bennett's f.
bimalleolar f.
blow-out f.
butterfly f.
capillary f.
closed f.
closed reduction of f.
Colles' f.
comminuted f.
complete f.
compound f.
compression f.

fracture *(continued)*
delayed union of f.
depressed f.
diastatic f.
direct f.
dislocation f.
displacement of f. fragments
double f.
Dupuytren's f.
Duverney's f.
fissure f.
fragment, f.
greenstick f.
hangman's f.
horizontal maxillary f.
impacted f.
incomplete f.
indirect f.
intercondylar f.
internal fixation of f.
interperiosteal f.
intertrochanter f.
intracapsular f.
intrauterine f.
lead pipe f.
Le Fort I f.
Le Fort II f.
Le Fort III f.
linear f.
Monteggia's f.
multiple f.
parry f.
pathologic f.
ping-pong f.
position and alignment of f.
Pott's f.
pyramidal f.
reduced f.
simple f.
site, f.

Additional Entries ______________________

fracture *(continued)*
- Smith's f.
- spiral f.
- spontaneous f.
- sprain f.
- stabilized f.
- stellate f.
- stress f. subcapital f.
- supracondylar f.
- tibial plateua, f.
- transvervical f.
- trimalleolar f.
- trophic f.
- Wagstaffe's f.

fractured
- capital femoral epiphysis, f.
- pelvis, f.
- skull, f.
- windpipe, f.

fragment
- antigen binding (FAB), f.
- crystallizable (Fc), f.

fragmentation
fragmented nodes
fragmentography
frame
framework
- sclcral f.
- uveal f.

francium (Fr)
Francke star method
Frankenhauser's ganglion
Frankfort horizontal plane
Franklin head stand
Frazier suction tube
free
- abdominal air, f.
- air chamber, f.
- area draped f.
- border of epiglottis, f.

free *(continued)*
- electron, f.
- floating fecalith, f.
- fluid, f.
- induction delay, f.(FID)
- nerve endings, f.
- pertechnetate, f.
- thyroxine index, f.

freely
- diffusible tracers, f.
- movable carina, f.
- movable joint, f.

fremitus
- bronchial f.
- pectoral f.
- pericardial f.
- pleural f.
- tactile f.
- tussive f.
- vocal f.

French catheter
frenoplasty
frenula
- colic valve f.

frenuloplasty
frenulum
- clitoris, f. of
- ileocolic valve, f. of
- labial f.
- labia minora, f. of
- lingual f.
- lip, f. of
- Morgagni, f. of
- prepuce of penis, f. of
- tongue, f. of
- veli, f.

frequency
- alpha f.
- beta f.
- delta f.
- theta f.
- urgency and f.

Additional Entries

French
catheter, F.
open-ended ureteral catheter
scale, F.
spring-eye needle, F.
fresh-tissue technique
fresnel zone plate
Freund adjuvant
friable
Fricke dosimetry
friction
murmur, f.
pericardial f. rub
Friedmann's vasomotor syndrome
Friedreich's ataxia
Friend's erythroleukemia
fringe magnetic field
Fritsch's catheter
frogleg
position, f.
view, f.
froglike position
Frommann's lines
frons
frontad
frontal
air sinuses, f.
artery, f.
bone, f.
calvarium, f.
convolution, f.
crest, f.
eminences, f.
gyri, f.
horn, f.
lobe, f.
nerve, f.
operculum, f.
plane, f.
process of maxilla, f.

frontal *(continued)*
sinus, f.
sulci, f.
suture, f.
tomography, f.
vein, f.
view, f.
frontipetal
frontoanterior position
frontoethmoidal
frontomalar
frontomaxillary
frontonasal
duct, f.
process, f.
fronto-occipital
view, f.
frontoparietal
frontopontile
fibers, f.
frontoposterior position
frontosphenoidal
process, f.
frontotemporal
frontotransverse position
frontozygomatic suture
Froriep's
ganglion, F.
induration, F.
frozen
biopsy submitted for f. section
section, f.
FS (focal spot)
FS (Fletcher-Suit)
applicator, FS
ovoid, FS
tandem, FS
FSD (focal skin distance)
fss (focal spot size)
Fuchs' coloboma
Fuchs' position

Additional Entries

fugax
  amaurosis f.
  hemianopia bitemporalis f.
fulguration
  cystoscoic f.
  excision f.
  indirect f.
  tubal f.
full-box bolus
full-intensity needle
full mammography
full wave
  rectification, f.w.
  rectified x-ray generator, f.w.
full width at half maximum (FWHM)
fully invasive
functional
  asplenia, f.
  bowel disease, f.
  overlay, f.
functioning adenoma
functionless tumor
fundal
fundi
fundic
fundiform
  ligament, f.
fundoplication
fundus
  gallbladder f.
  oculi, f. of
  stomach, f. of
  tympani, f. of
  uterus, f. of
  vagina, f. of
funduscope
funduscopy
fungate
fungating
fungemia
fungi
fungiform
  papillae of tongue, f.
fungistasis
fungistatic
fungoid
  phase, f.
fungous
fungus
  ball, f.
funiculi
  medulla spinalis, f. of
funiculitis
funiculoepididymitis
funiculopexy
funiculus
  separans, f.
  spermaticus, f.
funnel
  deformity, f.
  shaped infundibulum, f.
furosemide
furrow
  atrioventricular f.
  chordal f.
  dental f.
  digital f.
  genital f.
  gluteal f.
  mentolabial f.
  naso-optic f.
furuncle
furuncular
furunculoid
furunculosis
fused
  kidneys, f.
  vertebra, f.
fusible
fusiform
  aneurysmal widening, f.

Additional Entries

fusiform *(continued)*
- bone expansion, f.
- cataract, f.
- cells, f.
- deformity, f.
- dilatation, f.
- expansion, f.
- widening of abdominal aorta, f.

fusion
- defect, f.
- diaphyseal-epiphyseal f.
- disorder, f.

fusion *(continued)*
- joint f.
- multilevel spinal f.
- nerve f.
- reaction, f.
- spinal f.

fusocellular

fusospirillary

fusospirillosis

fusospirochetal

fusospirochetosis

FWHM (full width at half maximum)

Additional Entries

G

g. (gram or grams)
Ga (gallium)
    Ga 67 accumulation
    Ga 66, Ga 67, Ga 68 citrate
    Ga 67 gamma camera image
    Ga 67 isotope (galium citrate)
    48 hour posterior rectilinear 67 Ga scan
gadolinium (Gd) DTPA
gadolinium-enhanced T1 weighted image
gag
    Dingman mouth g.
    McIvor mouth g.
    reflex, g.
gain
galactoblast
galactocele
galactogenous
galactography
galactophlebitis
galactopoiesis
galactorrhea
    amenorrhea syndrome, g.
galactotherapy
galea
Galeati's glands
Galeazzi fracture
Galen
    vein of G.
gallbladder
    ampulla of g.
    bed, g.
    calculus, g.
    duplication, g.
    fossa, g.

gallbladder *(continued)*
    nonvisualization of g.
    series, g.
    shadow, g.
gallium (Ga)
    arsenide, g.
    citrate Ga 66, 67, 68, g.
    67 gamma camera image, g.
    scan, g.
    67 scintigraphy, g.
gallop
    atrial g.
    diastolic g.
    presystolic g.
    rhythm, g.
    ventricular g.
gallstone
galvanic
    cautery, g.
    response, g.
    stimulation, g.
galvanocautery
galvanogustometer
galvanometer
gamma
    camera, g.
    camera scintigraphy, g.
    decay, g.
    emission, g.
    emitting nuclide, g.
    knife, g.
    photon spectometry, g.
    photopeak, g.
    ray photon, g.
    ray source, g.
    scintillation camera, g.
    teletherapy unit, g.
    variage area-ratio method, g.

Additional Entries ______________________________

Gamma Med II c afterloading system
ganglia
ganglial
gangliform
ganglioblast
gangliocyte
ganglioglioma
gangliogliоneuroma
ganglion
accessory g.
acousticofacial g.
Acrel's g.
Andersch's g.
aorticorenal g.
aorticorenalia g.
Arnold's g.
auditory g.
Auerbach's g.
auricular g.
azygous g.
basal g.
Bezold's g.
Bidder's g.
Blandin's g.
Bochdalek's g.
Bochdalekii g.
Bock's g.
cardiac g.
carotid g.
celiac g.
cephalic g.
cerebrospinal g.
cervical g.
cervicale inferius g.
cervicale medium g.
cervicale superius g.
cervicothoracic g.
cervicothoracicum g.
cervicouterine g.
ciliare g.
ciliary g.

ganglion *(continued)*
Cloquet's g.
coccygeal g.
cochlear g.
collateral g.
compound g.
Corti's g.
Darkshevich's g.
diaphragmatic g.
diffuse g.
dorsal root g.
Ehrenritter's g.
extracraniale g.
false g.
Frankenhauser's g.
Froriep's g.
Ganser's g.
Gasser's g.
gasserian g.
geniculate g.
geniculi nervi facialis g.
glossopharyngeal nerve g.
habenulae, g. of
hepatic g.
hypogastric g.
hypoglossal g.
impar g.
inferius nervi glossopharyngei g.
inferius nervi vagi g.
inhibitory g.
intercarotid g.
intercraniale g.
intermedia g.
intermediate g.
interpenduncular g.
intervertebral g.
intervertebrale g.
jugular g.
jugulare nervi vagi g.
Kuttner's g.

Additional Entries

ganglion *(continued)*
Langley's g.
Laumonier's g.
Lee's g.
lingual g.
Lobstein's g.
Ludwig's g.
lumbalia g.
lumbar g.
Luschka's g.
lymphatica g.
maxillary g.
Meckel's g.
Meissner's g.
mesenteric g.
mesentericum inferius g.
mesentericum superius g.
Muller's g.
nephrolumbar g.
nervi splanchnici g.
nodose g.
nodusum g.
of glossopharyngeal nerve, g.
of habenulae, g.
of Meckel, g.
of Muller, g.
of sympathetic plexuses, g.
of sympathetic trunk, g.
of thalamus, anterior, f.
of trigeminal nerve, g.
of vagus nerve, g.
olfactory g.
ophthalmic g.
optic g.
orbital g.
otic g.
oticum g.
parasympathetic g.
pelvic g.

ganglion *(continued)*
pelvina g.
periosteal g.
petrosal g.
petrosum g.
petrous g.
phrenic g.
phenica g.
plexum autonomicorum g.
plexum sympathicorum g.
prevertebral g.
primary g.
prostatic g.
pterygopalatine g.
pterygopalatinum g.
Remak's g.
renal g.
renalia g.
retinae g.
Ribes' g.
sacral g.
sacralia g.
Scarpa's g.
Schacher's g.
Schmiedel's g.
semilunar g.
semilunare g.
sensory g.
simple g.
sinoatrial g.
sinus g.
Soemmering's g.
solar g.
sphenomaxillary g.
sphenopalatine g.
sphenopalatinum g.
spinal g.
spinale g.
spiral g.
spirale cochleae g.

Additional Entries

ganglion *(continued)*
spirale nervi cochleae g.
splanchnic g.
splanchnicum g.
stellate g.
stellatum g.
submandibular g.
submandibulare g.
submaxillare g.
submaxillary g.
superius g.
superius nervi glosso-pharyngei g.
superius nervi vagi g.
suprarenal g.
sympathetic g.
synovial g.
terminal g.
terminale g.
thoracalia g.
thoracic g.
thoracica g.
thoracicum primum g.
thyroid g.
trigeminal g.
trigeminale g.
Troisier's g.
trunci sympathici g.
tympanic g.
tympanicum g.
upper g.
vagal g.
vagus nerve g.
Valentin's g.
ventricular g.
vertebral g.
vertebrale g.
vestibular g.
vestibulare g.
Walther's g.
Wrisberg's g.
Wrisbergi g.

ganglioneuroblastoma
ganglioneurofibroma
ganglioneuroma
ganglionic
ganglionitis
ganglioplegic
gangliospore
gangliosympathectomy
gangrene
anaphylactic g.
angiosclerotic g.
circumscribed g.
cold g.
diabetic g.
dry g.
embolic g.
emphysematous g.
epidemic g.
Fournier's g.
fulminating g.
gas g.
gaseous g.
glycemic g.
hot g.
humid g.
inflammatory g.
mephitic g.
moist g.
oral g.
pressure g.
primary g.
progressive g.
progressive bacterial synergistic g.
Raynaud's g.
secondary g.
senile g.
static g.
symmetric g.
sympathetic g.
thrombotic g.
traumatic g.

Additional Entries

gangrene *(continued)*
  trophic g.
  venous g.
gangrenous
  appendix, g.
Ganser's ganglion
gantry
  angle, g.
  axis, g.
  rotation alignment, g.
  rotation range, g.
gap
  air-bone g.
  calculations, g.
  separation, g.
  technique, g.
Garceau catheter
Gardner's syndrome
Garland's curve
Garre's osteomyelitis
Gartner's
  cyst, G.
  duct, G.
  phenomenon, G.
gas
  containing abscess, g.
  density line, g.
  embolism, g.
  encephalography, g.
  feces, g. and
  filled detector, g.
  forming infection, g.
  gangrene, g.
  ionization, g.
  portal vein, g. in
  powdered injector, g.
  superimposed bowel g.
  tube, g. (roentgen-ray tube)
  ventriculography, g.
gaseous
  distention, g.
gasometer
gasometry
gasserian ganglion
Gasser's ganglion
gastradenitis
gastralgia
gastrectomy
  Hofmeister g.
  partial g.
  subtotal g.
  total g.
gastric
  air bubble, g.
  anacidity, g.
  analysis, g.
  antrum, g.
  arteries, g.
  aspirate, g.
  bull's eye lesion, g.
  carcinoma, g.
  cardia, g.
  contents, g.
  Crohn's disease, g.
  distention, g.
  diverticulum, g.
  emptying, g.
  glands, g.
  lavage, g.
  lymph nodes, g.
  mucosa, g.
  mucosa imaging, g.
  mucosal pattern, g.
  nerves, g.
  outlet, g.
  outlet obstruction, g.
  plexuses, g.
  polyps, g.
  pull-through segment, g.
  pylorus, g.
  reflux, g.
  resection, g.
  rugal folds, g.

Additional Entries

gastric *(continued)*
 secretion indicator, g.
 veins, g.
 washings, g.
gastrinoma
gastritis
 atrophic g.
 catarrhal g.
 erosive g.
 exfoliative g.
 hemorrhagic g.
 hypertrophic g.
 pseudomembranous g.
 radiating g.
 toxic g.
gastrocnemius
 muscle, g.
gastrocoele
gastrocolic
 ligament, g.
 omentum, g.
gastrocolitis
gastrocoloptosis
gastrocolostomy
gastrocolotomy
gastrocutaneous
gastrodermis
gastrodiaphane
gastrodiaphanoscopy
gastroduodenal
 artery, g.
gastroduodenectomy
gastroduodenitis
gastroduodenoscopy
gastroduodenostomy
gastrodynia
gastroenteric
 cyst, g.
gastroenteritis
 acute infectious g.
 eosinophilic g.
 viral g.
gastroenteroanastomosis
gastroenterocolitis
gastroenterocolostomy
gastroenteroplasty
gastroenterostomy
 Balfour g.
 Hofmeister g.
 Billroth I
 Billroth II
 stoma, g.
gastroenterotomy
gastroepiploic
 arteries, g.
 lymph node, g.
 veins, g.
gastroesophageal (GE)
 reflux, g.
 regurgitation, g.
gastroesophagitis
gastroesophagostomy
gastrofiberscope
gastrogastrostomy
gastrogavage
Gastrografin
gastrograph
gastrohepatic
 omentum, g.
gastrohepatitis
gastrohypertonic
gastroileac
gastroileitis
gastroileostomy
gastrointestinal (GI)
 bleed, g.
 bleeding scan, g.
 blood loss study, g.
 fat absorption study, g.
 fistula, g.
 hemorrhage, g.
 ischemia, g.
 lymphoma, g.
 mass, g.

Additional Entries

gastrointestinal *(continued)*
protein loss study, g.
tract (GI), g.
gastrojejunocolic
gastrojejunoesophagostomy
gastrojejunostomy
gastrokinesograph
gastrolienal
gastrolith
gastrolithiasis
gastrolysis
gastromalacia
gastromegaly
gastromycosis
gastromyotomy
gastromyxorrhea
gastropancreatic
fold, g.
gastropancreatitis
gastroparalysis
gastroparesis
gastroparietal
gastropathic
gastropathy
gastroperiodynia
gastroperitonitis
gastropexy
gastrophotography
gastrophrenic
ligament, g.
gastrophthisis
gastroplasty
gastroplegia
gastroplication
gastropneumonic
gastroptosis
gastropulmonary
gastropylorectomy
gastropyloric
gastroradiculitis
gastrorrhagia
gastrorrhaphy
gastrorrhea
gastrorrhexis
gastroschisis
gastroscope
fiberoptic g.
gastroscopy
gastrospasm
gastrosplenic
gastrostaxis
gastrostenosis
gastrostogavage
gastrostolavage
gastrostoma
gastrostomy
gastrotome
gastrotomy
gastrotonometer
gastrotonometry
gastrotropic
gated
blood pool study, g.
cardiac imaging, g.
motion study, g.
scintiphotography, g.
view, g.
wall-motion study, g.
wall-motion study, exercise g.
wall study, exercise g.
Gaucher's disease
gauge
gauss
gaussian
curve, g.
distribution, g.
line saturation, g.
mode profile laser beam, g.
gavage
Gavard's muscle
Gaynor-Hart position
gaze position changes

Additional Entries

GBq (gigabecquerel)
GD (given dose)
Gd (gadolinium) DTPA radioisotope
Ge (germanium)
GE (gastroesophageal)
GE-9800 high-resolution CT scanner
Geiger counter
Geiger-Mueller (GM)
 counter, GM
 tube, GM
Geissler's tube
Geissler-Pluecker tube
gelatinous
gelatin sponge
gel, coupling
Gelfilm
Gelfoam
Gellhorn pessary
gelometer
Geltabs
GE method
gemistocyte
gemistocytic
gemma
gemmule
 nerves, g. of
General Electric CT scanner
generalized
 fibromatosis, g.
 U shape, g.
general radiography
generator
 cardiac g.
 pulse g.
 unipolar pacemaker, g.
genetic disease
genicular
 arteries, g.
 ganglion, g.
 ligament, g.
geniculate
 bodies, g.
geniculum
 facial nerve, g. of
geniocheiloplasty
genioplasty
genital
 cord, g.
 corpuscles, g.
 glands, g.
 organs, g.
 ridge, g.
 tract, g.
 tubercle, g.
genitalia
genitocrural
 nerve, g.
genitofemoral
 nerve, g.
genitography
genitoplasty
genitourinary
Gennari's
 band, G.
 line, G.
genoblast
gentian
 violet, g.
geographical miss
genu
 capsulae internae, g.
 corporis callosi, g.
 corpus callosum, g. of
 extrorsum, g.
 facial canal, g. of
 facial nerve, g. of
 impressum, g.
 internal capsule, g. of
 (internum) radicus nervi facialis, g.
 introrsum, g.
 nervi facialis, g.

Additional Entries

genu *(continued)*
  recurvatum, g.
  valgum, g.
  varum, g.
genucubital position (knee-elbow)
genufacial position (knee-face)
genupectoral position (knee-chest)
Gerdy's fibers
Gerlach's
  network, G.
germanium (Ge)
germ centers
  lymph node g.c.
  dental g.c.
germicidal solution
germinal
  center, g.
  epithelium, g.
germinoma
germ layer tumor
geroderma
  osteodysplastica, g.
Gerota's
  capsule, G.
  fascia, G.
gestational trophoblastic neoplasm (GTN)
GeV (giga electron volts)
GFR (glomerular filtration rate)
Ghon-Sachs
  complex, G.
  primary lesion, G.
  tubercle, G.
Ghon's primary lesion
ghost nodes
GI (gastrointestinal)
Giacomini's
  band, G.
Giannuzzi's crescents
giant
  astrocytoma, g. cell
  cell reparative granuloma, g.
  cells of Betz, g.
  cell thyroiditis, g.
  cell tumor, g.
  fibroadenoma, g.
  ulcer, g.
Gianturco coil
Gianturco-Roehm filter
giardiasis
Gibbon's hernia
gibbous
Gibbs phenomenon
GI (gastrointestinal) bleeding scan
Gibson's murmur
Gidlung injector
Gierke's corpuscles
gigabecquerel (GBq.)
giga electron volts (GeV)
gigantism
Gilbert's
  disease, G.
  syndrome, G.
Gilchrist's disease
Gilles de la Tourette syndrome
Gimbernat's ligament
gingiva
  alveolar g.
  areolar g.
  buccal g.
  free g.
  labial g.
  lingual g.
  marginal g.
gingivae
gingival
gingivalgia

Additional Entries

gingivectomy
gingivitis
    atrophic senile g.
    herpetic g.
    hyperplastic g.
    necrotizing ulcerative g.
    senile atrohic g.
    ulceromembranous g.
gingivoaxial
gingivobuccoaxial
gingivoglossitis
gingivolabial
gingivolinguoaxial
gingivoplasty
gingivostomatitis
ginglymus (a/k/a hinge joint)
Giordano's sphincter
Giraldes' organ
girdle
    inferior extremity g.
    pelvic g.
    shoulder g.
    superior extremity g.
Giuffrida-Ruggieri stigma
given dose (GD)
glabella
glabellad
gladiolus
gladiomanubrial
gland
    accessory g.
    acinous g.
    adrenal g.
    alveolar g.
    apocrine g.
    areolar g.
    axillary g.
    Bartholin g.
    Blandin g.
    Bowman g.
    bronchial g.
    Bruch g.

gland *(continued)*
    Brunner g.
    buccal g.
    bulbocavernous g.
    bulbourethral g.
    cardiac g.
    ceruminous g.
    cervical g.
    ciliary g.
    circumanal g.
    closed gl
    Cobelli g.
    coccygeal g.
    compound g.
    conglobate g.
    Cowper g.
    Duverney g.
    Ebner g.
    eccrine g.
    endocrine g.
    excretory g.
    exocrine g.
    fundic g.
    Galeati g.
    gastric g.
    Gay g.
    genal g.
    glosspalatine g.
    gustatory g.
    guttural g.
    Harder g.
    haversian g.
    hematopoietic g.
    hemolymph g.
    holocrine g.
    intestinal g.
    jugular g.
    Krause g.
    lacrimal g.
    lingual g.
    Littre g.
    Luschka g.

Additional Entries

gland *(continued)*
- lymph g.
- mammary g.
- meibomian g.
- merocrine g.
- mixed g.
- Moll g.
- monoptychic g.
- Montgomery g.
- Morgagni g.
- mucous g.
- nabothian g.
- Nuhn g.
- oil g.
- olfactory g.
- parathyroid g.
- paraurethral g.
- parotid g.
- Peyer g.
- pineal g.
- pituitary g.
- preputial g.
- prostate g.
- pyloric g.
- racemose g.
- Rivinus g.
- saccular g.
- salivary g.
- sebaceous g.
- sentinel g.
- seromucous g.
- serous g.
- sex g.
- simple g.
- Skene g.
- solitary g.
- sublingual g.
- submandibular g.
- submaxillary g.
- sudoriferous g.
- suprarenal g.
- Suzanne g.

gland *(continued)*
- sweat g.
- target g.
- tarsal g.
- thymus g.
- thyroid g.
- tubular g.
- tubuloacinar g.
- Tyson g.
- unicellular g.
- urethral g.
- vaginal g.
- Virchow g.
- vulvovaginal g.
- Waldeyer g.
- Weber g.
- Zeis g.
- Zuckerlandl g.

glans
- clitoridis, g.
- clitoris, g. of
- penis, g.

glarometer

glaserian fissure

glass
- envelope, g.
- rays, g.
- syringe, g.
- wall of tube, g.

glassy cell carcinoma

Glenard's disease

Glenn shunt

glenohumeral

glenoid
- cavity, g.
- cavity of scapula, g.
- fossa, g.
- fossal, g.
- labrum, g.
- ligament of Cruveilhier, g.
- process, g.

Additional Entries ________________

glial cells
gliding joint
glioblastoma
    multiforme, g.
gliofibrillary
glioma
    butterfly-type g.
gliomatosis cerebri
gliomatous
glioneuroma
gliosis
Glisson's capsule
global ejection fraction
globe
    optic g.
globinometer
globular processes of HIS
globulomaxillary
globus
    hystericus, g.
    major (epididymis), g.
    minor (epididymis), g.
    pallidus, g.
glomangioma
glomectomy
glomera
glomerular
    afferent g. arterioles
    arterioles, g.
    basement membrane, g.
    capsule of kidney, g.
    filtration rate, g. (GFR)
    permeability, g.
    sclerosis, g.
glomeruli
glomerulitis
glomerulonephritis
    chronic membranous g.
    IgA g.
    lobular g.
    membranoproliferative g.
glomerulonephritis *(cont.)*
    mesangiocapillary g.
    rapidly progressive g.
glomerulonephropathy
glomerulopathy
glomerulosclerosis
glomerulus
glomus
    aorticum, g.
    caroticum, g.
    coccygeum, g.
    tumor, g.
glossa
glossal
glossalgia
glossanthrax
glossectomy
glossitis
glossocele
glossocoma
glossodynamometer
glossodynia
glossoepiglottic
    folds, g.
glossograph
glossohyal
glossopalatine
    arch, g.
    sulcus, g.
glossopalatinus
    muscle, g.
glossopathy
glossopexy
glossopharyngeal
    nerve, g.
    sympathetic afferent fibers, g.
glossopharyngeum
glossopharyngeus
glossoplasty
glossoptosis
glossopyrosis

Additional Entries

glossorrhaphy
glossoscopy
glossospasm
glossotilt
glossotomy
glossotrichia
glottal
glottic
  chink, g.
glottis
  respiratoria, g.
  vocalis, g.
glucagon
glucocorticoid
glucoheptonate
  flow study, g.
gluconate
glucose-6–phosphate-dehydrogenase
glutathione (GSH)
gluteal
  artery, g.
  lines of ilium, g.
  muscles, g.
  nerves, g.
  tuberosity, g.
  veins, g.
gluteofemoral
gluteoinguinal
gluteus
  maximus muscle, g.
  medius muscle, g.
  minimus muscle, g.
glycogen
  storage diseaase, g.
glycopolyuria
glycorrhachia
glycorrhea
glycosecretory
glycoside
glycosometer
glycosphingolipid
glycosuria
  renal g.
glycosylated
glycosyltransferase
glycotropic
Gm (gamma)
gm. (gram)
GM (Geiger-Mueller)
  counter, GM
  tube, GM
gnathodynamometer
gnathography
gnathoplasty
goiter
  aberrant g.
  adenomatous g.
  Basedow g.
  colloid g.
  cystic g.
  diffuse toxic g.
  diving g.
  exophthalmic g.
  fibrous g.
  follicular g.
  intrathoracic g.
  iodide g.
  lingual g.
  lymphadenoid g.
  multinodular g.
  nodular g.
  nontoxic g.
  parenchymatous g.
  simple g.
  substernal g.
  suffocative g.
  toxic g.
  toxic multinodular g.
  wandering g.
goitrous
  autoimmune thyroiditis, g.
Golay coil

Additional Entries

gold (Au)
  Au 198, g.
  ball, g.
  button, g.
  grain magazine, g.
  grain prostate implant, g.
  grains, g.
Goldblatt's clamp
Goldenhar syndrome
Goldflam's disease (myasthenia gravis)
Goldflam-Erb disease (myasthenia gravis)
Goldstein's
  disease, G.
  rays, G.
Golgi's
  cells, G.
  complex, G.
  corpuscles, G.
  organs, G.
Goll's
  column, G.
  tract, G.
GoLytely gastrointestinal lavage pump
Gombault-Philippe triangle
gomphosis
gonad
gonadal
  dysgenesis, g.
  shielding, g.
gonadoblastoma
gonadogenesis
gonadopathy
gonadotrope
gonadotropic
  hormone, g.
gonarthritis
gonarthromeningitis
gonatocele
gonecystitis
gonecystolith
gonepoiesis
gonepoietic
gonia
gonial
goniometer
gonion
goniopuncture
gonioscope
gonioscopy
goniosynechia
goniotomy
gonitis
gonorrhea
gonorrheal
gonyoncus
Goodpasture's
  stain, G.
  syndrome, G.
G0 phase
G1 phase
Gordon's bodies
Gorham disease
Gorlin's syndrome
Gosselin's fracture
Gottstein's fibers
gouge
gouging
Gouley's catheter
gout
  masked g.
  misplaced g.
  retrocedent g.
  rheumatic g.
  tophaceous g.
gouty
  arthritis, g.
Gower's
  column, G.
  tract, G.
Goyrand's hernia

Additional Entries

Graaff generator x-ray unit
graafian
  follicle, g.
  vesicle, g.
gracile nucleus
gracilis muscle
gradient
  coil, g.
  coil system, g.
  echo imaging, g.
  function, g.
  peak systolic g.
  pressure, g.
  pulmonic valve g.
  rephasing g.
  transplacental g.
Grafenberg's ring
graft
  allogenic g.
  aortofemoral g.
  autogenous g.
  autologous g.
  avascular g.
  bifurcation g.
  cancellous g.
  cortical g.
  Dacron g.
  defatted skin g.
  diamond inlay g.
  diced cartilage g.
  full-thickness g.
  island g.
  Marlex g.
  patch g.
  pedicle g.
  skin g.
  split-thickness g.
  Teflon g.
gram (gm.)
  atomic mass, g.
  atomic weight, g.
  molecular mass, g.
Gram's
  method, G.
  stain, G.
Grandry's
  corpuscles, G.
  tactile corpuscles, G.
Granger line
Granger view
granula
  iridica, g.
granular
  corpuscles, g.
  layer of dentin, g.
granulation
  arachnoid g.
  exuberant g.
granule
granuliform
granuloadipose
granulocyte
granuloctic
granulocytopathy
granulocytopathy
granulocytopenia
granulocytopoiesis
granulocytopoietic
granulocytosis
granuloma
  eosinophilic g.
  foreign body g.
  pyogenic g.
  septic g.
granulomatosis
  Wegener's g.
granulomatous
  angiitis, g.
  chronic g. disease
  colitis, g.
  disease, g.
  lymphoma, g.
  thyroiditis, g.
granulopoiesis

Additional Entries

granulovacuolar
graph
graphic
graphoanalysis
graphokinesthetic
graphoscopy
Graser's diverticulum
grasping forceps
Gratiolet's radiating fibers
Graves' disease
gravid
  uterus, g.
gravidarum
  hyperemesis g.
gravidocardiac
gravidopuerperal
gravimeter
gravis
  myasthenia g.
gravitational gradient
gravitometer
gravity
  dependent layering, g.
  drainage, g.
  specific g.
Grawitz's tumor
gray (Gy)
  central g.
  commissures of medulla spinalis, g.
  matter, g.
  matter edema, g.
  nerve fibers, g.
  perihypoglossal g.
  scale, g.
  scale band display, g.
  scale B-mode ultrasound image, g.
  scale echography, g.
  scale sonograaphy, g.
  scale ultrasonography, g.
  scale zone, g.

gray (Gy) *(continued)*
  silver g.
  steel g.
  substance of cerebellum, g.
Grawitz's tumor
great
  auricular nerve, g.
  cardiac nerve, g.
  cardiac vein, g.
  cerebral vein, g.
  longitudinal fissure, g.
  omentum, g.
  sacrosciatic ligament, g.
  saphenous vein, g.
  splanchnic nerve, g.
  transverse fissure of brain, g.
  vessel, g.
  wings of sphenoid, g.
greater
  cavernous nerve, g.
  curvature of stomach, g.
  multiangular bone, g.
  occipital nerve, g.
  omentum, g.
  palatine foramen, g.
  pelvis, g.
  peritoneal sac, g.
  sciatic foramen, g.
  sciatic notch, g.
  sigmoid cavity, g.
  splanchnic nerve, g.
  superficial petrosal nerve, g.
  trochanter, g.
  tuberosity g.
  vestibular glands, g.
  wing of sphenoid bone, g.
green
  acid g.

Additional Entries

green *(continued)*
  brilliant g.
  bromocresol g.
  Brunswick g.
  diazin g. S.
  ethyl g.
  fast acid g. N.
  Hoffman g.
  indocyanine g.
  iodine g.
  Janus g. B
  light g.
  malachite g.
  methyl g.
  methylene g.
  new solid g.
  Paris g.
  Schweinfurt g.
  solid g.
  Victoria g.
Greene
  biopsy set, G.
  needle, G.
Greenhow's disease
greenstick fracture
grenz ray
Greulich and Pyle scale
grid
  Bucky g.
  cassette, g.
  characteristics, g.
  controlled x-ray tube, g.
  focused g.
  function, g.
  interference, g.
  parallel g.
  penetration, g.
  Potter-Bucky g.
  stationary g.
Griesinger's disease
Gritti's amputation
Gritti-Stokes amputation
groin
Grollman pigtail catheter
groove
  atrioventricular g.
  auriculoventricular g.
  bicipital g.
  branchial g.
  carotid g.
  carpal g.
  chiasmatic g.
  costal g.
  Harrison's g.
  infraorbital g.
  interatrial g.
  intercondylar g.
  intercostal g.
  intertubercular g.
  labiogingival g.
  lacrimal g.
  laryngotracheal g.
  limbal g.
  medullary g.
  musculospiral g.
  mylohyoid g.
  neural g.
  obturator g.
  occipital g.
  olfactory g.
  optic g.
  palatine g.
  paracolic g.
  pectoral g.
  peroneal g.
  petrosal sinus g.
  pharyngeal g.
  popliteal g.
  primitive g.
  pterygopalatine g.
  sinus g.
  vertebral g.
  vomerine g.
Groshong catheter

Additional Entries

gross
anatomy, g.
appearance, g.
blood, g.
evidence, g.
hematuria, g.
sample count, g.
grossly displaced
Gross's disease
ground-glass appearance
ground state
Grove's cell
growth
arrest line, g.
plate, g.
Gruber's bougie
Gruber's fossa
Gruentzig (a/k/a Gruntzig) catheter
grunting
expiration, g.
respirations, g.
Grynfeltt's hernia
Grynfeltt-Lesgaft triangle
GSH (glutathione)
GTM classification (G-grade/T-tumor size & location/M-metastases)
GTN (gestational trophoblastic neoplasm)
GU (genitourinary)
guaiac
negative/positive stool, g.
guarding
involuntary g.
voluntary g.
Guarnieri's bodies
gubernaculum
dentis, g.
Hunter's g.
ovarii, g.
gubernaculum *(continued)*
testis, g.
Gubler's hemiplegia
Gudden's
commissure, G.
mammillo-tegmental bundle, G.
Gueneau de Mussy's point
Guerin's fold
guide wire
Bentson g.w.
J-curve movable core g.w.
Lunderquist exchange g.w.
Lunderquist-Ring torque g.w.
Newton g.w.
Guidi's canal
Guillain-Barre syndrome
guillotine
Guinon's disease
Guiteras' disease
gullet
Gull's disease
Gullstrand's slit lamp
gum
Gumprecht's shadow
Gunn's dots
Gunning's splint
Gunz's ligament
gurgling
rales, g.gusatory
calyculi, g.
cells, g.
hair, g.
pore, g.
gut
Guthrie's muscle
gutta
serena, g.
guttae

Additional Entries ______________________

____

____

gutta-percha
  baseplate, g.
guttural
Guyon's amputation
G value
gymnocyte
gymnoplast
gymnoscopic
GYN (gynecologic)
gynecogen
gynecogenic
gynecography
gynecologic
gynecological
gynecologist
gynecology
gynecomastia
gynoplasty
gyral enhancement
gyre
  medifrontal g.
  precentral g.
  subfrontal g.
  superfrontal g.
gyromagnetic ratio
gyrometer
gyrus
  angular g.
  Broca g.
  callosal g.
  central g.
  cerebral g.
  cingulate g.

gyrus *(continued)*
  dentate g.
  fornicatus g.
  frontal g.
  fusiform g.
  geniculi g.
  Heschl g.
  hippocampal g.
  infracalcarine g.
  lateral g.
  lingual g.
  longus insulae g.
  marginal g.
  medial g.
  occipital g.
  occipitotemoral g.
  olfactory g.
  orbital gyri
  paraterminal g.
  postcentral g.
  postparietal g.
  precental g.
  postparietal g.
  preinsular gyri
  precuneus g.
  quadrate g.
  rectus g.
  subcallosal g.
  supracallosal g.
  supramarginal g.
  temporal g.
  uncinate g.
  uncus g.

Additional Entries

H

H (Hounsfield unit)
H (hydrogen)
Haagensen's operability criteria
habenula
habenular commissure
habenulae
habitual
- abortion, h.
- dislocation, h.

Hadlock formula
Haering tube
Haff disease
Hagedorn's needle
Haglund's disease
hair
- bearing area, h.
- bulb, h.
- cuticle of h.
- follicle of h.
- gustatory h.
- olfactory h.
- on end pattern, h.
- root of h.
- scapus or shaft of h.

hairy
- nevus, h.

Hajdu-Chaney syndrome
Haldane chamber
Hales' piesimeter
half
- -axial, h.
- axial posteroanterior projection, h.
- beam, h.
- beam block, h.
- body irradiation, h. (HBI)
- circle, taper-point surgical needle, h.

half *(continued)*
- -cycle, h.
- field block, h.
- intensity needle, h.
- -life, h.
- moon marginal defect, h.
- value thickness, h. (HVT)
- -value layer, h. (HVL)

half-life
- antibody h.
- biological h.
- effective h.
- physical h.

half-wave
- rectification, h.

Hall band
Hallerman-Streiff syndrome
Hallevorden-Spatz disease
Hall's disease
Hall-Stone ring
Halle's point
Haller's
- ansa, H.
- vas aberrans, H.

Hallopeau's acrodermatitis
hallux
- dolorosa, h.
- flexus, h.
- malleus, h.
- rigidus, h.
- valgus, h.
- varus, h.

halo
- Fick's h.
- glaucomatous h.
- like clear space, h.
- senile h.

halodermia

Additional Entries ______________________

halometer
Halstead maneuver
hamarthritis
hamartoblastoma
hamartoma
hamartomatosis
hamartomatous
hamartoplasia
hamate
    bone, h.
    hook of h.
Hamberger's schema
Hamman's disease
Hamman-Rich syndrome
hammer
    toe correction, h.
    trip h. pulse
Hammond's disease
Hampton hump
hamstring
    inner h.
    outer h.
hamulus
    hamate bone, h. of
    lacrimal h.
    laminae spiralis h.
    pterygoid h.
hand
    articulations of h.
    claw h.
    cleft h.
    club h.
    drop h.
    fascia of h.
    foot-uterus syndrome, h.
    held syringe, h.
    muscles of h.
    phalanges of h.
handful of knuckles
Hand's disease
Hand-Schuller-Christian disease
Handley's lymphangioplasty
hanging
    block technique, h.
    cast, h.
hangman's fracture
Hannover's canal
Hanot's cirrhosis
haptic
haptometer
hard
    palate, h.
    rays, h.
Harder's glands
harelip
Harley's disease
Harrison's
    groove, H.
    sulcus, H.
harsh systolic murmur
Hartmann's pouch
Hashimoto's thyroiditis
Hasner's
    fold, H.
    valve, H.
Hassall's corpuscles
haustra
haustral
    fold, h.
    markings, h.
    pattern, h.
haustration
haustrum
haversian
    canal, h.
    system, h.
Hawkins needle
Hayem's corpuscles
Haygarth's node
Hb (symbol for hemoglobin)
HBI (hemi-body irradiation; half body irradiation)
HBO (hyperbaric oxygen)

Additional Entries

He (helium)
H42E hepatoma
head
- adjusted to true posteroanterior (PA) position, h.
- arteries of h.
- circumference, h.
- down tilting, h.
- femoral h.
- humeral h.
- hunter catheter, h.
- long h.
- lymphatics of h.
- mandible, h. of
- metatarsal h.
- muscles of h.
- radial h.
- rotated slightly toward affected side, h.
- scanning machine, h.
- short h.
- sparing, h.
- unit, h.
- veins of h.

Head's zones
headhunter catheter
healed
- infarct, h.
- wound h. per primam

healing
- first intention, h. by
- granulation, h. by
- phase, h.
- second intention, h. by
- stress fracture, h.
- third intention, h. by

Heaney retractor
heaped-up margins
hearing loss
- conductive h.l.
- patetoid h.l.

hearing loss *(continued)*
- paradoxic h.l.
- sensorineural h.l.
- transmission h.l.

heart
- apex, h.
- arteries, h.
- atrioventricular bundle of HIS, h.
- atrioventricular node, h.
- atrium, left/right, h.
- carcinoid disease of h.
- cradle, h.
- emission tomography of h.
- endocardium, h.
- fibers of ventricles of h.
- fibrous rings of h.
- lymphatic capillaries of h.
- lymphatic vessels of h.
- marginal veins of h.
- muscular structure, h.
- nerves, h.
- perfusion scintigraphy of h.
- shunt, h.
- sonogram, h.
- trigonum fibrosum, h.
- valves, h.
- veins, h.
- ventricle, left/right, of h.
- ventricular septum of h.

heart block
- arborization h.b.
- atrioventricular h.b.
- bundle-branch h.b.
- complete h.b.
- congenital h.b.
- incomplete h.b.
- interventricular h.b.
- intraventricular h.b.

Additional Entries

heart block *(continued)*
- Mobitz type I h.b.
- Mobitz type II h.b.
- partial h.b.
- sinoatrial h.b.
- Wenckebach h.b.

heart failure
- backward h.f.
- congestive h.f.
- forward h.f.
- high output h.f.
- left-sided h.f.
- left ventricular h.f.
- low output h.f.
- right-sided h.f.
- right ventricular h.f.

heat
- distribution, h.
- quantities, h.
- shock proteins, h.
- unit, h.

heated filament

heavy
- chain disease, h.
- chain disorder, h.
- charged particle therapy, h.
- ions, h.
- lipped facies, h.

Heberden's
- asthma, H.
- node, H.

Hebra's disease

hectoliter

hedrocele

heel effect

Heerfordt's disease

Hegar's dilator

Heidenhain's
- cells, H.
- demilunes, H.

Heilbronner's thigh

Heine-Medin disease

Heineke-Mikulicz pyloroplasty

Heinz bodies

Heinz-Ehrlich bodies

Heister's
- diverticulum, H.
- valve, H.

helical
- coil, h.
- intracavitary applicator, h.

helicotrema

heliotherapy

helium (He)
- nuclei, h.

helix
- alpha h.
- double h.
- Watson-Crick h.

Heller-Dohle disease

helmet
- field, h.

Helmholtz's
- coil, H.
- ligament, H.
- theory, H.

heloma

helotomy

Helweg's bundle

hemabarometer

hemacytometer

hemacytometry

hemadostenosis

hemadsorbent

hemadsorption

hemal
- nodes, h.

hemangiomatous pocket

hemangioameloblastoma

hemangioendothelioblastoma

hemangioendothelioma

Additional Entries

hemangiofibroma
hemangioma
  ameloblastic h.
  sclerosing h.
hemangiopericytoma
hemangiosarcoma
hematemesis
hematencephalon
hematinuria
hematocele
hematocephalus
hematochezia
hematochyluria
hematocoelia
hematocolpometra
hematocolpos
hematocrit
hematocyanin
hematocyst
hematocytopenia
hematocyturia
hematoencephalic
hematogenic
hematogenous
  dissemination, h.
hematohyaloid
hematoid
hematoidin
hematoma
  chronic subdural h.
  epidural h.
  pulsatile h.
  residual h.
hematometer
hematometry
hematomphalocele
hematomyelia
hematomyelitis
hematomyelopore
hematoncometry
hematonephrosis
hematoplastic
hematopoiesis
  extramedullary h.
hematopoietic
  depression, h.
hematorrhea
hematosalpinx
hematoscheocele
hematoscope
hematoscopy
hematospectroscope
hematospectroscopy
hematospermatocele
hematostatic
hematotropic
hematotympanum
hematuria
  gross h.
  intermittent h.
  microscopic h.
  painless h.
heme
hemiachromatopsia
hemiamblyopia
hemianencephaly
hemianopia
  absolute h.
  altitudinal h.
  binasal h.
  binocular h.
  bitemporal h.
  complete h.
  congruous h.
  crossed h.
  equilateral h.
  heteronymous h.
  homonymous h.
  horizontal h.
  lateral h.
  lower h.
  nasal h.
  quadrant h.
  temporal h.

Additional Entries

hemianopia *(continued)*
 true h.
 unilateral h.
 uniocular h.
 upper h.
 vertical h.
hemianopic
hemiapraxia
hemiarthroplasty
hemiarthrosis
hemiasynergia
hemiataxia
hemiathetosis
hemiatrophy
hemiautotroph
hemiautotrophic
hemiaxial
hemiazygos
 accessory vein, h.
 vein, h.
hemiballismus
hemibladder
hemiblock
hemibody irradiation (HBI)
hemicardia
hemicellulose
hemicentrum
hemicephalia
hemicephallus
hemicerebrum
hemichorea
hemichromatopsia
hemicolectomy
hemicorporectomy
hemicrania
hemicraniectomy
hemicraniosis
hemidecortication
hemidiaphragm
hemidisc
hemidystrophy
hemielastin
hemiencephalus
hemifacial
hemigastrectomy
hemigenesis
hemigeusia
hemigigantism
hemiglossal
hemiglossectomy
hemiglossitis
hemignathia
hemihepatectomy
hemihidrosis
hemihypalgesia
hemihyperesthesia
hemihypermetria
hemihyperplasia
hemihypertonia
hemihypertrophy
hemihypesthesia
hemihypometria
hemihypoplasia
hemihypotonia
hemilaminectomy
hemilaryngectomy
hemilateral
hemilesion
hemilingual
hemimacroglossia
hemimandibulectomy
hemimegalencephaly
hemimelia
heminephrectomy
heminephroureterectomy
hemineurasthenia
hemiobesity
hemiopalgia
hemiopia
hemiopic
hemiparanesthesia
hemiparaplegia
hemiparesis
hemiparesthesia

Additional Entries

hemiparetic
hemiparkinsonism
hemipelvectomy
hemiphalangectomy
hemiplacenta
hemiplegia
  alternate h.
  crossed h.
  facial h.
  spastic h.
  spinal h.
hemiplegic
hemiprostatectomy
hemipylorectomy
hemiarchischisis
hemisacralization
hemisection
hemiseptum
hemiskeleton centers
hemisoantibody
hemisphere
  cerebellar h.
  cerebral h.
  cortical atrophy, h.
  dominant h.
  focality, h.
hemispherectomy
hemispheric lesion
hemispheric width (HW)
hemispherical ball
hemispherium
Hemispora stellata
hemitetany
hemithorax
hemithyroidectomy
hemitremor
hemivagotomy
hemivertebra
hemizygosity
hemizygote
hemizygous
hemoblastosis
hemocatheresis
hemocatherectic
hemocholecyst
hemocholecystitis
hemochromatosis
hemochromatotic
hemochrome
hemochromogen
hemochromometer
hemochromometry
hemochromoprotein
hemoclasia
hemoclasis
hemoclastic
hemoclip
hemoconiosis
hemocrine
hemocrinotherapy
hemocryoscopy
hemoculture
hemocyte
hemocytoblast
hemocytoblastoma
hemocytocatheresis
hemocytoma
hemocytophagia
hemocytophagic
hemocytotripsis
hemodiagnosis
hemodialysis
hemodialyzer
hemodilution
hemodynamic
hemodynamometry
hemodystrophy
hemoendothelial
hemohistioblast
hemohydraulics
hemokinesis
hemolith
hemolutein
hemolymph

Additional Entries

hemolymph *(continued)*
    nodes, h.
hemolytic
    anemia, h.
    jaundice, h.
    splenomegaly, h.
    streptococci, h.
hemomanometer
hemomediastinum
hemopathology
hemopathy
hemoperfusion
hemopericardium
hemoperitoneum
hemophagocyte
hemophil
hemophilia
    A, h.
    B, h.
    C, h.
    classical h.
    vascular h.
hemophiliac
hemophilic
hemophotometer
hemophthalmia
hemophthisis
hemopneumopericardium
hemopneumothorax
hemoproctia
hemoptysis
hemorrhage
    cerebral h.
    concealed h.
    extradoral h.
    fibrinolytic h.
    intracerebral h.
    intraventricular h.
    petechial h.
    postpartum h.
    primary h.
    secondary h.

hemorrhage *(continued)*
    subarachnoid h.
    subdural h.
    uterine h.
hemorrhagic
    ascites, h.
    bronchitis, h.
    corpus luteum, h.
    cyst, h.
    disease, h.
    edema, h.
    infarction, h.
    lymphatics, h.
    regions, h.
    splenic cyst, h.
    thrombocythemia, h.
hemorrhoid
    external h.
    internal h.
    lingual h.
    strangulated h.
    thrombosed h.
hemorrhoidal
    artery, h.
    nerve, h.
    plexus, h.
    skin tags, h.
    vein, h.
    venous plexus, h.
hemorrhoidectomy
hemorrhoidolysis
hemoscope
hemosiderosis
    hepatic h.
    idiopathic pulmonary h.
    pulmonary h.
hemostasis
hemostat
hemostatic
    capillary h.
hemotherapeutics
hemotherapy

Additional Entries

hemothorax
spontaneous h.
traumatic h.
hemotoxic
hemotroph
hemotrophic
hemotropic
hemotympanum
hemoxometer
Henderson-Jones disease
Henke's space
Henle's
layer, H.
loop, H.
ligament, H.
Henoch's purpura
Henry, flexor knot of
Henschke
ovoid, H.
tandem, H.
Hensen's
canal, H.
canalis reuniens, H.
stripe, H.
supporting cells, H.
Hensing's ligament
hepar
adiposum, h.
capsula fibrosa, h.
facies, h.
lobatum, h.
margo anterior, h.
tunica serosa, h.
heparin
flush, h.
lock, h.
heparinemia
heparinize
hepatalgia
hepatatrophia
hepatectomize
hepatectomy
hepatic
adenoma, h.
arteriogram, h.
arteriography, h.
artery, h.
branches of vagus nerve, h.
cells, h.
coma, h.
cylinders, h.
cyst, h.
duct, h.
encephalopathy, h.
failure, h.
fibrosis, h.
flexure, h.
flow studies, h.
function study, h.
lobectomy, h.
lymph nodes, h.
metastases, h. (Mh)
parenchyma, h.
parenchymography, h.
plexus, h.
portal vein, h.
sinusoids, h.
steal pattern, h.
triad, h.
veins, h.
venography, h.
hepaticocholangiojejunostomy
hepaticocholedochostomy
hepaticodochotomy
hepaticoduodenostomy
hepaticoenterostomy
hepaticogastrostomy
hepaticojejunostomy
hepaticolithotomy
hepaticolithotripsy
hepaticopulmonary
hepaticostomy

Additional Entries

hepaticotomy
hepatitis
A, h.
anicteric, h.
B, h.
cholangiolitic, h.
chronic active h.
infectious h.
lupoid h.
neonatal h.
non-A h.
non-B h.
serum h.
transfusion h.
viral h.
hepatobiliary
function determination, h.
imaging, h.
scan, h.
scintigraphy, h.
hepatoblastoma
hepatobronchial
hepatocarcinogenesis
hepatocarcinoma
hepatocele
hepatocellular
hepatocholangeitis
hepatocholangioduodenostomy
hepatocholangioenterostomy
hepatocholangiogastrostomy
hepatocholangiostomy
hepatocholangitis
hepatocirrhosis
hepatocolic
hepatocuprein
hepatocystic
hepatodiaphragmatic interposition
hepatoduodenal
ligament, h.
hepatoduodenostomy
hepatodynia
hepatodystrophy
hepatoenteric
hepatoenterostomy
hepatofugal
hepatogastric
ligament, h.
hepatogenic
hepatogenous
hepatogram
hepatography
hepatohemia
hepatojugular
hepatolenticular
hepatolienal
hepatolienography
hepatolith
hepatolithectomy
hepatolithiasis
hepatology
hepatolysis
hepatoma
hepatomalacia
hepatomegalia
hepatomegaly
hepatomelanosis
hepatometry
hepatomphalocele
hepatomphalos
hepatonephric
hepatonephritis
hepatonephromegaly
hepatopancreas
hepatoperitonitis
hepatopetal
hepatopexy
hepatophage
hepatophlebitis
hepatophlebography
hepatophlebotomy
hepatophyma

Additional Entries ______________________________

hepatopleural
hepatopneumonic
hepatoportal
hepatoptosis
hepatopulmonary
hepatorenal
 ligament, h.
hepatorrhagia
hepatorrhaphy
hepatorrhea
hepatorrhexis
hepatoscan
hepatoscopy
hepatosis
hepatosplenitis
hepatosplenography
hepatosplenomegaly
hepatosplenometry
hepatosplenopathy
hepatostomy
hepatotherapy
hepatomy
hepatotoxemia
Herbst's corpuscles
Hering's
 law, H.
 nerve, H.
hernia
 abdominal h.
 Barth's h.
 Beclard's h.
 Birkett's h.
 bladder hernia
 Bochdalek's h.
 Cloquet's h.
 Cooper's h.
 diaphragm, h. of
 direct h.
 duodenojejunal h.
 epigastric h.
 esophagus, h. of
 femoral h.
hernia *(continued)*
 Gibbon's h.
 Goyrand's h.
 Gruber's h.
 Grynfeltt h.
 Hesselbach's h.
 Hey's h.
 hiatal h.
 Holthouse's h.
 incisional h.
 indirect h.
 inguinal h.
 internal h.
 interstitial h.
 Kronlein's h.
 Kuster's h.
 Laugier's h.
 Littre's h.
 lumbar h.
 Morgagni's h.
 paraumbilical h.
 Petit's h.
 reducible h.
 repair (Bassini-type; pants-over-vest type), h.
 retrocecal h.
 retrograde h.
 retroperitoneal h.
 Richter's h.
 Rieux's h.
 Rokitansky's h.
 root h.
 sciatic h.
 scrotal h.
 sliding h.
 sliding hiatal h.
 spigelian h.
 strangulated h.
 Treitz's h.
 umbilical h.
 Treitz's h.

Additional Entries

hernia *(continued)*
umbilical h.
Velpeau's h.
ventral h.
vesical h.
Von Bergmann's h.
W h.
hernial
herniated
brain, h.
disk or disc, h.
intervertebral disc, h.
nucleus pulposus, h. (HNP)
herniation
hernioappendectomy
hernioenterotomy
herniolaparotomy
hernioplasty
herniopuncture
herniorrhaphy
herniotomy
herpes
genital h.
simplex, h.
simplex encephalitis, h.
zoster, h.
herpetic
Herring bodies
Herter's disease
Herter-Heubner disease
Hertig-Rock ova
Hertwig's sheath
hertz (Hz)
hertzion rays
Heschl's
convolution, H.
gyri, H.
Hesselbach's
hernia, H.
ligament, H.
triangle, H.
heterochromia
heteroganglionic
heterogeneity
heterogeneous
uptake, h.
heterogenesis
heterogenic
heterogenous
heterograft
heterokinesis
heterolateral
heterologous
heterology
heterolytic
heterometaplasia
heterometropia
heteromorphosis
heteromorphous
heteronymous
diplopia, h.
hemianopia, h.
hemianopsia, h.
heteropancreatism
heteropathy
heterophagy
heterophasia
heterophoria
heterophthalmia
heterophyiasis
heteroplasia
heteroploidy
heteropodal
heteroscope
heteroscopy
heterotopic
bone formation, h.
gray matter, h.
ossification, h.
heterotransplantation
heterotropia
alternating h.
heterotropic ossification

Additional Entries

Heublein's irradiation
method
Heubner's disease
Heubner-Herter disease
Heuser's membrane
Hexabrix
Heyman
applicator, H.
capsules, H.
tube, H.
Heyman-Simon capsules
Hg (mercury)
203 Hg chlormerodrin
Hgb (hemoglobin)
H-1–H (headhunter) catheter
hiatal
hernia, h.
insufficiency, h.
sliding esophageal h.
hiatus
adductor h.
aortic h.
esophageal h.
facial canal, h. of
petrosal nerve, h. of
sacral h.
saphenous h.
semilunar h.
vertebrocostal h.
Hickey's position
Hickman catheter
HIDA (dimethyl derivative)
hidradenitis
suppurativa, h.
hidradenoid
hidradenoma
high
contrast, h.
density, h.
dose fractions, h.
dose radiation therapy,
h.
high *(continued)*
energy linear accelera-
tor, h.
energy photons, h.
field strength scanner, h.
field strength MR imag-
ing, h.
field surface coil MRI,
h.
frequency, h.
frequency generator, h.
frequency ultrasound, h.
grade chondrosarcoma,
h.
kilovoltage technique, h.
output failure, h.
power field, h. (HPF)
ratio grid, h.
resolution radiography,
h.
risk thyroid cancer, h.
spatial resolution, h.
speed bombarding elec-
trons, h.
voltage circuit, h.
voltage supply scintilla-
tor, h.
Z shield, h.
Z shielding block, h.
Highmore's antrum
hila
lungs, h. of
hilar
adenopathy, h.
dance, h.
density, h.
enlargement, h.
lymphadenopathy, h.
lymph node (s), h.
overlay sign, h.
mass, h.
node, h.

Additional Entries

Hildenbrand's disease
Hilgenreiner line
hilum
    kidney, h. of
    lung, h. of
    testicle, h. of
hindbrain
hindfoot
hindgut
hinge
    angle, h.
    joint, h.
    position, h.
hip
    arthrodesis of h.
    articulations, h.
    Austin-Moore h. prosthesis
    bone, h.
    nailing, h.
    pinning, h.
    prosthesis, h.
    replacement, total h.
    spica cast, h.
    total h. replacement
Hippel's disease
Hippel-Lindau disease
hippocampal
    commissure, h.
    fissure, h.
    gyrus, h.
hippocampus
Hippuran
Hirschfeld's canals
Hirschfeld's disease
Hirschsprung's disease
His'
    aortic spindle of H.
    atrioventricular bundle of H.
    bundle of H.
    bursa, H.
His' *(continued)*
    disease, H.
    globular processes of H.
    spindle of H.
    Werner disease, H.
Histalog
histiocyte
histiocytic
    lymphoma, h.
histiocytoma
histiocytosis
    lipid h.
    sinus h.
    X, h.
histochromatosis
histocompatibility
histocompatible
histodiagnosis
histodialysis
histodifferentiation
histofluorescence
histogenesis
histogenous
histogram
histography
histohematogenous
histohydria
histologic
histology
histolysis
histolytic
histoma
histometaplastic
histoplasmin
historadiography
histotroph
histrotropic
Hittorf tube
Hitzig's girdle
HL (half-life)
HLA B27 arthritides
Hoboken's nodules

Additional Entries

Hoche's bandelette
hockey-stick catheter
hockey-stick portal
Hodara's disease
Hodgen splint
Hodgkin's disease
Hodgson's disease
Hofbauer cells
Hoffa's disease
Hoffmann's atrophy
Hoffmann-Werdnig syndrome
Holden's line
hole
- bur h.
- drill h.

hollow
- needle guide, h.
- organ, h.
- plastic catheter, h.
- Sebileau's h.
- stainless steel guide, h.
- viscus, h.

Holmes's degeneration phenomenon
Holmes-Stewart phenomenon
hologram
holoprosencephaly
holosystolic
- murmur, h.

Holter-Heyman capsules
Holthouse's hernia
Holt-Oram syndrome
Holzknecht's chromoradiometer
homalocephalus
homalography
homeopathy
homeorrhesis
homeostasis
homeostatic control of growth
homeotherapy
homeotransplantation
homocentric
homochronous
homocystinuria
homogametic
homogamous
homogeneity
- coefficient, h.

homogeneous
- enhancement, h.
- lung perfusion, h.

homogenesis
homogenization
homogenous
homoiopodal
homoiothermy
homokeratoplasty
homolateral
- field, h.
- node, h.

homologous
homolysin
homolysis
homomorphosis
homonymous
- diplopia, h.
- hemianopia, h.
- hemianopsia, h.

homophil
homophilic
homoplastic
homoplasty
homosexual
homotropism
homotype
homozygosity for sickle cell disease
homozygous
honeycomb
- lung, h.
- pattern, h.

Additional Entries

- honeycombing
- hook of hamate
- hook-up
- Hopmann's polyp
- horizontal
  - beam arthrogram, h.
  - beam double contrast technique, h.
  - beam lateral, h.
  - beam technique, h.
  - blur, h.
  - cells of retina, h.
  - depression, h.
  - lie, h.
  - part of palatine bone, h.
  - plane, h.
  - position, h.
  - semicircular canal, h.
  - swivel plane, h.
- horizontally-oriented band
- hormone-binding proteins
- horn
  - cicatricial h.
  - lateral ventricles, h. of
  - spinal cord, h.
- Horner's
  - fold, H.
  - muscle, H.
  - syndrome, H.
- horseshoe kidney
- Hortega cell
- Horton's arteritis
- HORZ FNC (horizontal portion of facial nerve canal)
- host
  - compromised h.
- hot
  - cathode tube, h.
  - conization, h.
  - end needle, h.
  - nodule, h.
  - source, h.
- hot *(continued)*
  - spot, h.
  - spot infarct imaging, h.
- Hounsfield (H)
  - numbers, H.
  - unit, H.
- hourglass
  - bladder, h.
  - constriction, h.
- housing
  - codling curve, h.
  - heat storage capacity, h.
- Houston's
  - muscle, H.
  - valves of rectum, H.
- Hovius' canal
- Howell's bodies
- Howell-Jolly bodies
- Howship's lacuna
- HPF (high power field)
- HPO (hypertrophic pulmonary osteoarthropathy)
- HPS (hypertrophic pyloric stenosis)
- H rays
- 3HTdR triatiated thymidine
- HTLV (human T cell leukemia virus)
- HU (heat unit)
- HU (Hounsfield unit)
- Huchard's disease
- Hueck's ligament
- Hughes' reflex
- Hughston view
- Huguenin's edema
- Huguier's canal
- humeral
  - articulation, h.
  - circumflex arteries, h.
  - head, h.
  - nerves, h.
  - vessels, h.

Additional Entries

humerus
humor
  aqueous h.
  crystalline h.
  vitreous h.
Humphrey's ligament
Hunner's ulcer
Hunt's atrophy
Hunter's
  canal, H.
  ligament, H
  syndrome, H.
Hunter-Driffield (H-D) curve,
Huntington's
  chorea, H.
  disease,, H.
Hurler's syndrome
Hurler-Scheie compound syndrome
Hurthle cells
Huschke's canal
Hutchinson's
  disease, H.
  freckle, H.
Hutchinson-Gilford diseaase
Hutinel's disease
Huxley's layer
HVL (half-value layer)
HVL x-ray beam
5 HVL kidney shield
5 HVL liver shield
1 HVL spinal shield
5 HVL spinal shield
HVT (half-value thickness)
HW (hemispheric width)
hyaline
  articular cartilage, h.
  cartilage, h.
  cast, h.
  membrane disease, h. (HMD)
hyalitis
  asteroid h.
  suppurative h.
hyaloid
  artery, h.
  canal, h.
  membrane, h.
hyaloserositis
hydatid
  cyst, h.
  mole, h.
  Morgagni, h. of
hydatidiform
  mole, h.
hydatoid
hydraeroperitoneum
hydramnios
hydranencephaly
hydrargyrosis
hydrargyrum
hydrarthrosis
  intermittent h.
hydrate
hydrated
hydroappendix
hydrocalycosis
hydrocalyx
hydrocele
  cervical h.
  chylous h.
  colli h.
  communicating h.
  congenital h.
  diffused h.
  Dupuytren's h.
  encysted h.
  feminae h.
  funicular h.
  Gibbon's h.
  hernial h.
  Maunori's h.
  muliebris h.

Additional Entries ______________________________

hydrocele *(continued)*
 of neck, h.
 Nuck's h.
 renalis h.
 scrotal h.
 spinalis h.
hydrocelectomy
hydrocephalic
hydrocephalocele
hydrocephaloid
hydrocephalus
 acquired h.
 cerebrospinal fluid shunting, h.
 communicating h.
 ex vacuo, h.
 111 In-DTPA cisternography, h.
 low pressure h.
 noncommunicating h.
 normal-pressure h.
 obstructive h.
 otitic h.
hydrocolloid
 irreversible h.
 reversible h.
hydrocolpos
hydrocortisone sodium succinate
hydrodiffusion
hydrodiuresis
hydrodynamics
hydrogen (H)
 ion nuclei, h.
 nucleus, h.
hydrokinetic
hydrolymph
hydrolysis
hydromassage
hydromeningitis
hydromeningocele
hydrometer
hydrometry
hydromicrocephaly
hydromyelia
hydromyelomeningocele
hydromyoma
hydronephrosis
hydropancreatosis
hydroparotitis
hydropericarditis
hydropericardium
hydroperinephrosis
hydroperion
hydroperitoneum
hydropexic
hydrophilic
hydrophobic
hydrophorograph
hydrophthalmos
hydropic
 degeneration, h.
hydroplasma
hydropneumatosis
hydropneumogony
hydropneumopericardium
hydropneumoperitoneum
hydropneumothorax
hydrops
 folliculi, h.
hydropyonephrosis
hydrorachis
hydrorachitis
hydrorrhea
hydrosalpinx
hydroscheocele
hydroscope
hydrospirometer
hydrostabile
hydrothermic
hydrothorax
hydrotomy
hydrotubation
hydroureter

Additional Entries

hydrovarium
hydroxyzine
hydruria
hygroma
    colli, h.
    cystic h.
    subdural h.
hygromatous
hygrometry
hylergography
hymenal
    ring, h.
hyoepiglottic
hyoglossal
hyoglossus muscle
hyoid
    arch, h.
    bone, h.
    muscles of h. bone
hyothyroid
    ligaments, h.
    membrane, h.
Hypaque
    76, H.
    M-75, H.
    M-90, H.
    50%, H.
    60%, H.
hypalgesia
hypalgesic
hyparterial
    bronchi, h.
hypencephalon
hyperabsorption
hyperaeration
hyperaffectivity
hyperaldosteronism
hyperalimentosis
hyperbaric
    chamber, h.
    oxygen (HBO), h.
hyperbaric *(continued)*
    oxygen therapy, h.
hyperbarism
hypercalcemia
hypercapnia
hypercellular
hypercellularity
hypercementosis
hyperchromia
hyperchromic
hyperchylia
hypercoagulability
hypercoagulable
hypercryalgesia
hypercupremia
hypercupriuria
hypercythemia
hypercytochromia
hypercytosis
hyperdense
    infarct, h.
    lesion, h:
    nodule, h.
hyperdiuresis
hyperdynamia
hyperdynamic
hypereccrisia
hyperechema
hyperechoic
hyperemesis
    gravidarum, h.
hyperemetic
hyperemia
    active h.
    arterial h.
    collateral h.
    constriction h.
    leptomeningeal h.
    passive h.
    reactive h.
    venous h.
hyperemic

Additional Entries

hypergasia
hyperergic
hyperesthesia
acoustic h.
auditory h.
cerebral h.
gustatory h.
muscular h.
optic h.
tactile h.
hyperestrogenosis
hyperextended
hyperextension
fracture, h.
hyperfibrinogenemia
hyperfractionation
hypergenesis
hypergia
hyperglandular
hyperglycorrhachia
hyperhemoglobinemia
hyperheparinemia
hyperhepatia
hyperhydrosis
hyperimmunoglobulinemia
hyperinflation
hyperintensity
hyperinterrenal
hyperinterrenopathy
hyperirritability
hyperkeratinization
hyperkeratosis
hyperketonemia
hyperketonuria
hyperketosis
hyperkinemia
hyperkinesia
hyperkoria
hyperlipidemia
hyperliposis
hypermastia
hypermature
hypermelanotic
hypermenorrhea
hypermetria
hypernatremia
hypernephritis
hypernephroma
hyperopia
abdolute h.
axial h.
facultative h.
latent h.
manifest h.
relative h.
total h.
hyperopic
hyperostosis
ankylosing h. of spine
cranii, h.
frontal internal h.
frontalis interna, h.
general cortical h.
infantile cortical h.
Morgagni's h.
totalis, h.
hyperparathyroidism
hyperpathia
hyperphosphatemia
hyperpigmentation
hyperpituitarism
hyperplasia
adrenal cortical h.
cystic h.
endometrial h.
fibromuscular h.
gingival h.
intestinal h.
lymphoid h.
medial h.
neoplastic h.
proliferative h.
prostatic h.
stromal h.

Additional Entries ______________________

hyperplasia *(continued)*
subadventitial h.
hyperpnea
hyperprolactinemia
hyperpyrexia
malignant h.
hyperreactive
hyperreflexia
autonomic h.
hyperresonance
hypersecretion
hypersegmentation
hypersensitive
hypersensitivity angiitis
hypersphyxia
hypersplenism
hyperspongiosis
hypersthenia
hypersthenuria
hypertelorism
hypertension
accelerated h.
adrenal h.
benign h.
benign intracranial h.
borderline h.
essential h.
idiopathic h.
intracranial h.
labile h.
malignant h.
ocular h.
portal h.
primary h.
pulmonary h.
renal h.
renovascular h.
secondary h.
symptomatic h.
systemic venous h.
vascular h.
hypertensive
hypertensive *(continued)*
cardiovascular disease (HCVD), h.
crisis, h.
encephalopathy, h.
heart disease, h.
retinopathy, h.
hypertensor
hyperthermal
hyperthermalgesia
hyperthermia
hyperthermic bone cement
hyperthyroid
hyperthyroidism
factitial h.
hypertonia
hypertonic
bladder, h.
esophageal sphincter, h.
hypertonicity
hypertoxity
hypertrophic
cardiomyopathy, h.
gastritis, h.
IHSS (idiopathic h. subaortic stenosis)
lipping, h.
marginal spurring, h.
osteoarthropathy, h.
pulmonary osteoarthropathy (HPO), h.
pyloric stenosis, h.
spondylitis, h.
spurring, h.
subaortic stenosis, idiopathic h. (IHSS)
hypertrophy
atrial h.
benign prostatic (BPH) h.
BPH (benign prostatic h.)

Additional Entries

hypertrophy *(continued)*
  Brunner, h. of
  left ventricular (LVH) h.
  right ventricular (RVH) h.
  ventricular h.
hypervascular
  lesion, h.
  mass, h.
hyperventilation
hyperviscosity
hypesthesia
  stocking-and-glove h.
hyphema (suffused with blood)
hyphomycosis
hypnocinematograp
hypoactive
  bowel sounds, h.
  reflex, h.
hypoaeration
hypocalcification
hypocapnia
hypocellular
hypocellularity
hypochordal
  bar, h.
  brace, h.
hypodense
  center, h.
  extra-axial lesion, h.
  intra-axial lesion, h.
  periphery, h.
hypodermic
  needle, h.
hypodermis
hypodermoclysis
hypodipsia
hypodynamia
hypoechoic
  mass, h.
  structure, h.
hypoesthesia
hypoesthetic
hypoexophoria
hypoganglionosis
hypogastric
  arteriography, h.
  artery, h.
  lymph nodes, h.
  nodes, h.
  plexus, h.
  region, h.
  vein, h.
  zone, h.
hypogastrium
hypogenetic lung syndrome
hypoglossal
  canal, h.
  nerve, h.
  palsy, h.
hypoglottis
hypokinemia
hypokinesia
hypokinetic
hypolarynx
hypolemmal
hypolipemia
hypolipidemic
hypolymphemia
hypomagnesemia
hypomastia
hypomelanism
hypomelanosis
hypomenorrhea
hypometria
hypomicrosoma
hypomodal
hypomorph
hypomotility
hypomyxia
hyponeocytosis
hyponychium
hyponychon

Additional Entries

hypo-orchidia
hypo-orchidism
hypo-orthocytosis
hypo-osmolality
hypopancreatism
hypopancreorrhea
hypoparathyroidism
hypopepsia
hypoperfusion
hypopexia
hypopharyngeal mucosa
hypopharyngoscope
hypopharynx
hyphrenium
hypophysectomy
hypophysial
    arterry, h.
    fossa, h.
    vein, h.
hypophysis
    cerebri, h.
    pharyngeal h.
    sicca, h.
hypopigmentation
hypoplasia
hypoplastic
    anemia, h.
    annulus, h.
    left heaart syndrome, h.
    right heart syndrome, h.
    lung, h.
hypopnea
hypopraxia
hyporeactive
hyporeflexia
hyporeninemia
hyporrhea
hyposalemia
hyposensitive
hyposialadenitis
hypospadias
    balanitic h.
hyposplenism
hypostasis
hyposthenia
hyposthenuria
hypostomia
hypostosis
hyposystole
hypotelorism
hypotension
hypotensor
hypothalamic
hypothalamotomy
hypothalamus
    infundibulum, h.
    mamillary bodies of h.
    neurohypohysis of h.
    optic chiasma, h.
    subthalamic tegmental region, h.
    tuber cinerum, h.
hypothenar
    compartment, h.
    eminence, h.
hypothermal
hypothermia
hypothyroidism
hypotonia
hypotonic
    duodenography, h.
hypotropia
HYPOTYMP (hypotympanum)
hypotympanotomy
hypotympanum
hypouremia
hypoventilation
hypovolemia
hypovolemic
    shock, h.
hypoxemia
hypoxia
hypoxic

Additional Entries ______________________________

hypoxic *(continued)*
- cell marker, h.
- cells, h.
- gain factor, h.

hysterectomy
- abdominal h.
- cesarean h.
- complete h.
- partial h.
- radical h.
- subtotal h.
- supracervical h.
- total h.
- vaginal h.

hysteresis
hystereurynter
hysterocele
hysterocleisis
hysterocolpectomy
hysterocolposcope
hysterocystic
hysterocystocleisis
hysterogram
hysterograph
hysterolaparotomy
hysterolith
hysterology
hysterolysis
hysterometer
hysteromyomectomy
hysteromyotomy
hysteropathy
hysterpexy
hysterorrhaphy
hysterosalpingectomy
hysterosalpingogram
hysterosalpingography
hysterosalpingo-oophorectomy
hysterosalpingostomy
hysteroscope
hysteroscopy
hysterospasm
hysterostat
hysterotraumatic
hysterotraumatism
hysterotubogram
hysterovaginoenterocele
Hz (hertz)

Additional Entries

I

I (iodine)
I-123 (sodium iodide)
I-125 (sodium iodide)
iatrogenic
 hyperthyroidism, i.
IABP (intra-aortic balloon pump)
IADSA (intra-arterial digital subtraction angiography)
IBCA (isobutyl-2–cyanoacrylate)
I-cell disease
ichthyosis
 lamellar i.
 simplex, i.
 uteri i.
 vulgaris, i.
icterohepatitis
icteroid
icterus
IDA (iminodiacetic acid)
 analogs, IDA
 cholescintigraphy, IDA
 cholecystokinin administration in IDA
 hepatic accumulation of IDA
 renal excretion of IDA
idiopathic hypertrophic subaortic stenosis (IHSS)
idiopathic
 craniostenosis, i.
 disc calcification, i.
 dilatation, i.
 hypertrophic subaortic stenosis (IHSS), i.
 myocarditis, i.
 osteolysis, i.
 pulmonary hemosiderosis, i.

idiopathic *(continued)*
 purpura, i.
 skeletal hyperostosis, i.
 steatorrhea, i.
 thrombocytopenic purpura, i.
idioplasm
idioretinal
idiosome
IDIS (intraoperative digital subtraction angiography)
ID:OD (inside/outside diameter ratio)
125 I-fibrinogen uptake test
131 I-hippuran cortical renogram
131 I-hippuran images
131 I-hippuran renogram curves
IHSS (idiopathic hypertrophic subaortic stenosis)
131 I-human serum albumin
125 I-implantation
125 I-irradiation
125 I-isotope (seed)
131 I-isotope
IJC (internal jugular chain)
123 I-labeled amines
ileal
 atresia, i.
 bladder, i.
 conduit, i.
ileitis
 distal i.
 regional i.
 terminal i.
ileocecal
 junction, i.
 valve, i.
ileocecostomy

Additional Entries ______________________________

ileocecum
ileocolic
    artery, i.
    lymph nodes, i.
ileocolitis
ileocolonic intussusception
ileocolostomy
ileocolotomy
ileocystoplasty
ileocystostomy
ileoileostomy
ileoproctostomy
ileorectal
ileorrhaphy
ileosigmoid
ileosigmoidostomy
ileostogram
ileostomy
ileotomy
ileotransversostomy
ileum
    dilated i.
    distal i.
    lymphatic vessels of i.
    stenosed i.
    terminal i.
ileus
    adynamic i.
    intestinal i.
    paralytic i.
    postoperative i.
    spastic i.
Ilford, Inc.
ilia
iliac
    adenopathy, i.
    artery, i.
    artery aneurysm, i.
    bone, i.
    circumflex artery, i.
    colon, i.
    crest, i.

iliac *(continued)*
    disease, i.
    fascia, i.
    fossa, i.
    furrow, i.
    lesion, i.
    lymph nodes, i.
    nodes, i.
    spine, i.
    tuberosity, i.
    vein, i.
iliacus muscle
iliocapsularis muscle
iliococcygeal
iliococcygeus muscle
iliocolotomy
iliocostal
iliocostalis
    cervicis muscle, i.
    dorsi muscle, i.
    lumborum muscle, i.
iliofemoral
    ligament, i.
iliofemoroplasty
iliohypogastric
    nerve, i.
ilioinguinal
iliolumbar
    artery, i.
    ligament, i.
    vein, i.
iliometer
iliopectineal
    eminence, i.
    fascia, i.
iliopsoas
    bursitis, i.
    muscle, i.
iliopubic
iliosacral
iliosacralis muscle
iliosciatic

Additional Entries

iliospinal
iliotibial
- band, i.
- tract, i.

iliotrochanteric ligament
ilium
- ala of i.
- body of i.
- crest of i.
- dorsum of i.
- gluteal lines of i.
- spines of i.

ill-defined
- cardiac outline, i.
- diaphragm, i.
- lesion, i.
- limits, i.

illusion
illusional
I-loop
IM (intramuscular)
image
- addiction, i.
- amplifier, i.
- averaging, i.
- coronal i.
- degradation by scattered photons, i.
- delayed i.
- detail, i.
- dextrocardia mirror i.
- enhancement, i.
- formation, i.
- intensification, fluoroscopic system, i.
- manipulation, i.
- multi-echo i.
- noise, i.
- pixels, i.
- real-time i.
- reconstruction, i.
- reformatting, i.

image *(continued)*
- re-registration, i.
- parameters, i.
- scout i.
- smoothing, i.
- spin echo i.
- static i.
- subtraction, i.
- T1 weighted i.
- T1 weighted coronal i.
- T1 weighted sagittal i.
- T2 weighted i.

imaging
- bone i.
- cycle, i.
- 2D slice imaging
- 3D volume i.
- magnetic resonance (MRI) i.
- nuclear bone i.
- technique, i. (C15 02)

Imatron, Inc.
imbricated
imbricating
- layer, i.
- suture, i.

iminodiacetic-acid (IDA)
- cholescintigraphy, IDA
- hepatic uptake of IDA
- renal excretion of IDA

immature
- blood cells, i.
- cataract, i.

immiscibility
immobile cilia syndrome
immobilization device
immovable articulations
immune
- combined i. deficiency disease
- globulin, i.
- response, i.

Additional Entries

immunity
acquired i.
active i.
natural i.
nonspecific i.
passive i.
reaction, i.
specific i.
immunoadsorbent
immunoassay
immunoblastic
immunofiltration
immunofluorescence
immunologic typing
immunology
immunoparesis
immunopathogenesis
immunoprecipitation
immunoproliferative
immunoprophylaxis
immunosorbent
immunostimulation
immunosuppression
immunosympathectomy
immunotherapy
impact
impacted
cerumen, i.
fecal material, i.
fracture, i.
stool, i.
tooth, i.
impatency
impatent
impedance
plethysmography, i. (IPG)
impending
cord compression, i.
fetal distress, i.
myocardial infarction, i.
stroke, i.
imperforate
anus, i.
hymen, i.
impermeable
impetiiginous
impetigo
bullous, i.
contagiosa, i.
herpetiformis, i.
neonatorum, i.
vulgaris, i.
impingement
implant
endometrial i.
lens i.
Marlex mesh i.
metastatic i.
penile i.
radon seed i.
Silastic i.
Teflon i.
tendon i.
ureteral i.
implantation
pacemaker i.
impression
colic i.
duodenal i.
gastric i.
renal i.
rhomboid i.
suprarenal i.
trigeminal i.
impulse
apical i.
inguinal i.
point of maximal (PMI) i.
111 In (indium)
111 In window
in
situ, i.

Additional Entries

in *(continued)*
- situ lobular carcinoma, i.
- toto, i.
- utero, i.
- vitro, i.
- vivo, i.

inactive source
inarticulate
inborn error (s)
incandescent
incarcerated
- hernia, i.

incarceration
incident
- photon, i.
- rays, i.
- wave, i.

incidental
- agenesis, i.
- appendectomy, i.
- finding, i.
- hydronephrosis, i.
- nodules, i.

incipient
- cataract, i.
- gangrene, i.
- glaucoma, i.

incisive
- bone, i.
- canals, i.
- foramen, i.
- fossa, i.
- teeth, i.

incisolingual
incisoproximal
incisor
- crest, i.
- teeth, i.

incisura
- angularis, i.
- apicis cordis, i.
- cardiaca, i.

incisura *(continued)*
- fastigii, i.
- intertragica, i.
- radialis, i.
- semilunaris, i.
- temporalis, i.
- tentorii cerebelli, i.

incisure
inclination
- pelvic i.

incline
inclinometer
inclusion
- blenorrhea, i.
- bodies, i.
- cell, i.
- conjunctivitis, i.
- cyst, i.

incoagulable
incompatibility
incompatible
incompetence
- aortic i.
- cervical i.
- mitral i.
- pulmonary i.
- tricuspid i.
- urethral i.

incompetent
- cervix, i.
- esophageal sphincter, i.
- perforating vein, i.
- valve, i.

incomplete
- abortion, i.
- bundle branch block, i.
- resection, i.

incongruent distributions
incontinence
- fecal i.
- overflow i.
- stress i.

Additional Entries

incontinence *(continued)*
urinary i.
incontinent
feces, i. of
stool, i. of
urine, i. of
incremental lines of Salter
increased
abdominal girth, i.
activity, i.
bone length, i.
capillary permeability, i.
digital markings, i.
resting fluid, i.
vascularity, i.
increment
incretopathy
incretotherapy
incudomalleal
incudostapedial
incus
ligaments of i.
long process of i.
indeterminate
loop, i.
situs, i.
index
cardiac i.
free thyroxine i.
mean cardiac i.
stroke i.
therapeutic i.
thyroxin binding i.
vital i.
Indian Club needle
indicarmine
indicator dye
indigo carmine (a/k/a indigotindisulfonate sodium)
indigotindisulfonate sodium (a/k/a indigo carmine)
indirect

indirect *(continued)*
ballottement, i.
fluorescent antibody, i.
hernia, i.
indistinct
corticomedullary junction, i.
margins, i.
indium-111 (In-111)
autologous white blood cell scan, i.
isotope, i.
labeled leukocytes, i. (In 111)
oxine, i. (In 111)
oxyquinoline, i.
pentetate, i.
WBC (white blood cell) autologous scan, i.
indocyanine green
induction
inductive
heating, i.
radiofrequency, i.
indurated
induration
indurative
indwelling
Foley catheter, i.
inert
radioactive gas, i.
inertia
inevitable abortion
infantile
malignant histiocytosis, i.
uterus, i.
infarct
avid imaging, i.
avid scintigraphy, i.
necrosis, i.
infarction

Additional Entries

infarction *(continued)*
- anterior myocardial i.
- anterior wall i.
- anteroinferior myocardial i.
- anterolateral i.
- anterolateral myocardial i.
- anteroposterior i.
- anteroseptal myocardial i.
- atrial i.
- cardiac i.
- cerebral i.
- focal i.
- Freiberg's i.
- impending i.
- inferior myocardial i.
- inferior wall myocardial i.
- inferolateral myocardial i.
- intestinal i.
- lateral i.
- lateral myocardial i.
- lung, i. of
- mesenteric i.
- myocardial i.
- old inferior wall myocardial i.
- placenta, i. of
- posterolateral i.
- posterior myocardial i.
- pulmonary i.
- retina, i. of
- septal i.
- septal myocardial i.
- subendocardial i.
- transmural i.
- transmural myocardial i.

infection
- focus of i.

infection *(continued)*
- postoperative wound i.
- upper respiratory tract i.
- urinary tract i.

infectious mononucleosis

infective

inferior
- alveolar artery, i.
- articular arteries, i.
- calcaneonavicular ligament, i.
- cerebellar peduncles, i.
- constrictor muscle, i.
- dental artery, i.
- dental nerve, i.
- epigastric vein, i.
- fascia, i.
- ganglion, i.
- horn, i.
- labial artery, i.
- laryngeal nerve, i.
- longitudinal sinus, i.
- maxillary nerve, i.
- mesenteric arteriography, i.
- mesenteric artery, i.
- oblique muscle, i.
- petrosal sinus, i.
- profunda artery, i.
- pubic ligament, i.
- quadrigeminal body, i.
- sagittal sinus, i.
- stopper, i.
- striate veins, i.
- tarsal plate, i.
- thyroarytenoid ligaments, i.
- turbinated bone, i.
- vena cava, i.
- vena cavography, i.
- vesical artery, i.

inferodiaphragmatic

Additional Entries

inferolateral
inferomedian
inferoposterior
inferosuperior (occlusal) projection
infiltrate
basilar i.
confluent i.
hilar i.
interstitial i.
lower lobe i.
parenchymal i.
patchy pneumonic i.
pulmonary i.
residual i.
infiltrating
ductal cell carcinoma, i.
infiltration
fatty i. of liver
patchy i.
pneumonic i.
pulmonary i.
infiltrative
inflammation
catarrhal i.
chronic i.
exudative i.
fibrinous i.
granulomatous i.
hyperplastic i.
interstitial i.
parenchymatous i.
productive i.
pseudomembranous i.
purulent i.
serous i.
subacute i.
suppurative i.
inflammatory
adhesions, i.
bowel disease, i.
exudate, i.

inflammatory *(continued)*
mass, i.
pelvic i. disease (PID)
peritoneal i. reaction
reaction, i.
infracardiac
infraclavicular
branches of brachial plexus, i.
infracortical
infracostal
infraglenoid
tuberosity, i.
infrahepatic
infrahyoid
artery, i.
muscles, i.
inframamillary
inframammary
inframandibular
inframarginal
inframaxillary
inframesocolic
compartment, i.
region, i.
infraocclusion
infraorbital
artery, i.
canal, i.
foramen, i.
groove, i.
plexus, i.
infrapatellar
fat pad, i.
infrared
far i.
light, i.
long-wave i.
near i.
rays, i.
short-wave i.
thermal radiation, i.

Additional Entries ______________________________

infrascapular
artery, i.
infrasonic
infraspinous
fascia, i.
fossa, i.
muscle, i.
infrasternal
notch, i.
infrastructure
infratemporal
crest, i.
fossa, i.
surface of maxilla, i.
infratentorial
tumor, i.
infratrochlear
nerve, i.
infratubal
infraturbinal
infraumbilical
infraversion
infrequent voider
infundibula
infundibular
stenosis, i.
infundibulectomy
infundibuliform
fascia, i.
infundibulopelvic
ligament, i.
infundibulum
brain, i. of
ethmoid bone, i. of
hypothalamus, i. of
uterine tube, i. of
Infusaport catheter
infusion
excretory urogram, i.
intravenous i.
manometry test, i.
pyelography, i.
inguinal
adenopathy, i.
aponeurotic falx, i.
canal, i.
floor of i. canal
hernia, i.
impulse, i.
ligament, i.
lymphadenopathy, i.
lymph nodes, i.
node, i.
node dissection, i.
region, i.
ring, i.
inguinoabdominal
inguinocrural
inguinodynia
inguinolabial
inguinoscrotal
inhalational lung disease
inhomogeneity
inhomogeneous
appearance, i.
tracer distribution, i.
inion
injected
eardrum, i.
pharynx, i.
throat, i.
tympanic membrane, i.
injection
hypodermic i.
intracutaneous i.
intradermal i.
intramuscular i.
intravenous i.
subcutaneous i.
inlet
pelvic i.
thoracic i.
inner
catheter, i.

Additional Entries

inner *(continued)*
foil pouch, i.
needles, i.
shells, i.
innominate
artery, i.
bone, i.
fascia, i.
vein, i.
235 I nomogram
input-output
Insall-Salvati index
inscription
tendinous i.
inside/outside diameter ratio (ID:OD)
in situ
inspiration/expiration
radiograph, i/e.
study, i/e.
inspiratory
expiratory ratio, i.
flow rate, i.
reserve volume, i.
stridor, i.
vital capacity, i.
wheezing, i.
inspirometer
inspissated
cerumen, i.
inspissation
inspissator
instant thin-layer chromatography-silica gel (ITLC-SG)
instillation
instrument
defect, i.
failure, i.
instrumentation
urethral i.
insufficiency
adrenal i.

insufficiency *(continued)*
aortic i.
cardiac i.
coronary i.
hepatic i.
ileocecal i.
mitral i.
myocardial i.
placental i.
pulmonary i.
renal i.
thyroid i.
uterine i.
valvular i.
venous i.
vertebrobasilar i.
insufflation
tubal i.
insula
cerebral i.
circular sulcus of i.
gyri of i.
opercula of i.
Reil, i. of
intact ventricular septum
integral
dose, i.
exposure, i.
surface exposure, i.
integument
integumentum
interalveolar
cell islets, i.
interarticular
chondrosternal ligament, i.
costocentral ligament, i.
fibrocartilage, i.
sternocostal ligament, i.
interarytenoid
notch, i.
interatrial

Additional Entries

interatrial *(continued)*
groove, i.
septal defect, i.
intercalatum
intercapitular veins
intercarpal
articulations, i.
intercavernous
sinuses, i.
intercellular
biliary passages, i.
intercentral
ligaments, i.
intercerebral
interclavicular
interclinoid
ligament, i.
intercolumnar
fascia, i.
fibers, i.
intercondylar
intercondyloid
eminence of tibia, i.
fossa of femur, i.
fossa of tibia, i.
intercondylous
interconnecting lymphatics
intercostal
arteries, i.
fasciae, i.
lymph nodes, i.
membranes, i.
muscles, i.
nerves, i.
spaces, i.
veins, i.
intercostobrachial
nerve, i.
intercostohumeral
intercricothyroid needle
intercricothyrotomy
intercrural
intercrural *(continued)*
fascia, i.
fibers, i.
intercuneiform
articulations, i.
interface
acoustic i.
interfascicular
interferometer
interfoveolar ligament of Hesselbach
interfrontal
interganglionic
intergemmal
intergenic
interglobular
spaces, i.
intergluteal
fold, i.
intergonial
intergrade
interictal scan
interlobular
arteries, i.
fluid, i.
veins, i.
intermaxillary spine
intermediate
atrioventricular canal, i.
rays, i.
intermediolateral
intermedius
intermembranous
intermeningeal
intermetacarpal
articulations, i.
intermetatarsal
articulations, i.
intermittent
positive pressure breathing, i. (IPPB)
intermural

Additional Entries

intermuscular
internal
abdominal ring, i.
acoustic meatus, i.
arcuate ligament, i.
auditory canal, i.
calcaneal arteries, i.
calcaneal nerves, i.
calcaneoastragaloid ligament, i.
calcaneonavicular ligament, i.
canthus, i.
capsule, i.
carotid artery, i.
circumflex artery, i.
conversion, i. (IC)
cutaneous nerve, i.
derangement of knee, i.
electrode, i.
fixation, i.
geniculate body, i.
jugular chain lymph nodes, i.
iliac artery, i.
iliac lymph nodes, i.
iliac vein, i.
intercostal muscle, i.
jugular vein, i.
lateral ligament, i.
malleolar artery, i.
mammary artery, i.
mammary lymph nodes, i.
mammary pathway, i.
maxillary lymph nodes, i.
oblique muscle, i.
oblique projection, i.
os of uterus, i.
palpebral arteries, i.
plantar artery, i.
internal *(continued)*
plantar nerve, i.
popliteal nerve, i.
pterygoid muscle, i.
pudendal artery, i.
pudendal nodes, i.
pudendal veins, i.
pudic artery, i.
pudic nerve, i.
pudic veins, i.
resorption, i.
respiratory nerve of Bell, i.
ridges, i.
saphenous nerve, i.
saphenous vein, i.
semilunar fibrocartilage, i.
septate, i.
sphincter ani muscle, i.
International Imaging Electronics, Inc.
interocclusal
interolivary
interorbital
distance, i.
line, i.
interossei muscles
foot, i.m. of
hand, i.m. of
interosseous
arteries, i.
ligament, i.
membrane, i.
nerve, i.
interparietal
bone, i.
interparoxysmal
interpediculate
interpeduncular
distance, i.
fossa, i.

Additional Entries

interpeduncular *(continued)*
ganglion, i.
interpedunculate distance (IPD)
interphalangeal
articulations, i.
interpleural
space, i.
interpubic
disk, i.
fibrocartilaginous lamina, i.
interpupillary
interrenal
interruption of aortic arch
interscapilium
intersciatic
intersection
intersegmental
neurons, i.
septa, i.
interseptum
intersigmoid
fossa, i.
interspace
narrowing of i.
vertebral i.
intersperse
intersphincteric groove
interspinal
ligaments, i.
interspinales muscles
interspinous ligament
intersternal
interstitial
application, i.
brachytherapy, i.
calcification, i.
cystitis, i.
disease, i.
edema, i.
emphysema, i.
interstitial *(continued)*
fibrosis, i.
implant, i.
lung disease, i.
radiation therapy, i.
intertarsal
articulations, i.
intertragic notch
intertransverse
ligaments, i.
intertrochanteric
crest, i.
line, i.
ridge, i.
intertubercular plane
intertubular dentin
interureteric ridge
interventricular
disk, i.
foramen, i.
septal defect, i.
septum, i.
intervertebral
disk, i.
fibrocartilages, i.
foramina, i.
veins, i.
interventricular
heart block, i.
septal defect, i.
intervertebral
disc herniation, i.
disc space, i.
intervillous
intestinal
arteries, i.
glands, i.
ileus, i.
villi, i.
intestinal arcade:
arc of Buhler
arc of Burkow

Additional Entries ______________________

intestinal arcade: *(continued)*
arc of Riolan
intestine
large i.
lymphatic nodules of i.
lymphatics of i.
small i.
intestinum
caecum, i.
ileum, i.
jejunum, i.
rectum, i.
intima
intimal
fibroplasia, i.
tear, i.
intra-arterial
digital subtraction angiography (IADSA), i.
infusion of vasodilator, i.
intra-articular
disk or disc, i.
ligament, i.
intra-atrial
intra-aural
intra-axial
lesion, i.
mass, i.
nodule, i.
intrabronchial
intrabuccal
intracanalicular
intracapsular
intracartilaginous ossification
intracaval thrombosis
intracavitary
application, i.
brachytherapy, i.
insertion, i.
radiation therapy, i.
intracelial
intracellular
intracellular *(continued)*
siderophore, i.
intracephalic
intracerebellar
intracerebral
intracervical
intracolic
intraconal lesion
intracordal
intracorporeal
intracorpuscular
intracostal
intracranial
calcification, i.
hemorrhage, i.
intracrureus
intractable
intracutaneous
intracystic
intracytoplasmic
intradermal
intradermoreaction
intraductal
carcinoma, i.
intraduodenal
intradural
extramedullary mass, i.
intraepidermal
intraepiphyseal
intraepithelial
plexus of cornea, i.
intraerythrocytic
intrafascicular
intrafissural
intrafistular
intrafollicular
intrafusal
fasciculi, i.
fibers, i.
intraglandular
intraglobular
intragyral

Additional Entries

intrahepatic
intrahyoid
intraictal
intraintestinal
intrajugular
process, i.
intralamellar
intralaryngeal
intralesional
intraligamentous
intralingual
intralobar
intralobular veins
intralocular
intraluminal
brachytherapy technique, i.
filling defect, i.
radiation therapy, i.
intramammary
intramarginal
intramastoiditis
intramedullary
bone graft, i.
fixation device, i.
mass, i.
nailing, i.
intramembranous
ossification, i.
intrameningeal
intramural
aneurysm, i.
diverticulum, i.
fibroid, i.
hematoma, i.
injection, i.
intramuscular
intramyocardial
intranarial
intranasal
intraneural
intranuclear
intraocular
intraoperative
transluminal angioplasty, i. (IOTA)
intraoral
cone, i.
cone irradiation, i.
intraorbital
mass, i.
intraosseous
sarcoma, i.
venography, i.
intraovarian
intraovular
intraparenchymal
intraparenchymatous
intraparietal
sulcus, i.
intrapartum
intrapelvic
intrapericardial
intraperineal
intraperitoneal
abscess, i.
intraplacental
intrapleural
intrapontine
intrapulmonary
bronchi, i.
nodes, i.
intrarectal
intrarenal
intraretinal
intrascleral
intrascrotal
intrasellar
mass, i.
intraserous
intraspinal
mass lesion, i.
tumor, i.
veins, i.

Additional Entries

intrasplenic
intrasternal
intrastitial
intrastromal
intrasynovial
intratarsal
intrathecal
  imaging, i.
intrathenar
intrathoracic
intrathyroid cartilage
intratonsillar
intratrabecular
intratracheal
  catheter, i.
intraoperative
intrauterine
  device (IUD), i.
  gestation, i.
  growth rate, i.
  growth retardation, i. (IUGR)
  infection, i.
  pregnancy, i. (IUP)
  transfusion, i.
intravaginal
  cylinder, i.
intravasation
intravascular
  electrocoagulation, i.
  gas, i.
  thrombolysis, i.
intravenous (IV)
  angiography, i.
  cholangiography, i. (IVC)
  digital subtraction angiography, i. (IVDSA)
  drip, i.
  fluid, i.
  hydration, i.
intravenous (IV) *(continued)*
  infusion, i.
  intubation, i.
  line, i.
  Pitocin drip, i.
  pyelogram, (or pyelography) i. (IVP)
  urography, i.
intraventricular
  conduction delay, i.
  hemorrhage, i.
  tumor, i.
intravesical pressure
intrinsic
  angular spin, i.
  muscles, i.
introflexion
introgastric
intubation
  endotracheal i.
  nasal i.
  nasoendotracheal i.
  nasogastric i.
  oral i.
  orotracheal i.
intussusception
  ileocolonic i.
inulin H-3
invasion of adjacent structures
invasive
inversion position
inversion recovery
inversus
  situs i.
invertebrate
inverted-Y field
inverting papilloma
invertor
in vitro
in vivo
iobenzamic acid

Additional Entries

iocarmate meglumine
iocarmic acid
iocetamic acid
iodamide
  meglumine, i.
iodide
  metabolic pathway, i.
  uptake, i.
iodine (I)
  125, i. (I 125)
  131, i. (I 131)
  131 i. with triiodothyronine
  contrast oil, i.
  eye plaque, i. (I 125)
  fibrinogen uptake test, i. (I 125)
  hippuran cortical renogram, i. (I 131)
  hippuran images, i. (I 131)
  hippuran renogram curves, i. (I 131)
  implants, i. (I 125)
  isotope seed, i. (I 125)
  labeled amines, i. (I 123)
  orthoiodohippurate, i.
  thyroid scan, i.
  protein-bound i.
iodipamide
  meglumine, i.
  methylglucamine, i.
  sodium I 131, i.
iodized oil
iodoantipyrine I 131
iodocetylic acid I 123
iodocholesterol I 131
iodohippurate
  sodium I 123, i.
  sodium I 125, i.
  sodium I 131, i.
iodophthalein sodium
iodoprotein
iodopyracet I 125
iodopyracet I 131
iodoxamate meglumine
iodoxamic acid
iofetamine hydrochloride I 123
ioglicic acid
ioglucol
ioglucomide
ioglycamic acid
iomethin I 125
iomethin I 131
ion
  collection, i.
  dipolar i.
  gram i.
  hydrogen i.
  hydronium i.
ionization
  chamber, i.
ionize tissue
ionizing radiation
ionosphere
ionotherapy
iopamidol
iopanoic acid
iopentol
iophendylate
iophenoxic acid
iopydol
iopydone
131 I-orthoiodohippurate
iosefamic acid
ioseric acid
iosulamide meglumine
iosumetic acid
iotasul
IOTA (intraoperative transluminal angioplasty)
iotetric acid
iothalamate

Additional Entries

iothalamate *(continued)*
  meglumine, i.
  sodium, i.
  sodium I 125, i.
  sodium I 131, i.
iothalamic acid
iothyronine sodium
iotrolan
iotroxic acid
iotyrosine I 131
ioversol
IPD (interpedunculate distance)
IPG (impedance plethysmography)
ipodate calcium
ipodate sodium
ipratropium bromide
iprofenin
iproxamine hydrochloride
ipsilateral
  anhidrosis, i.
  appositional approach, i.
  eyeball, i.
  hilar, i.
  iliac nodes, i.
  lymph nodes, i.
  neck, i.
  side of the neck, i.
  structures, i.
  wedge pair portals, i.
Ir (iridium)
192 Ir afterloading tube
192 Ir eye plaque
iridectomize
iridectomy
iridectopia
iridemia
iridenclesis
irideremia
iridescence
iridescent
iridioplatinum
  sheath, i.
iridium (Ir)
  192, i. (Ir 192)
  afterloading tube, i. (Ir 192)
  eye plaque, i. (Ir 192)
  implant, i. (Ir 192)
  isodose display, i. (Ir 192)
  mold, i.
  needle, i.
  ribbon, i.
  seeds, i.
  wire, i.
iridoavulsion
iridocapsulitis
iridocele
iridochoroiditis
iridocoloboma
iridocyclectomy
iridocyclitis
  heterochromic i.
iridocyclochoroiditis
iridocystectomy
iridodialysis
iridodiastasis
iridodilator
iridokeratitis
iridokinesis
iridokinetic
iridopathy
iridoperiphakitis
iridoplegia
iridoptosis
iridopupillary
iridoschisis
iridosclerotomy
iridosteresis
iridotomy
iris
iron (Fe)

Additional Entries

192 Ir ribbon
131 I rose bengal scintigraphy
irradiate
irradiated
  bone, i.
  volume, i.
irradiation
  plaque, i.
  whole body i.
irregular
  edges, i.
  field technique, i.
  shaped fields, i.
irrigate
irrigated
  bladder i.
irrigation
  continuous i.
  Ringer's i.
irrigoradioscopy
irritability
  faradic i.
  galvanic i.
  gastric outlet i.
  mechanical i.
  myotatic i.
  tactile i.
irritable
  bowel syndrome, i.
  duodenal bulb, i.
192 Ir wire
IS (intercostal space; inferosuperior)
Isambert's disease
131 I scan
ischemia
  anterior wall i.
  myocardial i.
  transient cerebral i.
ischemic
  bowel disease, i.

ischemic *(continued)*
  heart disease, i.
  parenchymal degeneration, i.
  transient i. attack (TIA)
  zones, i.
ischiatic
ischial
  spine, i.
  tuberosity, i.
ischioanal
ischiobulbar
ischiocapsular
  ligament, i.
ischiocavernous
  muscle, i.
ischiorectal
  abscess, i.
  fossa, i.
ischiosacral
ischiovaginal
ischiovertebral
ischium
  body of i.
  rami of i.
  spine of i.
  tuberosity of i.
125 I seeds
island (s)
  blood i.
  bone i.
  Calleja i.
  graft, i.
  Langerhans, i's. of
  Reil, i. of
islet cell tumor
isobar
isobaric
isobutyl-2–cyanoacrylate (IBCA)
isocellular
isocentric

Additional Entries

isocentric *(continued)*
radiotherapy, i.
technique, i.
isochromosome
isodense
disc, i.
nodule, i.
rim, i.
isodose curve
isodynamic
isoechoic
isoeffect
line, i.
parameter, i.
plane, i.
isoelectric
electroencephalogram, i.
isoetharine
isofluorophate
isogamete
isogamous
isograft
isointense mass
isolated esophageal varix
isomerase
isomeric state
Isopaque 440
isophotometer
isoplastic
iso-power density curves
isoprel
isoproterenol
hydrochloride, i.
sulfate, i.
isopter
isopyknic
isopyknosis
ISO-SAR curves
isosulfan blue
isotone
isotope
brain scan, i.

isotope *(continued)*
radioactive i.
scan, i.
source, i.
stable i.
venogram, i.
ventriculogram, i.
Isotopen-Technik Gamma-Med II afterloader
Isovue
Isovue M
isthmectomy
isthmoplegia
isthmospasm
isthmus
aortic i.
auditory tube, i. of
eustachian tube, i. of
external auditory meatus, i. of
faucium, i. of
glandulae thyroideae, i.
glandular thyreoidea, i.
limbic lobe, i. of
oropharyngeal i.
rhombencephali, i.
thrombencephali i.
thyroid, i. of
uterine tube, i. of
IT (isomeric transition)
iterative
mathematical technique, i.
reconstruction, i.
iteroparity
iteroparous
ITLC-SG (instant thin-layer chromatography-silica gel)
ITP (idiopathic thrombocytopenic purpura)
I-transposition

Additional Entries

IU (international unit)
IUD (intrauterine device)
IUGR (intrauterine growth retardation)
IUP (intrauterine pregnancy)
IV (intravenous)
Ivalon
IVC (intravenous cholangiography)
IVCD (intrauterine contraceptive device)
IVDSA (intravenous digital subtraction angiography)
ivory
  epiphysis, i.
  teeth, i. of
  vertebra, i.
IVP (intravenous pyelogram)

Additional Entries

J

J (joule)
Jaboulay's amputation
jackknife position (Kraske position)
Jackson's membrane
Jacobsen's "Y" suture pusher
Jacob's membrane
Jacobson's
 anastomosis, J.
 cartilage, J.
 nerve of J.
 retinitis, J.
 vomeronasal organs of J.
Jacoud's arthritis
Jakob-Creutzfeldt disease
Jamshidi needle
Janet's diseae
Janeway lesion
Janeway's sphygmomanometer
Jansen's disease
Jarcho's pressometer
Jarjavay's muscle
jaundice
 cholestatic j.
 obstructive j.
 painless j.
 physiologic j.
Javal's ophthalmometer
Javid shunt
JB1 catheter
JB3 catheter
JB2 5 French catheter
J-curve
 movable core guide wire, J-c.
 wire, J-c.
Jefferson fracture
jejunal
jejunectomy
jejunitis
jejunocecostomy
jejunocolostomy
jejunoileal
jejunoileitis
jejunoileostomy
jejunojejunostomy
jejunorrhaphy
jejunostomy
jejunotomy
jejunum
 lymphatic vessels of j.
Jensen's sarcoma
jerk
 Achilles j.
 ankle j.
 elbow j.
 knee j.
jet
 collapse, j.
 phenomenon, j.
Jewett and Strong staging system
Jobert's fossa
Jod-Basedow phenomenon
Johne's disease
Johnson's position
Johnson-Stevens disease
joint (s)
 AC (acromioclavicular)
 acromioclavicular j. (AC)
 amphidiarthrodial j.
 ankle j.
 ankylosis, j.
 arthrodial j.
 ball-and-socket j.
 biaxial j.
 bilocular j.
 bleeders' j.

Additional Entries ______________________

____

____

joint (s) *(continued)*
- Brodie's j.
- Budin's j.
- cartilaginous j.
- Charcot's j.
- Chopart's j.
- Clutton's j.
- cochlear j.
- coffin j.
- composite j.
- compound j.
- condyloid j.
- Cruveilhier's j.
- diarthrodial j.
- DIP (distal interphalangeal) j.
- distal interphalangeal j. (DTP)
- dry j.
- elbow j.
- ellipsoidal j.
- enarthrodial j.
- facet j's.
- false j.
- fibrocartilaginous j.
- fibrous j.
- flail j.
- fluid, j.
- freely movable j.
- fringe j.
- ginglymoid j.
- gliding j.
- hemophilic j.
- hinge j.
- hip j.
- hysteric j.
- imaging, j.
- immovable j.
- intercarpal j.
- irritable j.
- knee j.
- ligamentous j.

joint (s) *(continued)*
- Lisfranc's j.
- metacarpophalangeal (MCP) j.
- metatarsophalangeal (MTP) j.
- midcarpal j.
- mixed j.
- multiaxial j.
- Luschka, j. of
- mouse, j.
- open j.
- peg-and-socket j.
- PIP (proximal interphalangeal) j.
- pivot j.
- plane j.
- polyaxial j.
- proximal interphalangeal (PIP) j.
- rotary j.
- sacrococcygeal j.
- sacroiliac j.
- saddle j.
- scapuloclavicular j.
- sellar j.
- shoulder j.
- SI (sacroiliac) j.
- simple j.
- socket j.
- spheroidal j.
- spiral j.
- stifle j.
- subtalar j.
- synarthrodial j.
- synovial j.
- tarsal j.
- tarsometatarsal j.
- temporomandibular j.
- through j.
- trochoid j.
- uniaxial j.

Additional Entries

joint (s) *(continued)*
- unilocular j.
- von Gies j.

Jolly's bodies
Jolly's reaction
Jones'
- fracture, J.

Jonston's arc
joule (J)
Jourdain's disease
J point
Judkins technique
jugal
jugomaxillary
jugular
- catheter, j.
- foramen, j.
- fossa, j.
- ganglion, j.
- nerve, j.
- notch of sternum, j.
- process, j.
- pressure, j.
- surface, j.
- tubercle, j.
- vein distention, j. (JVD)
- venous pulse, j.

jugulodigastric node
jugum sphenoidale
junction (s)
- cardioesophageal j.
- choledochoduodenal j.
- costochondral j.
- esophagogastric j.
- fibromuscular j.
- gastroesophageal j.

junction (s) *(continued)*
- ileocecal j.
- intermediate j.
- manubriogladiolar j.
- mucocutaneous j.
- mucogingival j.
- myoneural j.
- neuromuscular j.
- occluding j.
- osseous j.
- sclerocorneal j.
- tendinous j.
- ureteropelvic j.
- ureterovesical j.

junctional
- arrhythmia, j.
- beats, j.
- contractions, j.
- tachycardia, j.

Jung's muscle
juxta
juxta-articular bone lysis
juxtacortical osteosarcoma
juxtaepiphyseal
juxtaglomerular
- apparatus, j.

juxtangina
juxtaposing treatment fields
juxtaposition
juxtapyloric
juxtaspinal
juxtavesical
J-Vac drainage system
JVD (jugular venous distention)
JVP (jugular venous pulse)

Additional Entries

K

K (potassium)
K (kelvin)
k (kilo)
KA (King-Armstrong)
Kaes' line
Kahlbaum's disease
Kahler's disease
Kaplan technique
Kaposi's sarcoma
Karnofsky
    scale, K.
    score, K.
karyoreticulum
karyorrhexis
Katayama disease
katharometer
Kawasaki disease
Kayser's disease
kCi (kilocurie)
K-edge
keel
Keith's bundle
Keith-Flack node
keloid
Kelvin scale
Kent's bundle
Kent-His bundle
keratectomy
keratoacanthoma
keratocele
keratocentesis
keratoconjunctivitis
    epidemic k.
    phlycentular k.
    sicca k.
    viral k.
keratoiridocyclitis
keratoiridoscope
keratoleukoma
keratoma
keratomalacia
keratomata
keratome
keratometer
keratometry
keratomycosis
keratonosis
keratonosus
keratonyxis
keratopathy
    band k.
keratoplasty
    partial penetrating k.
keratoscleritis
keratoscope
keratoscopy
keratosis
    roentgen k.
    senile k.
Kerckring's
    folds, K.
    valves, K.
    ossicle, K.
    process, K.
Kerley's
    A lines, K.
    B lines, K.
    C lines, K.
kerma (acronym for "kinetic energy released in material")
Kernohan
    grading system, K.
    notch, K.
keV or kev (kilo electron volt)
keV boost
Key-Retzius foramen
kg. (kilogram)
kg.-cal. (kilogram-calorie)

Additional Entries ______________________________

____

____

kg.-m (kilogram-meter)
kHz (kilohertz)
kidney
  abscess, k.
  acidosis, k.
  acute tubular necrosis, k.
  adult polycystic disease, k.
  artery of k.
  asymmetry, k.
  bilateral cortical necrosis of k.
  blunt trauma of k.
  cadaver, k.
  calyces of k.
  congenital absence of k.
  dialysis, k.
  differential function of k.
  diuretic renography of k.
  duplication of k.
  failure, k.
  fascia of k.
  fatty capsule of k.
  floating k.
  67 Ga imaging of k.
  glomerular capsule of k.
  glomerular filtration rate (GFR), k.
  hilus, k.
  horseshoe-type k.
  131–I hippuran imaging, k.
  lower pole of k.
  lymphatic capillaries in k.
  lymphatic vessels of k.
  malpighian corpuscle k.
  medullary sponge k.
  nephrons, k.
  nerves of k.

kidney *(continued)*
  obstructive uropathy, k.
  paranephric body, k.
  pelvis of k.
  perfusion, k.
  perirenal abscess of k.
  polycystic k.
  ptotic k.
  punch, k.
  radiation effect on k.
  renal artery of k.
  renal artery occlusion, k.
  renal cell carcinoma, k.
  renal osteodystrophy, k.
  renal parenchyma, k.
  rest elevated, k.
  retention of bone scanning agents by k.
  scan, k.
  sonogram, k.
  tubules of k.
  urine sodium concentration, k.
  veins of k.
Kienbock atrophy
Kiernan's spaces
Kiesselbach's area
Kifa Catheter Mfg. Company
Kilian's line
kilo (K)
kilobecquerel (kBq)
kilocurie (kCi)
kilogram (kg)
kilogram-meter
kilohertz (kHz)
kiloliter (kl.)
kilomegacycle (kMc.)
kilometer (km)
kilovolt (Kv)
kilowatt (kW)
Kim-Ray Greenfield filter
kinematograph

Additional Entries

kineplasty
kinescope
kinesimeter
kinesthesiometer
kinetic energy
kinetocardiogram
kinetocardiography
kinetogenic
kinetographic
kinetonucleus
kinetoplasm
kinetoplast
kinetoscope
kinetoscopy
Kinevac
King-Armstrong (KA)
kinked
kinomometer
Kirchner's diverticulum
Kirschner wire
kl. (kiloliter)
Klatzkin's tumor
K-line
Klinefelter syndrome
Klippel's disease
Klippel-Feil syndrome
KLL Auger electron
Klumpke's paralysis
Klumpke-Dejerine paralysis
klystron (microwave power)
km. (kilometer)
kMc. (kilomegacycle)
kMcps (kilomegacycles per second)
K mesons
knee
 cap, k.
 chest position, k.
 joint, k.
 bursae of k.
 internal derangement of k.
knee *(continued)*
 jerk, k.
 medial compartment of k.
knee-chest position
knee-elbow position
kneeling-squatting position
Kneist syndrome
knob (s)
 aortic k.
knotted catheter
knuckle
 aortic k.
Kobak needle
Kobelt's tube
Koch's node
kocherization
Kohler's disease
Kohler-Freiberg disease
Kollmann's urethral dilator
konometer
Kopan's needle
Koranyi-Grocco triangle
Koshevnikoff's disease
Koster's nodule
Kovalevsky's canal
Koyter's muscle
Kr (krypton)
Krabbe's disease
Kraske position (jackknife position)
Krause
 end-bulbs of K.
 ligament, K.
Kretschmann's space
Krishaber's disease
Kristeller retractor
Krompecher's tumor
Kronecker's center
Kronig's field
Kronlein's hernia
81m Kr radioaerosol

Additional Entries

Krukenberg's hand
Krukenberg's veins
81m Kr gas
81m Kr ventilation
krypton (Kr)
clathrate Kr 85, k.
81m, k. (Kr 81m)
radioaerosol, k. (Kr 81m)
screening, k.
ventilation, k. (Kr 81m)
K shell
hydrogen, K s. of
tungsten, K s. of
KUB (kidney, ureter and bladder)
Kuhn's tube
Kuhne motor end-plates
Kulchitsky's cells
Kummell's disease
Kummell-Verneuil disease
Kuntscher nail
Kupffer's cells
Kupressoff's center
Kurloff's bodies
Kussmaul's
aphasia, K.
sign, K.
Kussmaul-Kien respiration
Kussmaul-Landry paralysis
Kussmaul-Maier disease
kV. (kilovolt)
kVp (kilovolt peak)
kVp measurement
kVp x-ray
KV smoothing
KV waveform
kw. (kilowatt)
kw.-hr. (kilowatt-hour)
kymogram
kymography
kyphoscoliosis
kyphosis

Additional Entries

L

La (lanthanum)
l (liter)
Labbe's
    posterior anastomotic triangle, L.
    triangle, L.
    vein, L.
label
    radioactive l.
labeled leukocytes
labia
    majora, l.
    minora, l.
    pudendi, l.
    oris, l.
labial
    arteries, l.
    commissures, l.
    fold, l.
    glands, l.
    grooves, l.
labioalveolar
labiocervical
labiochorea
labioclination
labiodental
    lamina, l.
labiogingival
labioglossolaryngeal
labioglossopharyngeal
labiograph
labioincisal
labiolingual
labiomental
labionasal
labiopalatine
labioplasty
labiotenaculum
labrum
    acetabulare, l.
labrum *(continued)*
    articularis, l.
    glenoidale, l.
labyrinth
    bony l.
    ethmoid l.
    membranous l.
    osseous l.
    perilymphatic l.
    vessels, l.
labyrinthus ethmoidalis
lacerated
    perineum, l.
lacertus
    cordis, l.
    fibrosus, l.
laciniate ligament
lacrima (pl. lacrimae)
lacrimal
    bone, l.
    canal, l.
    crest, l.
    duct, l.
    fold, l.
    gland, l.
    gland shield, l.
    nerve, l.
    papilla, l.
    punctum, l.
    reflex, l.
    sac, l.
    vein, l.
lactiferous
    ducts, l.
lacuna
    absorption, l.
    Blessig's l.
    bone, l.
    cartilage, l.
    Howship's l.

Additional Entries ______________________________

lacuna *(continued)*
intervillous l.
osseous l.
trophoblastic l.
lacunae
bone, l. of
cartilage, l. of
cerebral l.
urethra, l. of
venous l.
lacunar
infarct, l.
ligament, l.
skull, l.
lacus
lacrimalis, l.
lacy
bones in hand, l.
trabecular pattern, l.
Laennec's
catarrh, L.
cirrhosis, L.
Lafora's disease
lagena
lageniform
lagophthalmos
lake
contrast material, l. of
lacrimal l.
marginal l.
subchorial l.
Lake's pigment
Lallemand's bodies
Lalouette's pyramid
lambda
lambdoidal suture
lamella
circumferential l.
concentric l.
endosteal l.
ground l.
haversian l.
lamella *(continued)*
intermediate l.
interstitial l.
vitreous l.
lamina (pl. laminae)
alar, l.
basalis, l.
basilaris, l.
Bowman's l.
choriocapillaris l.
choroidocapillaris l.
cribrosa ossis ethmoidalis l.
cribrosa sclerae l.
dental l.
dorsal l.
elastic l.
elastica anterior l.
elastica posterior l.
epithelial l.
hypothalamus, l. of
labiodental l.
labiogingival l.
lingual l.
medullary l.
muscularis mucosae l.
nasal l.
papyracea, l.
perpendicularis l.
propria l.
reticularis l.
spiral l.
spiralis ossea l.
suprachoroid l.
terminalis l.
vasculosa l.
ventral l.
vertebrae, l. of
vertebral arch, l. of
vitreal l.
laminae
laminagraph

Additional Entries

laminar
air flow isolation room, l.
elastic tissue, l.
laminectomy
laminitis
laminogram
laminography
Lamino pad
laminotomy
Lancefield classification
Lancisi's nerves
Landeker-Steinberg light
Landing-Shirkey syndrome
landmark (s)
anatomical l.
bony l.
Landolt's bodies
Landouzy's disease
Landouzy-Dejerne dystrophy
Landry's paralysis
Landstrom's muscle
Lane's band
Langdon Down's disease
Langenbeck's amputation
Langer's axillary arch
Langerhans
centroacinar cells of L.
islands of L.
islets layer of L.
Langer's
axillary arch, L.
lines, L.
Langley's ganglion
lanthanic
lanthanum (La)
LAO (left anterior oblique)
laparocholecystotomy
laparocolectomy
laparocolostomy
laparocolotomy
laparocystectomy
laparocystidotomy
laparocystotomy
laparoenterostomy
laparoenterotomy
laparogastroscopy
laparogastrostomy
laparogastrotomy
laparohepatotomy
laparohysterectomy
laparohystero-oophorectomy
laparohysterosalpingo-oophorectomy
laparosalpingotomy
laparoscope
laparosplenectomy
laparosplenotomy
laparotome
Lardennois' button
large
angle scattering, l.
bore catheter, l.
bore needle, l.
bowel filling defect, l.
cavernous hemangioma, l.
cisterna magna, l.
duodenal cap, l.
field electron beams, l.
field irradiation, l.
field-of-view scintillation camera, l.
foramen magnum, l.
gauge core needle, l.
mass effect, l.
object film distance, l.
opacity, l.
radiation field, l.
Larkin position
Larmor
frequency, L.
precession, L.
Larsen's

Additional Entries ______________________

Larsen's *(continued)*
disease, L.
syndrome, L.
laryngeal
artery, l.
block, l.
dilator, l.
nerve, l.
saccule, l.
sinus, l.
laryngectomy
laryngendoscope
laryngismus
laryngitis
laryngocele
laryngocentesis
laryngofission
laryngofissure
laryngogram
anteroposterior l.
laryngography
laryngohypopharynx
laryngomalacia
laryngometry
laryngoparalysis
laryngopathy
laryngopharyngeal
laryngopharyngectomy
laryngopharyngeus
laryngopharyngitis
laryngopharyngoscope
laryngopharynx
laryngophony
laryngophthisis
laryngoplasty
laryngoplegia
laryngoptosis
laryngopyocele
laryngorhinology
laryngorrhagia
laryngorrhaphy
laryngorrhea
laryngoscleroma
laryngoscope
laryngoscopic
laryngoscopy
laryngospasm
laryngostasis
laryngostat
laryngostenosis
laryngostomy
laryngostroboscope
laryngotome
laryngotomy
laryngotracheal
laryngotracheitis
laryngotracheobronchitis
laryngotracheobronchoscopy
laryngotracheoscopy
laryngotracheotomy
laryngovestibulitis
larynx
cartilages of l.
conus elasticus of l.
elastic membrane of l.
glands of l.
inferior of l.
ligaments of l.
lymphatic vessels of l.
mucous membrane of l.
muscles of l.
nerves of l.
ventricle of l.
ventricular folds of l.
vessels of l.
vestibule of l.
vocal cords of l.
vocal folds of l.
Lasegue's disease
laser
argon l.
carbon-dioxide l.
dye l.
helium-neon l.

Additional Entries

laser *(continued)*
 ion l.
 krypton l.
 neodynium:yttrium-aluminum-garnet (Nd:YAG) l.
 statio l.
late film
latent image
late phase arteriogram
laterad
lateral
 bending projection, l.
 cartilage, l.
 cerebrospinal fasciculus, l.
 compression of bladder, l.
 cricoarytenoid muscle, l.
 decubitus position, l.
 disc, l.
 electron beam ports, l.
 hyothyroid ligament, l.
 inferior genicular artery, l.
 nasal cartilage, l.
 oblique projection, l.
 olfactory gyrus, l.
 olfactory stria, l.
 position, l.
 projection, l.
 recess, l.
 recumbent position (a/k/a English position), l.
 relaxation time, l.
 simulation film, l.
 sinuses of dura, l.
 spinothalamic fasciculus, l.
 superior genicular artery, l.
 thyrohyoid ligament, l.

lateral *(continued)*
 ventricle, l.
 ventricular compression, l.
 ventricular width, l. (LVW)
 vertebral muscles, l.
 view, l.
 vibrations, l.
 wedged field, l.
lateroabdominal
lateroaortic nodes
lateroconal fascia
laterodeviation
lateroduction
lateroflexion
lateroposition
lateropulsion
laterotorsion
lateroversion
lattice
 relaxation time, l.
 vibrations, l.
latissimus dorsi muscle
latitude film
Laugier's hernia
Laumonier's ganglion
Laveran's bodies
lawrencium (Lr)
Law's position
Law's view
layer (s)
 bacillary l.
 basal l.
 blastodermic l.
 buffy l.
 clear l.
 columnar l.
 compact l.
 enamel l.
 fascial l.
 functional l.

Additional Entries

layer (s) *(continued)*
ganglionic l.
germ l.
germinative l.
granular l.
half-value l.
Henle's l.
horny l.
imbricating l.
keratohyaline l.
malpighian l.
mantle l.
mucosal l.
muscular l.
of rods and cones, l.
Ollier's l.
osteogenetic l.
prickle-cell l.
Rauber's l.
serosal l.
spinous l.
spongy l.
subcutaneous fat l.
subendocardial l.
layering of contrast material
LD (lethal dose)
LDA (left dorsoanterior)
LDM (low-dose plain film myelography)
LDP (left dorsoposterior)
LE (lupus erythematosus)
lead (s) (Pb)
AVF l.
AVL l.
AVR l.
bipolar l.
electrocardiographic l.
encephalopathy l.
I, l.
II, l.
III, l.
limb l.

lead (s) (Pb) *(continued)*
precordial l.
unipolar l.
V1 l.
V2 l.
V3 l.
V4 l.
V5 l.
V6 l.
lead (Pb)
button, l.
marker, l.
mask, l.
protective apron, l.
rubber backing sheet, l.
shield, l.
shot, l.
leaflet
aortic l.
excursion, l.
mitral valve l.
prolapse, l.
leakage radiation
leaking aortic aneurysm
least squares technique (LST)
leaves
broad ligament, l. of
diaphragm, l. of
Lefort I, II, III fractures
left
anterior oblique (LAO) projection, l.
atrial angiography, l.
atrial myxoma, l.
axillary catheterization, l.
crux of diaphragm, l.
heart catheterization, l.
lateral depth, l.
lateral position, l.
lateral view, l.

Additional Entries

left *(continued)*
posterior oblique (LPO), l.
-to-right shift, l.
-to-right shunt, l.
-to-right shunting, l.
ventricular aneurysm, l.
ventricular ejection fraction, l.
ventricular hypertrophy (LVH), l.
ventriculography, l.
Legal's disease
Legg's disease
Legg-Calve-Perthes disease
leg length study
Leiner's disease
leiodermia
leiodystonia
leiomyoblastoma
leiomyofibroma
leiomyoma
submucous l.
uteri, l.
leiomyosarcoma
Leksell
stereotactic gamma unit, L.
stereotaxic device, L.
stereotaxic system, L.
Leloir's disease
lemniscus
lateralis, l.
medial, l.
spinal, l.
Lenard rays
length
crown-heel l.
crown-rump l.
lengthening
heel cord l.
tendon l.
LEN PR (lenticular process)
lenticular
degeneration, l.
ganglion, l.
glands of stomach, l.
process of incus, l.
lenticulo-optic
lenticulothalamic
lentiform
nucleus, l.
lentiginosis
progressive cardiomyopathic l.
lentiginous
lentiglobus
lentigo maligna
Leonard cathode-ray tube
lepidoma
leptomeningeal
cyst, l.
metastases, l.
leptomeninges
leptomeningitis
leptoscope
Leri syndrome
Leriche's disease
lesion
annular l.
apple-core like l.
margin, l.
polypoid l.
sessile l.
space-occupying l.
wedge-shaped l.
lesser
cavernous nerve, l.
curvature of stomach, l.
lacrimal bone, l.
multangular bone, l.
omentum, l.
pelvis, l.
peritoneal sac, l.

Additional Entries

lesser *(continued)*
    sac, l.
    saphenous system,, l.
    sciatic foramen, l.
    sciatic notch, l.
    sigmoid cavity, l.
    splanchnic nerve, l.
    trochanter, l.
    tubercle, l.
    tuberosity, l.
    wing of sphenoid, l.
LET (linear energy transfer)
Letterer-Siwe disease
leukemogenesis
leukocyte
    agranular l.
    basophilic l.
    endothelial l.
    eosinophilic l.
    granular l.
    hyaline l.
    lymphoid l.
    neutrophilic l.
    nongranular l.
    polymorphonuclear l.
    typing serum, l.
leukocytogenesis
leukocytoma
leukocytopenia
leukocytosis
    basophilic l.
    eosinophilic l.
    lymphocytic l.
    mononuclear l.
    pathologic l.
leukoderma
leukodermatous
leukodystrophy
    metachromatic l.
leukoencephalitis
leukoencephalopathy
leukoencephaly
leukogram
leukoma
leukomatous
leukomyelitis
leukomyelopathy
leukonychia
leukopathy
leukopenia
    basophilic l.
    malignant l.
    pernicious l.
leukopenic
leukopheresis
leukoplakia
leukosarcoma
leukosarcomatosis
leukoscope
leukosis
LeVeen shunt
level
    air fluid l.
    stability, l. of
Levin tube
levocardia
levogram
levoscoliosis
Levy-Amplatz transthoracic needle
Lewis position
LFA (left frontoanterior)
LFP (left frontoposterior)
LFT (left frontotransverse)
LHRH (luteinizing hormone releasing hormone)
Libman-Sacks disease
Lichtheim's aphasia
lidofenin
lie
    horiizontal l.
    longitudinal l.
Liebel-Flarsheim-Angiomat 3000 injector

Additional Entries

Liebel-Flarsheim Company
Lieberkuhn's
ampulla, L.
crypts, L.
Liebermeister's furrows
lien
accessorius, l.
lienal (pertaining to spleen)
artery, l.
plexus, l.
vein, l.
LiF (lithium fluoride)
ligament
accessory l.
acromioclavicular l.
alar l.
annular l.
anococcygeal l.
apical odontoid l.
Arantius l.
arcuate l., lateral
arcuate l, medial
auricularis l.
axis l.
Bardinet l.
Barkow l.
Bellini l.
Berry l.
Bertin l.
Bichat l.
bifurcated l.
Bigelow l.
Botallo l.
Bourgery l.
broad l.
Brodie l.
Burns' l.
calcaneocuboid l.
calcaneofibular l.
calcaneonavicular l.
calcaneotibial l.
Caldani l.

ligament *(continued)*
Campbell l.
Camper l.
capsular l.
cardinal l.
caroticoclinoid l.
carpal dorsal l.
carpal palmar l.
carpometacarpal l. (dorsal)
carpometacarpal l. (palmar)
caudal l.
cervical l.
check l.
ciliary l.
Civinini l.
Clado l.
collateral l.
Colles' l.
conoid l.
Cooper l.
coracoacromial l.
coracoclavicular l.
coracohumeral l.
corniculopharyngeal l.
coronary l.
costoclavicular l.
costocolic l.
costotransverse l.
costoxiphoid l.
cotyloid l.
cricoarytenoid posterior l.
cricopharyngeal l.
cricosantorinian l.
cricothyroid l.
cricotracheal l.
crucial l.
cruciate l.
cruciform l.
Cruveilhier l.

Additional Entries

ligament *(continued)*
- cubonavicular l.
- cuneocuboid l.
- cystoduodenal l.
- deltoid l.
- dental l.
- denticulate l.
- Denuce l.
- diaphragmatic l.
- epihyal l.
- external lateral l.
- falciform l.
- fallopian l.
- Ferrein l.
- fibular collateral l.
- flava l.
- Flood l.
- fundiform l.
- gastrolienal l.
- gastrophrenic l.
- gastrosplenic l.
- Gerdy l.
- Gillette l.
- Gimbernat l.
- gingivodental l.
- glenoid l.
- glossoepiglottic l.
- Gunz l.
- Helmholtz l.
- Henle l.
- Hensing l.
- hepatocolic l.
- hepatoduodenal l.
- hepatogastric
- hepatorenal l.
- Hesselbach l.
- Holl l.
- Hueck l.
- Humphry l.
- Hunter l.
- hyoepiglottic l.
- iliofemoral l.

ligament *(continued)*
- iliolumbar l.
- iliopectineal l.
- iliotrochanteric l.
- infundibulo-ovarian l.
- infundibulopelvic l.
- inguinal l.
- inguinal reflex l.
- intercarpal l.
- interchondral l.
- interclavicular l.
- interclinoid l.
- intercornual l.
- intercostal l.
- intercuneiform l.
- interfoveolar l.
- intermetacarpal l.
- intermetatarsal l.
- internal lateral l.
- interspinous l.
- intertransverse l.
- intra-articular l.
- ischiofemoral l.
- jugal l.
- Krause l.
- laciniate l.
- lacunar l.
- lateral l.
- Lauth l.
- lienophrenic l.
- Lisfranc l.
- Lockwood l.
- longitudinal l.
- lumbocostal l.
- Luschka l.
- Mackenrodt l.
- malleolar l.
- Mauchart l.
- Meckel l.
- metatarsophalangeal collateral l.
- nuchal l.

Additional Entries ______________________

ligament *(continued)*
nuchae l.
occipitoaxial l.
odontoid l.
orbicular l.
ovarian l.
palpebral l.
pectinate l.
pectineal l.
perineal l.
Petit l.
phrenicocolic l.
phrenicosplenic l.
phrenogastric l.
phrenosplenic l.
pisiunciform l.
pisohamate l.
pisometacarpal l.
plantar l.
popliteal arcuate l.
popliteal oblique l.
Poupart l.
pterygospinous l.
pterygomandibular l.
pubic l.
pubocapsular l.
pubofemoral l.
puboprostatic l.
pubovesical l.
pulmonary l.
quadrate l.
radial collateral l.
radiate l.
radiocarpal l.
Retzius l.
rhomboid l.
Robert l.
round l.
sacrococcygeal l.
sacroiliac (anterior) l.
sacroiliac (interosseous)
sacroiliac (posterior l.

ligament *(continued)*
sacrosciatic l.
sacrospinous l.
sacrotuberous l.
Sappey l.
sheath l.
sphenomandibular l.
spinoglenoid l.
spiral of cochlea l.
spring l.
stellate l.
sternoclavicular l.
sternocostal l.
sternopericardial l.
stylohyoid l.
stylomandibular l.
suprascapular l.
supraspinous l.
suspensory l.
sutural l.
synovial l.
talocalcaneal l.
talofibular l.
talonavicular l.
talotibial l.
tarsal l.
tarsometatarsal l.
tarsotibial l.
tarsotibial l.
temporomandibular l.
teres (of liver) l.
Teutleben l.
thyroepiglottic l.
thyrohyoid l.
tibial collateral l.
tibiofibular l.
tibionavicular l.
transverse l.
trapezoid l.
Treitz l.
triangular l.
ulnar collateral l.

Additional Entries

ligament *(continued)*
umbilical l.
uterosacral l.
vaginal l.
Valsalva l.
ventricular l.
vertebropelvic l.
Vesalius l.
vesicouterine l.
vesicoumbilical l.
vestibular l.
vocal l.
Weitbrecht l.
Winslow l.
Wrisberg l.
Y-shaped l.
yellow l.
Zinn l.
ligamentopexis
ligamentopexy
ligamentous
ligamentum
arteriosum, l.
flavum, l.
teres, l.
ligand
ligate
ligation
ligature
light
chain disorder, l.
field, l.
isotope, l.
localizing collimator, l.
wave length, l.
limb
anacrotic l.
catacrotic l.
lead, l.
length, l.
motion absent, l.
overgrowth, l.

limb *(continued)*
pelvic l.
phantom l.
thoracic l.
limbal
groove, l.
incision, l.
suture, l.
limbic system
limbus
acetabuli, l.
cornea, l. of
laminae spiralis osseae, l.
surgical l.
vertebra, l. of
limey bile
limitation
extension, l. of
flexion, l. of
limited view
linac
Lindau's disease
Lindau-von Hippel disease
line
anterior axillary l.
arcuate l.
axillary l.
cleavage l.
colored l.
curved l.
CVP (central venous pressure)
dentate l.
fat l.
fracture l.
gas density l.
gluteal l.
iliopectineal l.
incision l.
incremental l. (of Salter)
intercondyloid l.

Additional Entries ______________________________

line *(continued)*
- intertrochanteric l.
- Kerley A l.
- Kerley B l.
- Kerley C l.
- Langer's l.
- low intensity l.
- medial joint l.
- midaxillary l.
- midclavicular l.
- midcostal l.
- midsternal l.
- mucocutaneous l.
- mylohyoid l.
- Nelaton's l.
- nuchal l.
- oblique l.
- pacing, l.
- pectate l.
- pectinate l.
- pectineal l.
- popliteal l.
- posterior axillary l.
- saturation, l.
- scan, l.
- spiral l.
- Schreger l.
- supracondylar l.
- suture l.
- temporal l.
- tension l.
- voltage, l.
- voltage compensator, l.
- white l. (of Toldt)
- width, l.
- Z-line

linea
- alba, l.
- aspera, l.
- nigra, l.
- quadrata, l.

linea *(continued)*
- semicircularis, l.
- splendens, l.

lineae semilunares

linear
- accelerator, l.
- amplification, l.
- array, l.
- attenuation coefficient, l.
- coefficient, l.
- energy transfer (LET), l.
- grid, l.
- irridium wire source, l.
- phased arrays, l.
- quadratic (LQ) formula, l.
- ribbon array, l.
- scanning, l.
- strands, l.
- tomography, l.

linearity

lined gloves

lingua
- apex of l.
- dorsum of l.
- musculi l.
- papillae l.
- tunica mucosa, l. of

linguae

lingual
- artery, l.
- bone, l.
- branches, l.
- gyrus, l.
- lamina, l.
- lymph nodes, l.
- nerve, l.
- papillae, l.
- tonsil, l.
- veins, l.
- tonsil, l.

Additional Entries

lingula
cerebellum, l. of
mandibulae l.
sphenoid, l. of
lingulae
lingular
lingulectomy
linguoaxial
linguocervical
linguodistal
linguogingival
linguoincisal
linguomesial
linguo-occlusal
linguopapillitis
linguoplacement
linguopulpal
linguoversion
liothyronine
lip
hare l.
tympanic l.
vestibular l.
liparocele
lipectomy
lipid deposition
Lipiodol 28%
Lipiodol 40%
lipoadenoma
lipoarthritis
lipoatrophy
lipoblastoma
lipocardiac
lipochondroma
lipodystrophy
lipogranulomatosis
lipohemarthrosis
lipolipoidosis
lipolytic activity
lipoma
lipomatosis
lipomatosis *(continued)*
renal l.
lipomatous
lipomeningocele
lipomyoma
lipomyxoma
liponecrosis
lipopathy
liposarcoma
Lipowitz's metal
Lippes loop (intrauterine device IUD)
lipping
osteoarthritic l.
liquefaction
liquid crystal thermogram
liquid embolic media
liquid scintillator
liquified hematoma
Lissauer
fasciculus, L.
tract, L.
lissencephaly
Lister's tubercle
liter (l)
lithiasis
lithium borate
lithium fluoride (LiF)
lithotomy position
lithotriptoscope
little mass effect
Little's area
Little's disease
Littre's
crypts, L.
urethral glands, L.
liver
abscess, l.
arteries, l.
bare area, l.
bed, l.

Additional Entries ______________________

liver *(continued)*
- bile ducts, l.
- biopsy, l.
- capsule, l.
- computed tomography of l.
- echinococcal cyst, l.
- edge palpable, l.
- edge smooth, l.
- exretory apparatus, l.
- fatty infiltration of l.
- fossae, l.
- IDA compound uptake by l.
- imaging, l.
- ligaments, l.
- lobe, l.
- lobules, l.
- longitudinal fissures, l.
- lymphatic capillaries, l.
- mass lesion, l.
- metastases, l.
- nerves, l.
- portal vein, l.
- scan, l.
- scintiphoto, l.
- scintiscanning correlation, l.
- spleen scan, l.
- vessels, l.

LL (left lateral)

LML (lateral malleolar ligament)

lobar
- agenesis, l.
- bronchi, l.
- collapse, l.
- consolidation, l.
- emphysema, l.
- lesion, l.
- nephronia, l.
- resection, l.

lobe
- azygous l.
- brain, l. of
- cardiac l.
- caudate l.
- cerebellar l.
- cerebral hemisphere l.
- cuneate l.
- ear l.
- frontal l.
- hepatic l.
- hypophysis, l. of
- kidney, l. of
- liver l.
- lower l.
- lung l.
- median l. decompression
- middle l.
- occipital l.
- parietal l.
- prostate l.
- Riedel's l.
- spigelian l.
- temporal l.
- thyroid gland, l. of
- upper l.

lobular invasive carcinoma

lobule
- auricle, l. of
- cerebellum, l. of
- epididymis, l. of
- hepatic l.
- kidney, l. of
- lung, l. of
- mammary gland, l. of
- paracentral l.
- parietal l.
- pituitary gland, l. of
- portal l.
- testis, l. of
- thymus, l. of
- thyroid gland, l. of

Additional Entries

lobuli glandulae thyreodeae
lobulus
auriculae, l.
parietalis inferior, l.
parietalis superior, l.
lobus
caudatus, l.
frontalis, l.
hepatis dexter, l.
hepatis sinister, l.
occipitalis, l.
parietalis, l.
quadratus hepatis, l.
temporalis, l.
local
anesthesia, l.
application, l.
autoregulation disturbance, l.
circulation, l.
efficiency factor, l.
excision, l.
infiltration, l.
involvement, l.
recurrence, l.
spasm, l.
localization
film, l.
needle l.
tumor l.
localized cystic osteolytic lesion
localizing cone
Lockwood's
tendon, L.
ligament, L.
locoregional
control, l.
failure (LF-RF), l.
progression, l.
loculated
abscess, l.
loculated *(continued)*
empyema,, l.
fluid, l.
pleural effusion, l.
loculi
loculus
locus
caeruleus, l.
Loevit's cell
Loffler's
pneumonia, L.
syndrome, L.
logarithmic
amplification, l.
scales, l.
value, l.
log cell kill
logoscope
Lohlein-Baehr lesion
Lohlein's diameter
loin (a/k/a lumbus)
lollipop system
long
buccal nerve, l.
calcaneocuboid ligament, l.
ciliary nerves, l.
external lateral ligament, l.
field, l.
narrow field, l.
plantar ligament, l.
saphenous nerve, l.
saphenous vein, l.
subscapular nerve, l.
thoracic artery, l.
thoracic nerve, l.
longilineal
longipedate
longiradiate
longissimus
longitudinal

Additional Entries

longitudinal *(continued)*
axis of mandibular body, l.
groove, l.
heating length, l.
magnetization, l.
section, l.
sonographic imaging, l.
tomography, l.
wrinkling of dura, l.
longitudinalis
longus
capitis muscle, l.
colii muscle, l.
loop
afferent l.
bowel l.
closed l.
colostomy, l.
duodenal l.
efferent l.
Henle's l.
loopogram
loose
body in joint, l.
watery stools, l.
looser zones (pseudofracture)
LOP (left occipitoposterior)
lordosis
flattening of l.
lumbar l.
lordotic
curve, l.
projection, l.
view, l.
Lorentzian line saturation
loss of carrying angle
LOT (left occipitotransverse)
Louis's angle
Low-Beers projection
Low-Beers view
low
attachment of tentorium, l.
attenuation area, l.
contrast film, l.
density lesion, l.
density structure, l.
dose film, l.
dose plain film myelography (LDM), l.
flow state, l.
frequency, l.
intestinal obstruction, l.
jugular lymph nodes, l.
mA setting, l.
parity, l.
peak energy, l.
ratio grid, l.
sampling rate, l.
Z material, l.
Lowe's ring
Lowenberg's canal
Lowenthal's tract
lower
end of humerus, l.
esophageal ring, l.
moiety, l.
pole of patella, l.
zone vessels, l.
Lower's rings
Lowitt's bodies
LP (long process)
LPO (left posterior oblique)
LQ (linear quadratic) formula
Lr (lawrencium)
LSA (left sacroanterior)
LSC (lateral semicircular canal)
L-shaped appearance
L-shell of tungsten

Additional Entries

LSP (left sacroposterior)
LST (left sacrotransverse; least squares technique)
lucency
lucent defect
lucite plate
Ludwig's angle
Ludwig's ganglion
Luer-Lok fitting
Luer-Lok syringe
lues
 hepatis, l.
 syphilitica, l.
Lugol's solution
LUL (left upper lobe)
lumbar
 approach, l.
 arteriogram, l.
 artery, l.
 canal stenosis, l.
 curvature, l.
 disc herniation, l.
 laminectomy, l.
 myelogram, l.
 puncture, l.
 scoliosis, l.
 spinal canal stenosis, l.
 spine, l.
 spurring, l.
 sympathectomy, l.
 transverse process, l.
 vertebra, l.
lumboabdominal
lumbocolostomy
lumbocolotomy
lumbocostal
lumbocrural
lumbodorsal
 fascia, l.
lumbodynia
lumboiliac
lumboinguinal
lumboperitoneal shunt
lumbosacral
 joint, l.
 plexus, l.
 spine, l.
 trunk, l.
lumbricales
 muscles, l.
lumen
 bowel l.
 vein l.
 patent l.
 triple l. catheter
lumina
luminal
luminescence
luminosity of light
luminous
 rays, l.
 surface, l.
lumniferous
lunate
 bone, l.
 surface of acetabulum, l.
Lunderquist exchange guide wire
Lunderquist-Ring torque guide wire
lung
 aerosol imaging, l.
 apices, l.
 base, l.
 capacity, l.
 chronic obstructive l. disease (COLD)
 coin lesion of l.
 collapse of l.
 decortication of l.
 diffusing capacity of l.
 disease, l.

Additional Entries ______________________

lung *(continued)*
- field, l.
- 67 Ga imaging, l.
- hernia, l.
- infarction, l.
- infiltrate, l.
- lobe of l.
- parenchyma, l.
- perfusion, l.
- perfusion scan, l.
- perfusion scintigraphy, l.
- scintiscan, l.
- 201 Tl accumulation by l.
- ventilation scan, l.

lunulae
- nails, l. of
- semilunar valves, l. of

lupus
- arteritis, l.
- erythematosus (LE), l.

Luschka
- body of L.
- crypts, L.
- foramina of L.
- gland of L.
- glomus of L.

luteal

lutein
- cyst, l.

luteinizing
- hormone, l.
- hormone releasing hormone (LHRH), l.

Lutembacher disease

luteoma

luteum
- hemorrhagic corpus l.

Luys'
- body, L.
- nucleus, L.

LVH (left ventricular hypertrophy)

LVW (lateral ventricular width)

L x-rays

lymphadenography

lymphadenopathy

lymphangiectasia

lymphangiographic injector

lymphangiography

lymphangioma

lymph
- channel, l.
- duct cannulator, l.
- duct holder, l.
- duct occluder, l.

Lymphazurin

lymph node (s)
- abdominal l.n.
- aortic l.n.
- auricular l.n.
- axillary l.n.
- buccinator l.n.
- cervical l.n.
- capsule l.n.
- Cloquet l.n.
- cortex of l.n.
- deltoideopectoral l.n.
- diaphragmatic l.n.
- epigastric l.n.
- facial l.n.
- gastric l.n.
- gastroepiploic l..n.
- head, l.n. of
- hepatic l.n.
- hilum of l.n.
- hypogastric l.n.
- ileocolic l.n.
- iliac l.n.
- infraorbital l.n.
- inguinal l.n.

Additional Entries

lymph node (s) *(continued)*
intercostal l.n.
internal mammary l.n.
lingual l.n.
lower extremity l.n.
lumbar l.n.
mastoid l.n.
maxillar l.n.
mediastinal l.n.
medulla l.n.
mesenteric l.n.
mesocolic l.n.
neck, l.n. of
obturator l.n.
occipital l.n.
pancreaticoduodenal l.n.
pancreaticolienal l.n.
pararectal l.n.
paratracheal l.n.
parieetal l.n.
parotid l.n.
pelvic l.n.
popliteal l.n.
preauricular l.n.
receptacles, l.n.
retropharyngeal l.n.
Rosenmuller l.n.
sacral l.n.
splenic l.n.
Stahr l.n.
sternal l.n.
subinguinal l.n.
submaxillary l.n.
submental l.n.
suprahyoid l.n.
supramandibular l.n.
supratrochlear l.n.
thorax, l.n. of
tibial l.n.
tongue, l.n. of
tracheobronchial l.n.

lymph node (s) *(continued)*
upper extremity, l.n.
visceral, l.n.
lymphadenectomy
lymphadenhypertrophy
lymphadenitis
mesenteric l.
lymphadenocele
lymphadenocyst
lymphadenogram
lymphadenography
lymphadenoma
lymphadenomatosis
lymphadenopathy
axillary l.
giant follicular l.
hilar l.
palpable l.
lymphadenosis
lymphangiectasia
lymphangiectasis
lymphangiectomy
lymphangioendothelioma
lymphangiofibroma
lymphangiogram
lymphangiography
lymphangioma
cavernous l.
cystic l.
lymphangiomyomatosis
lymphangiophlebitis
lymphangioplasty
Handley's l.
lymphangiosarcoma
lymphangitic
carcinomatosis, l.
spread, l.
lymphangitis
lymphatic
capillaries, l.
chain, l.

Additional Entries

lymphatic *(continued)*
channels, l.
drainage, l.
leukemia, l.
metastases, l.
nodules, l.
pathways, l.
sump, l.
system, l.
trunks, l.
vessels, l.
lymphatolysis
Lymphazurin
lymphectasia
lymphedema
lymphoblast
lymphoblastic
leukemia, l.
lymphosarcoma, l.
lymphoblastoma
lymphoblastomatosis
lymphoblastomatous
lymphoblastomid
lymphoblastosis
lymphocele
lymphocytapheresis
lymphocyte
activated l.
atypical l.
B l.
killer l.
null l.
predominance, l.
reticular l.
T l.
lymphocytic
depletion, l.
thyroiditis, l.
lymphocytoma
cutis, l.
lymphocytomatosis
lymphocytomatous
lymphocytopenia
lymphocytosis
lymphocytotoxicity
lymphocytotoxin
lymphodermia
lymphoepithelioma
lymphogenous
lymphogenous
lymphogram
lymphogranuloma
inguinale, l.
venereum, l.
lymphogranulomatosis
lymphography
lymphoid
hyperplasia, l.
lymphoidectomy
lymphoidocyt e
lymphoma
Burkitt's l.
diffuse lymphocytic l.
gastric l.
giant follicular l.
granulomatous l.
histiocytic l.
implant, l.
lymphoblastic l.
lymphocytic l.
malignant l.
mixed cell l.
non-Hodgkin's l.
poorly-differentiated l.
stem cell l.
undifferentiated l.
well-differentiated l.
lymphomatosis
lymphomatous
lymphomyxoma
lymphopathy
ataxic l.
lymphopoiesis
lymphopoietic

Additional Entries

lymphoproliferative
lymphoreticular
lymphoreticulosis
 benign, l.
lymphorrhea
lymphorrhoid
lymphosarcoma
 lymphoblastic l.
 lymphocytic l.
lymphosarcomatosis
lymphoscintigram
lymphoscintigraphy
lymphostasis
lymphotaxis
lymphotome
lymphotoxemia
lymphotrophy
lymphous
lyra of fornix
lysis
 adhesions, l. of
lytic
 area, l.
 change, l.
 lesion, l.
 neuroblastoma, l.
 shift defect, l.

Additional Entries

M

M (distant metastases)
m. (meter)
ma. (milliampere)
Macewen's
  operation, M.
  suprameatal triangle, M.
Mackenrodt's ligament
Mackenzie's
  disease, M.
  ligament, M.
  syndrome, M.
MacLean-Maxwell disease
MacLeod's syndrome
Mackler tube
macrencephaly
macroadenoma
macroblast
  Naegeli, m. of
macrocephaly
macrodactyly
macrodystrophia
macroencephaly
macroerythroblast
macroglobulinemia
  Waldenstrom's m.
macroglossia
macrognathia
macrography
macroleukoblast
macrolymphocyte
macrolymphocytosis
macronormoblast
macrophage
  alveolar m.
  armed m.
  cytoxicity, m.
  fixed m.
  free m.
  inflammatory m.
macrophagocyte
macrophthalmous
macropromyelocyte
macroscopic
  agglutination, m.
  anatomy, m.
  lymph node involvement, m.
macroscopy
macrosigmoiid
macrosomatia
  adiposa congenita, m.
macrosomia
macrospore
macula (pl. maculae)
  acustica sacculi m.
  adherens, m.
  atrophicae, m.
  caeruleae, m.
  cerebral m.
  cribrosa media, m.
  cribrosa superior, m.
  densa, m.
  flava, m.
  folliculi, m.
  germinativa, m.
  lutea retinae, m.
  retinae, m.
  sacculi, m.
  utriculi, m.
macular
  atrophy, m.
  degeneration, m.
macule
maculocerebral
maculopapular
  rash, m.
maculovesicular
Maddox rods
Madelung's deformity
Maffucci's syndrome

Additional Entries ______________________

____

____

Magendie's foramen
Magitot's disease
magnesium (Mg)
magnetic
  coil, m.
  dipole, m.
  field, m.
  moments, m.
  nuclei, m.
  pole, m.
  relaxation rates, m.
  resonance imaging, m. (MRI)
magnetization vector
magnetocardiograph
magnetoencephalograph
magnetogyric ratio
magnetometer
magnetotherapy
Magnetrode system
magnetron
Magnevist
magnification
  high-powered m.
  radiography, m.
  technique, m.
magnifying
  loupe, m.
magnum
  foramen, m.
Maher's disease
Maier's sinus
main
  bronchus, m.stem
Maisonneuve's amputation
Maissiat's band
Majocchi's disease
malabsorption
  syndrome, m.
malacoplakia
  vesical m.
malacosarcosis
malalignment
malar
  bone, m.
  eminence, m.
  flush, m.
  process of maxilla, m.
Malassez's disease
Malecot catheter
malformation
  congenital m.
Malgaigne's
  amputation, M.
  fracture, M.
  hook, M.
malignant
  effusion, m.
  growth, m.
  hypertension, m.
  melanoma, m.
  process, m.
  tumor, m.
  zone, m.
MA linearity
malinterdigitation
malleability
malleable
malleation
malleoincudal
malleolar
  arteries, m.
  folds, m.
  sulcus, m.
malleoli
malleolus
  external m.
  inner m.
  internal m.
  lateral m.
  medial m.
  outer m.
  radial m.
  tibial m.

Additional Entries

malleolus *(continued)*
ulnar m.
malleotomy
mallet
toe, m.
malleus
ligaments of m.
Mallinkrodt Chemical Works
Mallory's bodies
Mallory-Weiss syndrome
malocclusion
malpighian
bodies, m.
corpuscles, m.
pyramid of kidney, m.
Malpighi's pyramids
Malpighi's vesicles
malposition
malrotation
kidney, m. of
malum
articulorum senilis, m.
coxae senilis, m.
vertebrale suboccipitale, m.
malunion
mamillae
mamillary
process, m.
mamilliplasty
mamma
mammae
nipple of m.
papilla of m.
mammary
arteries, m.
dysplasia, m.
fold, m.
gland, m.
internal lymph node, m.
process, m.
prosthesis, m.

mammary *(continued)*
veins, m.
mammogenesis
mammogram
mammography
mammoplasia
mammoplasty
augmentation m.
McKissock m.
reduction m.
Manchester
approach, M.
style interstitial single-plane implant, M.
style ovoid, M.
system, M.
mandible
angle of m.
articulations of m.
body of m.
condyle of m.
condyloid process of m.
coronoid process of m.
ramus of m.
semilunar notch of m.
symphysis of m.
mandibula
mandibulae
mandibular
arch, m.
branches of facial nerve, m.
canal, m.
foramen, m.
fossa, m.
nerve, m.
notch, m.
ridge, m.
mandibularis
mandibulopharyngeal
manganese (Mn)
Mangoldt's epithelial grafting

Additional Entries

Mani catheter
maniphalanx
manipulation
  closed m.
  open m.
Mann-Bollman fistula
mannitol
  hexanitrate, m.
Mann-Williamson ulcer
manometer
manometric
  measurement, m.
  pressure measurement, m.
manoptoscope
manoscopy
Manson's disease
mantle
  blocks, m.
  brain m.
  field, m.
  radiation therapy, m.
mantra
manual
  exploration, m.
  reduction of fracture, m.
  variation of flow, m.
MANUB.IN TM (manubrium within tympanic membrane)
manubria
manubrium
  mallei, m.
  malleus, m. of
  sterni, m.
  sternum, m. of
manudynamometer
Manz's glands
marasmic
Marchand's accessory adrenal bodies
Marchifava-Bignami disease
Marcus Gunn pupil
marfanoid
  habitus, m.
Marfan syndrome
margin
  ciliary m.
  dentate m.
  gingival m.
  indistinct m.
  intercostal m.
  lesion, m.
  psoas m.
  well-demarcated m.
  wound m.
marginal
  filling defect, m.
  fracture, m.
  misses, m.
margination
marginoplasty
Marie's ataxia
Marie-Bamberger disease
Marie-Strumpell disease
Marie-Tooth disease
Marine-Lenhart syndrome
Mariotte's spot
Marjolin's ulcer
mark
  display, m. (grid and scale)
marked
  enlargement, m.
  granularity, m.
  medicine glass, m.
marker
markings
  bronchovesicular m.
  haustral m.
  linear m.
  lung m.
  pulmonary vascular m.
Marlex mesh

Additional Entries

Maroteaux-Lamy syndrome
marrow
  aspiration, b. marrow
  biopsy, b. marrow
  depression, b. marrow
  transplant, b. marrow
Marsh's disease
Marshall's
  ligament, M.
  modification, M.
  oblique vein, M.
  vein, M.
  vestigial fold, M.
mAs (tube milliampere seconds)
mask film
mass
  atomic m.
  attenuation coefficient, m.
  cell m.
  coefficient, m.
  defect, m.
  density, m.
  effect, m.
  energy duality, m.
  energy transfer coefficient, m.
  lean body m.
  lesion, m.
  number, m.
massa intermedia
massage
  cardiac m.
  carotid m.
  vibratory m.
masseter
  nerve, m.
  muscle, m.
  vein, m.
masseteric
  artery, m.
masseteric *(continued)*
  fascia, m.
  nerve, m.
  sling, m.
mastatrophy
mastication
  muscles, m.
mastitis
  chronic cystic m.
  periductal m.
  plasma cell m.
  neonatorum, m.
mastocarcinoma
mastochondroma
mastocyte
mastocytoma
mastocytosis
mastodynia
mastogram
mastography
mastoid
  air cells, m.
  antrum, m.
  bone, m.
  canaliculus, m.
  cells, m.
  foramen, m.
  fossa, m.
  lymph nodes, m.
  notch, m.
  portion of temporal bone, m.
  process, m.
  sinus, m.
  tip, m.
mastoidal
mastoidectomy
mastoideocentesis
mastoiditis
mastoidotomy
mastoidotympanectomy
masto-occipital

Additional Entries

mastoparietal
mastopathy
mastopexy
mastoplastia
mastoptosis
mastorrhagia
mastoscirrhus
mastosquamous
mastostomy
mastotomy
matachromic leukodystrophy
match
    focal V/Q match
matched peripheral dose (MPD)
mater
    dura m.
    pia m.
material
    mass, m.
    volume, m.
Mathieu's disease
matrices
matrix
    bone m.
    cartilage m.
    dimension, m.
    nail m.
    size, m.
    unguis m.
matter
    gray m.
    white m.
maturation of ovum
mature
    cataract, m.
matured placenta
Mauchart's ligament
Maunoir's hydrocele
Maurer's dots
Maxcy's disease
maxilla
maxilla *(continued)*
    frontal process of m.
    lacrimal notch of m.
    LeFort's fracture of m.
maxillae
maxillary
    antrum, m.
    artery, m.
    lymph nodes, m.
    nerve, m.
    process, m.
    ridge, m.
    sinus, m.
    tuberosity, m.
    vein, m.
maxillectomy
maxillitis
maxillodental
maxilloethmoidectomy
maxillofacial
maxillojugal
maxillolabial
maxillomandibular
maxillopalatine
maxillopharyngeal
maxillotomy
maxima
maximal
    breathing capacity, m.
    expiratory flow, m.
    heart rate, m.
    inspiratory flow, m.
    mass effect, m.
maximum
    dose, (Dmax), m.
    energy (Emax), m.
    permissible dose (MPD), m.
    permission concentration (MPC), m.
    permissible dose equivalent (MPDE), m.

Additional Entries

maximum *(continued)*
slope, m.
target absorbed dose, m.
tolerated dose (MTD)
Maxwell's ring
Mayer's
position, M.
view, M.
Mays vein
Mazer stent
Mb (brain metastases)
MBq (megabecquerel)
MCB Reagents
mcg (microgram)
mCi (millicurie)
mCid (millicurie days)
mCih (millicurie hours)
McGregor's line
3 M Company
McKesson mouth prop
McLeod's syndrome
MCP (metacarpophalangeal) joint
mcU (microunit)
McWhirter's method
Md (mendelevium)
MDA (minimum detectable activity)
MDF (multiple daily fractionation)
MDP (99mTc-methylene-diphosphonate)
meal
barium m.
fatty m.
mean
arterial pressure, m.
ionization, m.
latency period, m.
life, m.
pulmonary artery pressure, m.

mean *(continued)*
pulmonary wedge pressure, m.
sac size, m.
standard deviation of the m.
stopping power, m.
meatal stenosis
meatometer
meatorrhaphy
meatoscope
meatoscopy
meatotome
meatotomy
meatus
acoustic m.
auditory m.
external acoustic m.
internal acoustic m.
nose, m. of
urethral m.
urinarius m.
urinary m.
MEC (multiplicative expanding cell compartment)
mechanical
implant, m.
isocenter, m.
scanning, m.
mechanism
body temperature m.
deglutition m.
quadriceps m.
sphincter m.
swallowing m.
Meckel's
band, M.
cartilage, M.
diverticulum, M.
ganglion, M.
meconium
aspiration, m.

Additional Entries

meconium *(continued)*
cyst, m.
ileus, m.
peritonitis, m.
plug, m.
staining, m.
stool, m.
media
acute otitis m.
adhesive otitis m.
tunica m.
mediad
medial
collateral ligament, m.
compartment, m.
cuneiform, m.
deviation, m.
femoral condyle, m.
fibroplasia, m.
geniculate body, m.
inferior genicular artery, m.
joint space, m. (MJS)
lemniscus, m.
longitudinal fasciculus, m.
malleolus, m.
meniscus, m.
palatine, m.
superior genicular artery, m.
tarsal arteries, m.
wall of nasal cavity, m.
medialis
medially rotated
median
antebrachial vein, m.
basilic vein, m.
cleft face, m.
nerve, m.
olfactory gyrus, m.
olfactory stria, m.

median *(continued)*
plane, m.
raphe, m.
sagittal plane (MSP), m.
sulcus, m.
target absorbed dose, m.
mediastinal
adenopathy, m.
arteries, m.
lymphadenopathy, m.
lymph nodes, m.
lymphoma, m.
mass, m.
node, m.
pleura, m.
shift, m.
structures. m.
widening, m.
mediastinitus
mediastinography
mediastinogram
mediastinopericarditis
mediastinoscope
mediastinoscopic
mediastinoscopy
mediastinotomy
mediastinum
widening of superior m.
medicine
cup, m.
glass, m.
medifrontal
gyre, m.
Medin's disease
mediolateral
episiotomy, m.
oblique view, m.
projection, m.
view, m.
medionecrosis
aorta, m. of
mediotarsal

Additional Entries

Mediport
Medi-Tech catheter
Medi-Tech, Inc.
mediscalenus
medium
bore catheter, m.
contrast m.
culture m.
dispersion m.
fine metal file, m.
opaque m.
radiopaque m.
voltage x-rays, m.
Medrad Mark II injector
Medrad Mark III injector
Medrad Mark IV oscilloscope module
Medrad Mark IV injector
Medrad Mark V injector
Medrad, Inc.
medulla
adrenal m.
anterior district of m. oblongata
arcuate fibers of m. oblongata
central canal of spinalis m.
columns of spinalis m.
fissures and sulci of m. oblongata
fissures of spinalis m.
gray commissures of spinalis m.
gray substance of m. oblongata
lateral district of m. oblongata
lateral district of m. oblongata
meninges of m. spinalis
nephrica, m.

medulla *(continued)*
oblongata m.
ossium, m.
posterior column of m. spinalis
posterior district of m. oblongata
pyramid of m. oblongata
restiform bodies of m. oblongata
spinalis, m.
substance of m. spinalis
sulci of m. spinalis
spinalis, m.
thymus, m. of
veins of spinalis m.
white commissure of m. spinalis
medullae
medullary
artery, m.
bone graft, m.
canal, m.
carcinoma, m.
cystic kidney, m.
lamina, m.
membrane, m.
nail, m.
portion of suprarenal gland, m.
pyramids, m.
rays, m.
segments of nerves, m.
sheath of nerve fibers, m.
spaces of bone, m.
sponge kidney, m.
stenosis, m.
substance of kidney, m.
velum, m.
medulated nerve fibers
medullectomy

Additional Entries

medulloadrenal
medulloarthritis
medulloblast
medulloblastoma
medulloepithelioma
megabecquerel (MBq)
megabladder
megacalycosis
megacardia
megacecum
megacisterna magna
megacolon
 acquired m.
 congenital m.
 idiopathic m.
 toxic m.
megacurie (MCi)
megacycle (Mc)
megahertz (MHz)
megakaryoblast
megakaryocyte
megakaryocytopoiesis
megakaryocytosis
megalencephalon
megaloblast
megaloblastoid
megalobulbus
megalocephaly
megalocornea
megalocyte
megalophthalmos
 anterior m.
megalosyndactyly
megaloureter
megarectum
megasigmoid
megasoma
megasporangium
megaspore
megaunit
megaureter
megavolt
megavoltage
 apparatus, m.
 external beam radiation, m.
 irradiation, m.
 moving strip technique, m.
 photon irradiation, m.
 photon radiation, m.
 radiation, m.
 unit, m.
 x-ray dosimetry, m.
Meglin's point
meglumine
 cation, m.
 diatrizoate, m.
 iothalamate, m.
 medium, m.
 salts, m.
megophthalmos
meibomian
 cyst, m.
 foramen, m.
 gland, m.
 stye, m.
Meige's disease
Meigs'
 capillaries, M.
 syndrome, M.
meiosis
Meissner's
 ganglion, M.
 plexus, M.
 tactile corpuscles, M.
melanin
melanoacanthoma
melanomeloblastoma
melanoblast
melanoblastoma
melanoblastosis
melanocarcinoma
melanocyte

Additional Entries

melanocytic
melanocytoma
melanodermatitis
melanoepithelioma
melanoglossia
melanoleukoderma
melanoma
    cutaneous malignant m.
    juvenile m.
    malignant m.
melanomatosis
melanomatous
melanonychia
melanophage
melanoplakia
melanosarcoma
melanosis
    coli, m.
    sclerae, m.
melanosome
melanotic
    carcinoma, m.
    stool, m.
Meleda disease
melena
membrana
    abdominis, m.
    adventitia, m.
membranaceous
membranae
membrane (s)
    amniotic m.
    arachnoid m.
    artificial rupture of m.
    basement m.
    basilar m.
    Bichat's m.
    Bowman's m.
    Bruch's m.
    Brunn's m.
    cell m.
    chorionic m.
membrane (s) *(continued)*
    cloacal m.
    Corti's m.
    croupou m.
    decidual m.
    Descemet's m.
    diphtheritic m.
    drum m.
    elastic m.
    embryonic m.
    enamel m.
    extraembryonic m.
    false m.
    fenestrated m.
    fetal m.
    fibroelastic m.
    germinal m.
    glomerular m.
    hyaline m.
    hyaloid m.
    Jackson's m.
    keratogenous m.
    limiting m.
    medullary m.
    mucous m.
    nictitating m.
    nuclear m.
    olfactory m.
    ovular m.
    perforated tympanic m.
    peridental m.
    periodontal m.
    placental m.
    plasma m.
    premature rupture of m.
    prolonged rupture of m.
    pupillary m.
    Reissner's m.
    reticular m.
    rupture of m.
    Ruysch's m.
    ruyschian mm.

Additional Entries

membrane (s) *(continued)*
- Scarpa's m.
- schneiderian m.
- serous m.
- Shrapnell's m.
- spontaneous rupture of m.
- striated m.
- synaptic m.
- synovial m.
- tectorial m.
- tympanic (TM) m.
- Zinn's m.

membranectomy
membraniform
membranocartilaginous
membranolysis
membranous
- cochlea, m.
- cranium, m.
- glomerulonephritis, m.
- labyrinth, m.
- portion of urethra, m.
- semicircular canals, m.
- subaortic stenosis, m.
- urethra, m.
- vertebral column, m.

mendelevium (Md)
mendosal suture
Menetrier's disease
Mengert's index
Menghini needle
Meniere's disease
meningeal
- accessory artery, m.
- anterior artery, m.
- artery, m.
- hemorrhage, m.
- inflammation, m.
- irritation, m.
- middle artery, m.
- posterior artery, m.

meningematoma
meningeocortical
meningeorrhaphy
meninges
meninghematoma
meningioma
meningiomatosis
meningitic
meningitis
- acute m.
- aseptic m.
- bacterial m.
- basilar m.
- cerebral m.
- meningococcal m.
- occlusive m.
- ossificans, m.
- otitic m.
- pyogenic m.
- septicemia m.
- serous m.
- spinal m.
- sterile m.
- tubercular m.
- viral m.

meningoarteritis
meningoblastoma
meningocele
meningococcemia
meningococci
meningococcidal
meningococcin
meningococcosis
meningococcus
meningocortical
meningocyte
meningoencephalitis
meningoencephalocele
meningoencephalomyelitis
meningoencephalomyelopathy
meningoencephalopathy

Additional Entries

meningofibroblastoma
meningogenic
meningomalacia
meningomyelitis
meningomyelocele
meningomyeloencephalitis
meningomyeloradiculitis
meningo-osteophlebitis
meningopathy
meningopneumonitis
meningoradicular
meningoradiculitis
meningorrhagia
meningorrhea
meningovascular
meniscal
    cyst, m.
    degeneration, m.
    tear, m.
meniscectomy
menisci
meniscitis
meniscocyte
meniscocytosis
meniscosynovial
meniscus
    bucket handle tear of m.
    detachment of medial m.
    dislocated medial m.
    lateral m.
    medial m.
    posterior horn of medial m.
    torn m.
Menkes syndrome
mensuration technique
mentoanterior
mentolabial
mentoplasty
mentoposterior
mentotransverse
mEq. (milliequivalent)
meralgia
    paresthetica, m.
Mercier's catheter
mercury (Hg.)
    203 chlormerodin, m.
meridian
meridianus
meridional
merisoprol acetate Hg 197
merisoprol acetate Hg 203
merisoprol Hg 197
Merkel
    cells, M.
    muscle, M.
    Ranvier cells, M.
    tactile disks of M.
Merseburg triad
Merzbacher-Pelizaeus disease
mesad
mesangial
mesangiocapillary
mesangium
mesaortitis
mesarteritis
mesectoderm
mesencephalitis
mesencephalohypophyseal
mesencephalon
mesencephalotomy
mesenchyma
mesenchymal
    anlage, m.
mesenchyme
mesenchymoma
mesenterectomy
mesenteric
    adenitis, m.
    cyst, m.
    ischemia, m.
    lymphadenitis, m.
mesenteriole of vermiform process

Additional Entries

mesenteriolum
mesenteriopexy
mesenteriorrhaphy
mesenteritis
mesenterium
mesentery
    root, m.
mesentoderm
mesiad
mesial
    occlusion, m.
    surface, m.
mesially
mesiobuccal
mesiobucco-occlusal
mesiobuccopulpal
mesiocervical
mesioclination
mesioclusion
mesiodistal
mesiogingival
mesioincisodistal
mesiolabial
mesiolabioincisal
mesiolingual
mesiolinguoincisal
mesiolinguo-occlusal
mesiolinguopulpal
mesio-occlusal
mesio-occlusodistal
mesiopulpal
mesiopulpolabial
mesiopulpolingual
mesioversion
meso-aortitis
mesoappendicitis
mesoappendix
mesoatrial
mesobacterium
mesoblast
mesoblastema
mesoblastic
mesobronchitis
mesocardia
mesocardium
mesocaval
mesocecum
mesocele
mesocephalic
mesochondrium
mesochoroidea
mesocolic
    lymph nodes, m.
mesocolon
    ascending m.
    descending m.
    transverse m.
    sigmoid m.
mesocolopexy
mesocoloplication
mesocornea
mesocranic
mesocuneiform
mesocyst
mesocytoma
mesoderm
mesodermal
mesodermopath
mesoduodenal
mesoduodenum
mesoepididymis
mesoesophagus
mesogastrium
mesoglea
mesoglia
mesoglioma
mesogluteal
mesogluteus
mesognathous
mesoileum
mesojejunum
mesomelic dwarfism
mesomere
mesomeric

Additional Entries

mesometrium
mesonasal
mesonephric
mesonephroma
mesonephros
meso-omentum
mesophile
mesophilic
mesophlebitis
mesophragma
mesorchium
mesorectum
mesoretina
mesosalpinx
mesosigmoid
mesosigmoidopexy
mesosoma
mesosome
mesosternum
mesostroma
mesosystolic
mesotarsal
mesotendineum
mesothelioma
mesothelium
mesothenar
mesothorium
mesotropic
mesotympanum
mesovarium
metabolic trapping
metacarpal
- arteries, m.
- bones, m.
- head, m.
- neck of m.

metacarpectomy
metacarpophalangeal
- articulations, m.
- joint, m. (MCP)

metacarpus
metachromatic leukodystrophy
metagastrula
metal fatigue fracture
metallic
- button, m.
- clip, m.
- density, m.
- electrodes, m.
- femoral component, m.
- foreign body, m.
- inserter, m.
- long screw, m.
- sound, m.
- stylet, m.

metalloscopy
metaphyseal
- dysplasia, m.
- fracture, m.
- lesion, m.

metaphyses
metaphysis (pl. metaphyses)
metaphysitis
metaplasia
- myeloid m.
- patchy m.
- squamous m.

metaplasm
metaplastic
metaplexus
metaraminol
metastable
metastases (sg. metastasis)
- advanced m.
- axillary m.
- bone m.
- brain m.
- chest wall m.
- distant m.
- generalized m.
- liver m.

Additional Entries

metastases *(continued)*
    local m.
    lung m.
    lymphangitic m.
    osseous m.
    pelvic m.
    pleural m.
    pulmonary m.
    skeletal m.
    widespread m.
metastasis (pl. metastases)
metastasize
metastatic
    adenocarcinoma, m.
    bone lesion, m.
    calcification, m.
    disease, m.
    foci, m.
    implants, m.
    involvement, m.
    lesion, m.
    node, m.
    nodule, m.
    site, m.
    spread, m.
metasternum
metasynapsis
metasyncrisis
metatarsal
    artery, m.
    bone, m.
    cuneiform joint, m.
    head, m.
    osteotomy, m.
    vein, m.
metatarsophalangeal
    articulation, m.
    joint, m. (MPJ)
metathalamus
metatrophic dworfism
metencephalon
metencephalospinal
meter (m)
methacrylate
    methyl m.
methiodal sodium
methylglucamine compound
methylglucamine diatrizoate
methyl methacrylate
methylene blue
methoxsalen
methysergide effect
meticulous radiation protection
metoclopramide
metopic
    suture, m.
metopism
metopopagus
metoposcopy
metralgia
metrectomy
metriocephalic
metritis
metrizamide
    CT cisternogram, m.
    enhanced CT study, m.
    myelography, m.
metrizoate
    sodium, m.
metrocarcinoma
metrocele
metrocolpocele
metrocystosis
metrocyte
metrodynia
metroendometritis
metrofibroma
metroleukorrhea
metrolymphangitis
metromalacia
metromenorrhagia

Additional Entries ______________________

____

____

metronoscope
metroparalysis
metropathia
hemorrhagica, m.
metropathy
metroperitoneal
metroperitonitis
metrophlebitis
metroplasty
metroptosis
metrorrhagia
metrorrhea
metrorrhexis
metrosalpingitis
metrosalpingography
metrostasis
metrostaxis
metrostenosis
metrotherapy
metrotoxin
metyrapone tartrate
MeV (megaelectron volt)
MeV electron beam
MeV photon
25–MeV single x-ray beam
4–MeV Varian accelerator
Meyer's
disease, M.
organ, M.
Meynert's
bundle, M.
fasciculus retroflexus, M.
fountain decussation, M.
nodes, M.
Meynet's nodes
MF tumeurs d'emblee
mf (microfarad)
mg. (milligram)
Mg (magnesium)
MG (multigate) Doppler flow imaging
mgh (milligram hours)
Mh (hepatic metastases)
mHg. (millimeters of mercury)
mHz. (megahertz)
Mick applicator
micrangium
micrencephalon
micrencephalous
micrencephaly
microabscess
microadenoma
microadenopathy
microaerophile
microaerophilic
microaerotonometer
microaggregate
microaleuriospore
microammeter
microanalysis
microanastomosis
microanatomy
microaneurysm
microangiopathic
microangiopathy
diabetic m.
thrombotic m.
microbacterium
microblast
microcalcification
microcalix
microcardia
microcentrum
microcephalic
microcephalus
microcephaly
microcinematography
microcirculation
microcolloid
microcolon
microcolony
microconidia

Additional Entries ____________________

microconidium
microcoria
microcornea
microcoulomb
microcrania
microcrith
microcrystal
microcurie
microcurie-hour
microcyst
microcystometer
microcytase
microcyte
microcythemia
microcytotoxicity
microdactyly
microdensitometer
microdermatome
microdetermination
microdissection
microdosage
microdose
microembolus
microenvironment
microfarad (mf)
microfibrillar collagen
microfilament
microfilaremia
microfilaria
microfilm
microgastria
microgenesis
microgenia
microglia
microgliocyte
microglioma
microgliomatosis
microglobulin
microgram (mcg)
micrograph
    electron m.
micrography
microgyria
microinfarct
microinjector
microinvasion
microinvasive
microkinematography
microliter
microlith
microlithiasis
    pulmonary alveolar m.
microlymphoidocyte
micromandible
micromanipulation
micromanipulator
micromanometer
micromanometric
micromastia
micromaxilla
micromegalopsia
micromelia
micromelus
micromere
micrometastasis
micrometer
    diffraction m.
    eyepiece m.
    filar m.
    ocular m.
    stage m.
micrometry
micromicrocurie
micromicrogram
micromicron
micromilligram
micromillimeter
micromolecular
micromyelia
micromyeloblast
micromyelolymphocyte
micron
microneedle
micronodular

Additional Entries ____

micronormoblast
micronucleus
micronutrient
microorganic
microorganism
microperfusion
microphage
microphakia
microphone
microphonic
microphotograph
microphthalmia
microphthalmos
microphthalmoscope
microphthalmus
micropinocytosis
microplasia
microplating
microplethysmography
micropolariscope
microprecipitation
microprobe
    laser m.
microprojection
microprojector
micropuncture
    peel-away introducer, m.
microradiogram
microrefractometer
microrespirometer
microscope
    acoustic m.
    operating m.
    scanning electron m.
    slit lamp m.
    Zeiss operating m.
microscopic
    agglutination, m.
    anatomy, m.
    diagnosis, m.
    hematuria, m.
    section, m.
microscopy
    electron m.
    fluorescence m.
    light m.
    transmission electron m.
microsecond
microsection
microseme
microslide
microsoma
microsomal
microsomatia
microsome
microsomia
microspectrophotometer
microspectroscope
microsplanchnic
microsplenia
microsplenic
microsporangia
microsporangium
microspore
microstat
microsthenic
microstomia
microstrabismus
microsurgery
microsyringe
microthelia
microthrombosis
microthrombus
microtomy
microtonometer
microtransfusion
microtron
microunit (mU)
microvascular
microvasculature
microvillus
microviscosimeter
microvolt (mV)
microvoltomete

Additional Entries

microwatt (mW)
microwave
    power source, m.
microxycyte
midaortic
midaxilla
midaxillary
    line, m.
midbody
midbrain
midcarpal
midclavicular
    line, m.
midconvexity
middle genicular artery
middlepiece
midfoot
midfrontal
midgut
midjugular lymph nodes
midline
    block, m.
    brain, m. of
    episiotomy, m.
    lethal granuloma, m.
    shift of m. structures
    trachea, m.
midlung
    field, m.
midoccipital
midperiphery
midpiece
midplane
    dose, m.
    depth, m.
midpole
midriff
midsection
midsternum
midstream aortogram
midsystolic click
midtarsal
midtegmentum
midtrimester
    bleeding, m.
migraine
    abdominal m.
    cluster m.
    headache, m.
    ophthalmoplegic m.
migrating intervertebral disk
migratory
    osteoporosis, m.
    pain, m.
    pathway, m.
    polyarthritis, m.
miliaria
    rubra, m.
miliary
    aneurysm, m.
    embolism, m.
    pattern, m.
    plaque, m.
    pneumonia, m.
    sclerosis, m.
    tuberculosis, m.
milk
    alkali syndrome, m.
    calcium bile, m. of
Milkman's fracture
Milkman's syndrome
milky
    ascites, m.
    cataract, m.
    fluid, m.
Miller-Abbott tube (Abbott-Miller)
Miller position
milliammeter
milliampere (mA)
    minutes, m.
    seconds, m.(mAs)
millibar
millicoulomb (mC)

Additional Entries

millicurie (mCi)
millicurie-day (mCi-d)
millicurie-hour (mCi-h)
milliequivalent (mEq.)
milligamma
milligram (mg.)
milligram hours (mgh)
milliinternational unit (mIU)
millijoule
Millikan rays
millilambert
milliliter (ml.)
millimeter (mm.)
millimeters of mercury (mm.Hg.)
millimicrogram (mmg)
millimicron (mu.)
millimole (mmol)
millimole/liter (mmol/l)
millinormal (mN.)
milliosmole (mOsm.)
milliosmoles/liter (mOsm/l)
millipede
milliphot
millirad (mrad)
millirem (mrem)
milliroentgen (mr.)
millisecond (ms)
  CT scan, m.
milliunit (mU.)
millivolt (mV.)
Mills' disease
Milroy's disease
Milton's edema
miniscule
Minamata disease
minicoil
minicolpostat
minification gain
minilaparotomy
minimantle
minimum acceptable distance
minimum detectable activity (MDA)
minimum target absorbed dose
minin
  lamp, m.
  rays, m.
mini-silicone balloon
mini-template
minitraumatic implant
Minkowski-Chauffard syndrome
monochromatic light
Minor's disease
miocardia
miodidymus
miosis
miotic
mirror image branching
miscibility
miscible
mismatch
  single moderate V/Q m.
  single segment V/Q m.
mismatched perfusion scan defect
misonidazole
missing tissue compensator
missile effect
mitosis
mitral
  atresia, m.
  commissurotomy, m.
  configuration, m.
  first sound, m. (M1)
  gradient, m.
  incompetence, m. (MI)
  insufficiency, m. (MI)
  murmur, m.
  orifice, m.
  reflux, m.
  regurgitation, m.

Additional Entries

mitral *(continued)*
 second sound, m. (M2)
 stenosis, m.
 valve, m.
 valve prolapse, m.
 valve prosthesis, m.
mIU (milliinternational unit)
mixed
 abscess, m.
 aphasia, m.
 beam, m.
 cataract, m.
 cellularity, m.
 culture, m.
 density, m.
 enhancement, m.
 flora, m.
 hemorrhoids, m.
 phase, m.
 situs, m.
mixing bowl effect
MJS (medial joint space)
ml. (milliliter)
MLS (multiparameter light-scattering device)
mm. (millimeter)
mm.Hg. (millimeters of mercury)
M-mode display
M-mode echocardiography
mmol (millimole)
mmol/l (millimoles per liter)
Mn (manganese)
Mo (molybdenum)
 Mo-99
mobile
 echogenic foci, m.
 tongue implant, m.
mobilization
 stapes, m. of
mobilometer
Mobin-Uddin umbrella filter
mode
 A m.
 B m.
 blink m.
 multiplanar m.
moderator
 band, m.
modified
 anteroposterior vies, m.
 lateral projection, m.
modiolus of cochlea
Moeller's glossitis
Moeller-Barlow disease
Mohrenheim's fossa
Mohs' chemosurgery
moiety
moist desquamation
molar
 glands, m.
 teeth, m.
mold
molded polypropylene syringe
molding
mole
 hairy m.
 hydatidiform m.
 pigmented m.
 vesicular m.
molecular
 layer of cortex, m.
molecule
Moll's glands
Molnar disc
molybdenosis
molybdenum (Mo)
Monakow
 rubrospinal fasciculus of M.
 syndrome, M.
monarthric
monarthritis

Additional Entries ______________________

monathetosis
monaural
    hearing loss, m.
Monckeberg's arteriosclerosis
Mondor's disease
Monel cups
monitor
    apnea m.
    cardiac m.
    fetal heart m.
    Holter m.
    telemetry m.
    video m.
monoanesthesia
monoarthritis
monoblastoma
monochromatism
    cone m.
    rod m.
monocular
    diplopia, m.
    dressing, m.
    microscope, m.
    vision, m.
monocyte
monocytic
    leukemia, m.
monocytopenia
monodermoma
monoenergetic
    beam, m.
    photons, m.
    x-rays, m.
monoexponential
monofilament
    suture, m.
    wire, m.
monofilm
monoganglial
monogastric
monograph
monolocular
monomaxillary
monometallic
monomorphic
monomorphous
mononeural
mononuclear phagocyte system
mononucleosis
    cytomegalovirus m.
    infectious m.
monoparesis
monoparesthesia
monopathy
monoplast
monoplegia
monoplegic
monopodia
monopodial
monorchidic
monorchism
monospasm
monospecific
monostratal
monostratified
monozygotic twins
Monro's
    bursa, M.
    foramen, M.
Monte Carlo technique
mons
    pubis, m.
    ureteris, m.
    veneris, m.
Monteggia's
    dislocation, M.
    fracture, M.
    fracture-dislocation, M.
Montgomery
    follicles, M.
    glands, M.
    tubercles, M.
monticulus

Additional Entries

monticulus *(continued)*
cerebelli, m.
moon
face, m.
facies, m.
Mooren's ulcer
Moore's fracture
Morand's
foramen, M.
spur, M.
Morax-Axenfeld conjunctivitis
morbus
coxae senilis, m.
moniliformis, m.
morcellation
Morel-Kraepelin disease
Morgagni's
appendix, M.
fossa, M.
hydatid, M.
rectal columns, M.
sinus, M.
morgagnian cyst
moribund
Morison's
pouch, M.
space, M.
morphogenesis
morphogenetic
morphography
morphology
morphometric measurements
morphometry
Morquio syndrome
Morquio-Ullrich disease
mortise
ankle m.
Morton's disease
morula
morular
morulation
moruloid
mOsm.(milliosmol)
mosquito forceps
Moss'
classification, M.
fibers, M.
Mousseau-Barbin tube
moth-eaten pattern
motility
esophageal m.
motion
arthrography, m.
blurring, m.
imaging (M-mode), m.
modulation, m. (M-mode)
peristaltic m.
pill rolling m.
range of m.
study, m.
motoneuron
lower m.
peripheral m.
upper m.
motor
activity, m.
ataxia, m.
behavior, m.
cell, m.
conduction studies, m.
end-plates, m.
nerve, m.
neuron, m.
tract, m.
unit, m.
unusual m. activity
mottled
mottling
extremities, m. of
mouse
joint m.
peritoneal m.

Additional Entries

mouth
bath, m.
gag, m.
movable core spring guide
movement
ameboid m.
artifact m.
associated m.
athetoid m.
bronian m.
choreiform m.
dystonic m.
peristaltic m.
rapid m.
saccadic eye m.
vermicular m.
moving
field, m.
strip therapy, m.
Moya-Moya disease
MP (metacarpophalangeal/ metatarsophalangeal)
MPC (maximum permissible concentration)
MPD (maximum permissible dose)
MPDE (maximum permissible dose equivalent)
mrad. (millirad)
MR (magnetic resonance)
angiography, MR
enhanced Gd-DTPA, MR
mrem (millirem)
MRI (magnetic resonance imaging)
MRS (magnetic resonance spectroscopy)
Ms (skin metastases)
msec. (millisecond)
MSP (median sagittal plane)
MTD (maximum tolerated dose)
MTF (modulation transfer function)
MTP (metatarsophalangeal joint)
mU. (milliunit)
muciform
mucigen
mucigenous
mucilaginous
mucin
mucinoid
mucinosis
mucinous
carcinoma, m.
tumor, m.
mucocartilage
mucocele
mucoclasis
mucocolitis
mucocolpos
mucocutaneous
hemorrhoid, m.
junction, m.
mucocyte
mucoderm
mucoenteritis
mucoepidermoid
mucofibrous
mucoflocculent
mucoglobulin
mucoid
impaction, m.
mucolipid
mucolipidosis
mucolytic
mucomembranous
mucoperichondrium
mucoperiosteal
flap, m.

Additional Entries

mucoperiosteum
mucopolysaccharide
mucopurulent
    discharge, m.
    drainage, m.
    exudate, m.
    sputum, m.
mucosa
mucosal
    atrophy, m.
    coarsening, m.
    cuff, m.
    erosions, m.
    fold, m.
    gastric m. erosions
    ischemia, m.
    pattern, m.
    thickening, m.
mucosanguineous
mucoserous
mucosin
mucositis
mucosocutaneous
mucous
    membrane, m.
    plug, m.
    threads, m.
mucoviscidosis
mucus
MUGA (multiple gated acquisition) scan
    nitro MUGA
    stress MUGA
mulberry-like mass
Muller's
    capsule, M.
    maneuver, M.
    muscle, M.
mullerian
    duct, m.
    eminence, m.
mullerian *(continued)*
    tumor, m.
mullerianoma
multangular
multangulum
    majus, m.
    minus, m.
multiallelic
multiarticular
multibacillary
multicapsular
multicell
multicellular
multicellularity
multicentric
    hepatoma, m.
    tumor, m.
multicontaminated
multicrystal
    camera, m.
    ring detector system, m.
    scanner, m.
multicuspid
    teeth, m.
multicuspidate
multicystic
    disease, m.
    dysplastic kidney, m.
    kidney, m.
multidentate
multi-echo imaging
multi-exposure limit
multifid
multifidus muscle
multifield technique
multifocal
    form, m.
    leukoencephalopathy, m.
    type, m.
multiform
    display, m.

Additional Entries

multiform *(continued)*
imaging device, m.
multiforme
erythema, m.
multiganglionic
multigated
multigravida
multihole collimator
multi-infarct dementia
multilobar
multilobular
multilocular
multiloculated
cyst, m.
multinodular
goiter, m.
thyroiditis, m.
multiparameter light-scattering device (MLS)
multiplanar
multiplane
electrodes, m.
tomographic scanner, m.
multiple
coarctation, m.
coin lesions, m.
daily fractionation (MDF), m.
endocrine adenomata syndrome, m.
enhancing lesions, m.
epiphyseal dysplasia, m.
fields, m.
gated acquisition (MUGA) scan, m.
line scanning method, m.
myeloma, m.
niches, m.
phase bone imaging, m.
plane imaging, m.

multiple *(continued)*
sclerosis, m.
segmental perfusion, m.
sensitive point method, m.
spike complex, m.
unilateral mass effect, m.
multiplicative expanding cell compartment (MEC)
multipolar
multirooted
multisection tomography
multislice
imaging, m.
spin echo technique, m.
multitarget inactivation
multiterminal
multivaned collimator
multivessel disease
multi-view splenic scintigraphy
Mu mesons
Munchmeyer's disease
Munk's disease
Munro-Richter line
Munro's point
mural
aneurysm, m.
mass, m.
thrombus, m.
murmur
aneurysmal m.
aortic m.
apical m.
arterial m.
blowing m.
cardiac m.
cooing m.
crescendo m.
diastolic m.
dissection, m.

Additional Entries

murmur *(continued)*
- ejection m.
- end-diastolic m.
- end-systolic m.
- friction m.
- functional m.
- harsh m.
- holosystolic m.
- mitral m.
- musical m.
- organic m.
- pansystolic m.
- pericardial m.
- prediastolic m.
- pulmonic m.
- systolic m.
- thrombus, m.
- vascular m.
- venous m.
- vesicular m.

Murphy's sign

Murri's disease

muscle (s)
- abductor (of great toe) m.
- abductor (of little finger) m.
- abductor (of little toe) m.
- abductor (of thumb) m.
- adductor (great) m.
- adductor (long) m.
- adductor (short), m.
- adductor (smallest) m.
- adductor (of great toe) m.
- adductor (of thumb) m.
- Aeby's m.
- agonistic m.
- Albinus' m.
- anconeus m.
- anconeus (lateral) m.

muscle (s) *(continued)*
- anconeus (medial) m.
- anconeus (short) m.
- antagonistic m.
- antigravity m.
- appendicular m's.
- arrector (of hair) m's.
- articular m.
- articular (of elbow) m.
- articular (of knee) m.
- aryepiglottic m.
- arytenoid (oblique) m.
- arytenoid (transverse) m.
- auricular (anterior) m.
- auricular (posterior) m.
- auricular (superior) m.
- Bell's m.
- biceps (of arm) m.
- biceps (of thigh) m.
- bipennate m.
- Bowman's m.
- brachial m.
- brachioradial m.
- bronchoesophageal m.
- Brucke's m.
- buccinator m.
- buccopharyngeal m.
- bulbocavernous m.
- caninc m.
- cardiac m.
- Casser's m.
- casserian m.
- ceratocricoid m.
- ceratopharyngeal m.
- Chassaignac's axillary m.
- choncroglossus m.
- chondropharyngeal m.
- ciliary m.
- coccygeal m's.
- compressor (of naris) m.
- congenerous m's.

Additional Entries

muscle (s) *(continued)*
constrictor of pharynx m.
coracobrachial m.
Crampton's m.
cremaster m.
cricoarytenoid (lateral) m.
cricoarytenoid (posterior) m.
cricopharyngeal m.
cricothyroid m.
cutaneous m.
dartos (of scrotum)
deltoid m.
depressor (superciliary) m.
depressor (of angle of mouth) m.
depressor (of lower lip) m.
depressor (of septum of nose) m.
detrusor m.
diaphragmatic m.
digastric m.
dilator m.
dilator (of pupil) m.
emergency m's.
epicranial m.
epimeric m.
epitrochleoanconeus m.
erector (of penis) m.
erector (of spine) m.
eustachian m.
extensor(of digits common) m.
extensor (of fingers) m.
extensor (of fifth digit proper) m.
extensor (of great toe, long) m.

muscle (s) *(continued)*
extensor (of great toe, short) m.
extensor (of index finger) m.
extemsor (of thumb, long) m.
extensor (of toes, long) m.
extensor (of toes, short) m.
extraocular m's.
extrinsic m.
femoral m.
fibular (long) m.
fibular (short) m.
fibular (third) m.
fixation m's.
fixator m's.
fixator (of base of stapes) m.
flexor (accessory) m.
flexor (of fingers) m.
flexor (of great toe) m.
flexor (of little finger) m.
flexor (of little toe) m.
flexor (of thumb) m.
flexor (of toes) m.
Folius' m.
frontal m.
fusiform m.
gastrocnemius m.
gastrocnemius (lateral) m.
gastrocnemius (medial) m.
Gavard's m.
gemellus (inferior)
gemellus (superior)
genioglossus m.
geniohyoid m.

Additional Entries ______________________________

____

____

muscle (s) *(continued)*
glossopalatine m.
glossopharyngeal m.
gluteal (lease) m.
gracilis m.
Guthrie's m.
hamstring m's.
Hilton's m.
Horner's m.
Houston's m.
hyoglossal m.
hyoglossus m.
hypaxial m's.
hypomeric m.
iliac m.
iliococcygeal m.
iliocostal m's.
iliopsoas m.
incisive (of inferior lip) m.
incisive (of lower lip) m.
incisive (of superior lip) m.
incisive (of upper lip) m.
infrahyoid m's.
infraspinous m.
inspiratory m's.
intercostal (external) m.
intercosal (innermost) m.
intercostal (internal) m.
interfoveolar m.
interosseous (of foot) m's.
interosseous (of hand) m's.
interosseous (palmar) m's.
interosseous (plantar) m's.
interosseous (volar) m's.
interspinal m's.

muscle (s) *(continued)*
interspinal (of thorax) m.
intertransverse m's.
intertransverse (anterior) m.
intertransverse (of neck) m.
intertransverse (of thorax) m.
intraauricular m's.
intraocular m's.
intrinsic m.
involuntary m.
iridic m's.
ischiocavernous m.
Jarjavay's m.
Jung's m.
Koyter's m.
Landstrom's m.
Langer's m.
latissimus dorsi m.
levator (of angle of mouth) m.
levator ani m.
levator (of prostate) m.
levator (of ribs) m.
levator (of scapula) m.
levator (of thyroid gland) m.
levator (of upper eyelid) m.
levator (of upper lip and ala of nose) m.
levator (of velum palatini) m.
longissimus m.
longissimus (of back) m.
longissimus (of head) m.
longissimus (of neck) m.
longissimus (of thorax) m.

Additional Entries

muscle (s) *(continued)*
longissimus (of tongue) m.
lumbrical (of foot) m.
lumbrical (of hand) m.
Luschka's m's.
masseter m.
Merkel's m.
mesothenar m.
Muller's m.
multifidus m's.
mylohyoid m.
mylopharyngeal m.
nasal m.
nonstriated m.
oblique (of abdomen) m.
oblique (of auricle) m.
oblique (of eyeball) m.
obturator (external) m.
obturator (internal) m.
occipital m.
occipitofrontal m.
Ochsner's m.
ocular m's.
Oddi's m.
of antitragus, m's.
of auditory ossicles, m's.
of eye, m's.
of fauces, m's.
of hyoid bone, m's.
of palate and fauces, m's.
of tragus, m.
of Treitz, m.
of uvula, m.
omohyoid m.
opposing (of little finger) m.
opposing (of thumb) m.
orbicular m.
orbicular (of eye) m.

muscle (s) *(continued)*
orbicular (of mouth) m.
orbital m.
organic m.
palatoglossus m.
palatopharyngeal m.
palmar (long) m.
palmar (short) m.
papillary m's.
papillary (of left ventricle) m.
papillary (of right ventricle) m.
papillary (of right ventricle, septal) m.
pectinate m's.
pectineal m.
pectoral (greater) m.
pectoral (smaller) m.
penniform m.
perineum, m's. of
peroneal (long) m.
peroneal (short) m.
peroneal (third) m.
pharyngopalatine m.
Phillips' m.
piriform m.
plantar m.
platysma m.
pleuroesophageal m.
popliteal m.
postaxial m.
preaxial m.
procerus m.
pronator (quadrate) m.
pronator (round) m.
psoas (greater) m.
psoas (smaller) m.
pterygoid (external) m.
pterygoid (internal) m.
pterygoid (lateral) m.

Additional Entries

muscle (s) *(continued)*
pterygoid (medial) m.
pterygopharyngeal m.
pubicoperitoneaal m.
pubococcygeal m.
puboprostatic m.
puborectal m.
pubovaginal m.
pubovesical m.
pyramidal m.
pyramidal (of auricle) m.
quadrate (of lower lip) m.
quadrate (of sole) m.
quadrate (of thigh) m.
quadrate (of upper lip) m.
quadriceps (of thigh) m.
rectococcygeus m.
rectourethral m.
rectouterine m.
rectovesical m.
red m.
Reisseisen's m.
rhomboid (greater) m.
rhomboid (lesser) m.
ribbon m's.
rider's m's.
Riolan's m.
risorius m.
rotator m's.
rotator (long) m.
rotator (short) m.
rotator (of neck) m.
rotator (of thorax) m.
Rouget's m.
Ruysch's m.
sacrococcygeal (anterior) m.
sacrococcygeal (dorsal) m.

muscle (s) *(continued)*
sacrococcygeal (posterior) m.
sacrococcygeal (ventral) m.
sacrospinal m.
salpingopharyngeal m.
Santorini's m.
Santorini's (circular) m.
sartorius m.
scalene (anterior) m.
scalene (middle) m.
scalene (posterior) m.
scalene (smallest) m.
semimembranous m.
semispinal m.
semispinal (of head) m.
semispinal (of neck) m.
semispinal (of thorax) m.
semitendinous m.
serratus (anterior) m.
serratus (posterior) m.
skeletal m's.
slow m.
smooth m.
soleus m.
somatic m's.
sphincter m.
sphincter (of anus) m.
sphincter (of bile duct) m.
sphincter (of hepatopancreatic ampulla) m.
sphincter (of membranous urethra) m.
sphincter (of pupil) m.
sphincter (of pylorus) m.
sphincter (of urinary bladder) m.
spinal m.

Additional Entries

muscle (s) *(continued)*
- splenius (of head) m.
- splenius (of neck) m.
- stapedius m.
- sternal m.
- sternocleidomastoid m.
- sternohyoid m.
- sternohyoid m.
- sternomastoid m.
- sternothyroid m.
- strap m's.
- striated m.
- striped m.
- styloglossus m.
- stylohyoid m.
- stylopharyngeus m.
- subclavis m.
- subcostal m's.
- subscapular m.
- subvertebral m's.
- supinator m.
- suprahyoid m's.
- supraspinous m.
- suspensory (of duodenum) m.
- synergic m's.
- synergistic m's.
- tarsal (inferior) m.
- tarsal (superior) m.
- temporal m.
- temporoparietal m.
- tensor (of fascia lata) m.
- tensor (of tympanic membrane) m.
- tensor (of velum palatini) m.
- teres major m.
- teres minor m.
- thenar m's.
- thyroarytenoid m.
- thyroepiglottic m.
- thyrohyoid m.

muscle (s) *(continued)*
- thyropharyngeal m.
- tibial (anterior) m.
- tibial (posterior) m.
- tonic m.
- tracheal m.
- trachelomastoid m.
- transverse (of abdomen) m.
- transverse (of auricle) m.
- transverse (of chin) m.
- transverse (of nape) m.
- transverse (of perineum) m.
- transverse (of thorax) m.
- transverse (of tongue) m.
- transversospinal m.
- trapezius m.
- triangular m.
- triceps (of arm) m.
- triceps (of calf) m.
- twitch m.
- unipennate m.
- unstriated m.
- vertical (of tongue) m.
- vestigial m.
- visceral m.
- vocal m.
- voluntary m.
- white m.
- Wilson's m.
- yoked m's.
- zygomatic m.
- zygomatic (greater) m.
- zygomatic (lesser) m.

muscular
- dystrophy, m.

musculature
- cervical m.
- lumbar m.

Additional Entries

musculature *(continued)*
paravertebral m.
musculoaponeurotic
musculocutaneous
musculodermic
musculoelastic
musculointestinal
musculomembranous
musculospiral
groove, m.
nerve, m.
musculospiralis
musculotendinous
musculotonic
musculotropic
musculus
abductor digiti minimi manus m.
abductor digit minimi pedis m.
abductor hallucis m.
abductor pollicis brevis m.
abductor pollicis longus m.
accelerator urinae m.
adductor brevis m.
adductor hallucis m.
adductor longus m.
adductor magnus m.
adductor minimus m.
adductor obliquus pollicis m.
adductor pollicis m.
adductor transversus hallucis m.
anconeus m.
antitragicus m.
arrectores pilorum m.
articularis cubiti m.
articularis genu m.
aryepiglotticus m.

musculus *(continued)*
arytenoideus obliquus m.
artenoideus transversus m.
aryvocalis m.
attollens aurem m.
attrahens aurem m.
auricularis anterior m.
auricularis posterior m.
auricularis superior m.
azygos uvulae m.
biceps brachii m.
biceps femoris m.
biceps flexor cruris m.
bipennatus m.
biventer mandibulae m.
brachialis m.
brachioradialis m.
bronchoesophageus m.
buccinator m.
buccopharyngeus m.
bulbocavernosus m.
caninus m.
cephalopharyngeus m.
ceratocricoideus m.
ceratopharyngeus m.
cervicalis ascendens m.
chondroglossus m.
chondropharyngeus m.
ciliaris m.
cleidoepitrochlearis m.
cleidomastoideus m.
cleidooccipitalis m.
coccygeus m.
complexus m.
complexus minor
compressor naris m.
compressor urethrae m.
constrictor pharyngis inferior m.
constrictor pharyngis medius m.

Additional Entries

musculus *(continued)*
- constrictor pharyngis superior m.
- constrictor urethrae m.
- coracobrachialis m.
- corrugator cutis ani m.
- corrugator supercilii m.
- cremaster m.
- cricoarytenoideus lateralis m.
- cricoarytenoideus posterior m.
- cricopharyngeus m.
- cricothyreoideus m.
- crureus m.
- cucullarius m.
- deltoideus m.
- depressor anguloris m.
- depressor labii inferioris m.
- depressor septi nasi m.
- depressor supercilii m.
- depressor urethrae m.
- detrusor urinae m.
- diaphragma m.
- digastricus (digastric) m.
- dilator naris m.
- dilator pupillae m.
- ejaculator seminis m.
- epicranius m.
- epitrochleoanconeus m.
- erector clitoridis m.
- erector penis m.
- erector spinae m.
- extensor brevis pollicis m.
- extensor carpi radialis longus m.
- extensor carpi ulnaris m.
- extensor coccygis m.
- extensor communis digitorum m.
- extensor digiti minimi m.

musculus *(continued)*
- extensor digitorum m.
- extensor digitorum brevis m.
- extensor digitorum brevis manus m.
- extensor digitorum longus m.
- extensor hallucis brevis m.
- extensor hallucis longus m.
- extensor indicis m.
- extensor longus digitorum m.
- extensor longus pollicis m.
- extensor minimi digiti m.
- extensor ossis metacarpi pollicis m.
- extensor pollicis brevis m.
- extensor pollicis longus m.
- flexor accessorius digitorum m.
- flexor brevis digitorum m.
- flexor brevis hallucis m.
- flexor brevis minimi digiti m.
- flexor carpi radialis m.
- flexor carpi ulnaris m.
- flexor digiti minimi brevis m.
- flexor digitorum brevis m.
- flexor digitorum profundus m.
- flexor digitorum superficialis m.
- flexor hallucis brevis m.
- flexor hallucis longus m.

Additional Entries

musculus *(continued)*
flexor longus digitorum m.
flexor longus hallucis m.
flexor longus pollicis m.
flexor pollicis brevis m.
flexor pollicis longus m.
flexor profundus digitorum m.
flexor sublimis digitorum m.
frontalis m.
gastrocnemius m.
gemellus inferior m.
genellus superior m.
genioglossus m.
geniohyoideus m.
glossopalatinus m.
glossopharyngeus m.
gluteus maximus m.
gluteus medius m.
gluteus minimus m.
gracilis m.
helicis major m.
helicis minor m.
hyoglossus m.
hyopharyngeus m.
iliacus m.
iliacus minor m.
iliocapsularis m.
iliococcygeus m.
iliocostalis m.
iliocostalis cervicis m.
iliocostalis dorsi m.
iliocostalis lumborum m.
iliocostalis thoracis m.
iliopsoas m.
incisivus labii inferioris m.
incisivus labii superioris m.
incisurae helicis m.
infracostalis m.

musculus *(continued)*
infraspinatus m.
intercostalis externus m.
intercostalis internus m.
intercostalis intimus m.
interosseus dorsalis manus m.
interosseus dorsalis pedis m.
interosseus palmaris m.
interosseus plantaris m.
interosseus volaris m.
interspinalis m.
intertransversarius m.
ischiocavernosus m.
ischiococcygeus m.
keratopharyngeus m.
laryngopharyngeus m.
latissimus dorsi m.
levator alae nasi m.
levator anguli oris m.
levator anguli scapulae m.
levator ani m.
levator costae m.
levator glandulae thyroideae m.
levator labii inferioris m.
levator labii superioris m.
levator labii superioris alaeque nasi m.
levator palati m.
levator palpebrae superioris m.
levator prostatae m.
levator scapulae m.
levator veli palatini m.
longissimus capitis m.
longissimus cervicis m.
longissimus thoracis m.
longitudinalis dorsi m.
longitudinalis inferior m.

Additional Entries ___

musculus *(continued)*
longitudinalis superior m.
longus capitis m.
longissimus cervicis m.
longissimus thoracis m.
longitudinalis dorsi m.
longitudinalis inferior m.
longitudinalis superior m.
longus capitis m.
longus colli m.
lumbricalis manus m.
lumbricalis pedis m.
masseter m.
mentalis m.
multifidus m.
mylohyoideus m.
mylopharyngeus m.
nasalis m.
obliquus auriculae m.
obliquus capitis inferior m.
obliquus capitis superior m.
obliquus externus abdominis m.
obliquus inferior m.
obliquus internus abdominis m.
obliquus superior m.
obturatorius externus m.
obturatorius internus m.
occipitalis m.
occipitofrontalis m.
omohyoideus m.
opponens digiti minimi m.
opponens digiti quinti m.
opponens minimi digiti m.
opponens pollicis m.

musculus *(continued)*
orbicularis oculi m.
orbicularis oris m.
orbicularis palpebrarum m.
orbitalis m.
orbitopalpebralis m.
palatoglossus m.
palatopharyngeus m.
palatosalpingeus m.
palatostaphylinus m.
palmaris brevis m.
palmaris longus m.
papillaris m.
pectinatus m.
pectineus m.
pectoralis major m.
pectoralis minor m.
peroneocalcaneous m.
peroneus brevis m.
peroneus longus m.
peroneus tertius m.
petropharyngeus m.
petrostaphylinus m.
pharyngopalatinus m.
piriformis m.
plantaris m.
platysma m.
pleuroesophageus m.
popliteus m.
procerus m.
pronator pedis m.
pronator quadratus m.
pronator teres m.
prostaticus m.
psoas major m.
psoas minor m.
pterygoideus externus m.
pterygoideus internus m.
pterygoideus lateralis m.
pterygoideus medialis m.
pterygopharyngeus m.

Additional Entries

musculus *(continued)*
pterygospinosus m.
pubococcygeus m.
puboprostaticus m.
puborectalis m.
pubovesicalis m.
pyramidalis m.
pyramidalis auriculae m.
pyramidalis nasi m.
pyriformis m.
quadratus femoris m.
quadratus labii inferioris m.
quadratus labii superioris m.
quadratus lumborum m.
quadratus menti m.
quadratus plantae m.
quadriceps femoris m.
rectococcygeus m.
rectourethralis m.
rectouterinus m.
rectovesicalis m.
rectus abdominis m.
rectus capitis anterior m.
rectus capitis anticus major m.
rectus capitis lateralis m.
rectus capitis posterior major m.
rectus capitis posterior minor m.
rectus externus m.
rectus femoris m.
rectus inferior m.
rectus internus m.
rectus lateralis m.
rectus medialis m.
rectus superior m.
rectus thoracis m.
retrahens aurem m.
rhomboatloideus m.

musculus *(continued)*
rhomboideus major m.
rhomboideus minor m.
risorius m.
rotatores mm.
rotatores breves mm.
rotatores cervicis mm.
rotatores lumborum mm.
rotatores thoracis mm.
sacrococcygeus anterior m.
sacrococcygeus dorsalis m.
sacrococcygeus posterior m.
sacrococcygeus ventralis m.
sacrolumbalis m.
sacrospinalis m.
salpingopharyngeus m.
sartorius m.
scalenus anterior m.
scalenus medius m.
scalenus minimus m.
scalenus posterior m.
scansorius m.
semimembranosus m.
semispinalis capitis m.
semispinalis cervicis m.
semispinalis colli m.
semispinalis dorsi m.
semispinalis thoracis m.
semitendinosus m.
serratus anterior m.
serratus magnus m.
serratus inferior posterior m.
serratus posterior superior m.
soleus m.
sphenosalpingostaphylinus m.

Additional Entries

musculus *(continued)*
sphincter ampullae hepatopancreaticae m.
sphincter ani externus m.
sphincter ani internus m.
sphincter oris m.
sphincter pupillae m.
sphincter pylori m.
sphincter urethrae m.
sphincter urethrae membranaceae m.
sphincter vaginae m.
sphincter vesicae m.
spinalis capitis m.
spinalis cervicis m.
spinalis colli m.
spinalis dorsi m.
spinalis thoracis m.
splenius capitis m.
splenius cervicis m.
splenius colli m.
stapedius m.
staphylinus externus m.
staphylinus internus m.
staphylinus medius m.
sternalis m.
sternochondroscapularis m.
sternoclavicularis m.
sternocleidomastoideus m.
sternofascialis m.
sternohyoideus m.
sternothyroideus m.
styloauricularis m.
styloglossus m.
stylohyoideus m.
stylolaryngeus m.
stylopharyngeus m.
subclavis m.
subcostalis m.

musculus *(continued)*
subcrureus m.
subscapularis m.
supinator m.
supinator longus m.
supraclavicularis m.
supraspinalis m.
supraspinatus m.
suspensorius duodeni m.
tarsalis inferior m.
tarsalis superior m.
temporalis m.
tensor fasciae latae m.
tensor palati m.
tensor tarsi m.
tensor tympani m.
tensor veli palatini m.
teres major m.
teres minor m.
thyreoarytenoideus m.
thyreoarytenoideus externus m.
thyreoarytenoideus internus m.
thyreoepiglotticus m.
thyreohyoideus m.
thyreopharyngeus m.
tibialis anterior m.
tibialis gracilis m.
tibialis posterior m.
tibialis secundus m.
tibiofascialis anterior m.
trachealis m.
tracheloclavicularis m.
trachelomastoideus m.
tragicus m.
transversalis abdominis m.
transversalis capitis m.
transversalis cervicis m.
transversalis nasi m.
transversospinalis m.

Additional Entries

musculus *(continued)*
transversus abdominis m.
transversus auriculae m.
transversus linguae m.
transversus menti m.
transversus nuchae m.
transversus perinei profundus m.
transversus perinei superficialis m.
transversus thoracis m.
trapezius m.
tiangularis m.
triangularis labii inferioris m.
triangularis labii superioris m.
triangularis sterni m.
triceps brachii m.
triceps surae m.
triticeoglossus m.
uvulae m.
vastus externus m.
vastus intermedius m.
vastus internus m.
vastus lateralis m.
vastus medialis m.
ventricularis m.
verticalis linguae m.
vocalis m.
zygomaticus major m.
zygomaticus minor m.
mushroom worker's lung
Mv (magnetization vector)
Mv. (millivolt)
4–6 MV linear accelerator
M x-rays
Mya's disease
myalgia
myasthenia
gastrica, m.
myasthenia *(continued)*
gravis, m.
gravis pseudoparalytica, m.
neonatal, m.
myasthenic
myatonia
congenita, m.
myatrophy
mycelial
mycelium
mycetogenic
mycetoma
mycoderma
mycodermatitis
mycomyringitis
mycoplasma
mycosis
fungoides, m.
mycotic
aneurysm, m.
endocarditis, m.
phase, m.
myelencephalitis
myelencephalon
myelencephalospinal
myelin
sheath, m.
myelinated
myelinic
myelinization
myelinoclasis
myelinogenetic
myelinolysin
myelinolysis
myelinopathy
myelinosis
myelitic
myelitis
bulbar m.
compression m.
myeloblast

Additional Entries

myeloblastemia
myeloblastic
  leukemia, m.
myeloblastoma
myeloblastomatosis
myeloblastosis
myelocele
myeloclast
myelocoele
myelocone
myelocyst
myelocystic
myelocystomeningocele
myelocyte
myelocythemia
myelocytic
  anemia, m.
  leukemia, m.
myelocytoma
myelocytomatosis
myelocytosis
myelodysplasia
myeloencephalic
myeloencephalitis
  epidemic m.
myelofibrosis
myelofugal
myelogenesis
myelogenous
  leukemia, m.
myelogram
myelography
  cervical m.
  thoracic m.
  lumbar m.
  negative contrast (gas) m.
  positive contrast m.
  water-soluble m.
  pantopaque m.
myelohyoid
  artery, m.

myelohyoid *(continued)*
  groove, m.
  line, m.
  muscle, m.
  muscle, m.
  nerve, m.
myeloid
  erythroid ratio, m.
  leukemia, m.
  metaplasia, m.
myelolipoma
myelolymphangioma
myelolysis
myelolytic
myeloma
  giant cell m.
  malignant m.
  multiple m.
  nephropathy, m.
  osteosclerotic m.
myelomalacia
myelomatoid
myelomatosis
myelomenia
myelomeningitis
myelomeningocele
myelomere
myelomyces
myelon
myeloneuritis
myelonic
myelo-opticoneuropathy
myelopathic
myelopathy
  sclerosing m.
  spondylitic cervical m.
  transverse m.
myelopetal
myelophage
myelophthisis
myeloplast
myeloplegia

Additional Entries

myelopoiesis
myelopore
myeloproliferative
myeloradiculitis
myeloradiculodysplasia
myeloradiculopathy
myelorrhagia
myelosarcoma
myelosarcomatosis
myeloschisis
myeloscintogram
myelosclerosis
myelosis
  erythremic m.
myelospasm
myelospongium
myelosuppressive
myelosyringosis
myelotherapy
myelotome
myelotomy
Mylar portion
myoblast
myoblastic
myoblastoma
  granular cell m.
myobradia
myocardial
  conduction defect, m.
  fibrosis, m.
  focal m. fibrosis
  hypertrophy, m.
  imaging, m.
  infarction, m.
  insufficiency, m.
  ischemia, m.
  necrosis, m.
  perfusion, m.
  revascularization, m.
  rupture, m.
  tear, m.
  thinning, m.
myocardiogram
myocardiograph
myocardiolysis
myocardiopathy
myocardiorrhaphy
myocarditis
  acute bacterial m.
  idiopathic m.
  interstitial m.
  rheumatic m.
  tuberculous m.
myocardium
myocardosis
myocele
myocelialgia
myoclonia
myoclonic
  jerks, m.
myoclonus
myocoele
myocolpitis
myocytolytic degeneration
myocytoma
myodegeneration
myodemia
myodiastasis
Myodil
myodiopter
myodynamometer
myodynia
myodystonia
myodystrophia
myoedema
myoelastic
myoelectric
myoendocarditis
myoepithelial
myoepithelioma
myoepithelium
myofacitis
myofibroblast
myofibroma

Additional Entries ____________

myofibrosis
myofibrositis
myofilament
myogenous
myogram
myography
myoid
myoidism
myokinesimeter
myolipoma
myolysis
myoma
myomagenesis
myomalacia
myomata
  submucous m.
  uteri m.
myomatosis
myomatous
myomectomy
myomelanosis
myometer
myometritis
myometrium
myoneural
myopathy
  centronucleaar m.
  late distal m.
  myotubular m.
  nemaline m.
  ocular m.
myopericarditis
myopia
  axial m.
  indicial m.
  pernicious m,.
  prodromal m.
myopic
  astigmatism, m.
myoplasm
myoplastic
myoplasty
myopolar
myosalpingitis
myosalpinx
myosarcoma
myoscope
myositis
  epidemic m.
  fibrosa m.
  lumbar m.
  multiple m.
  ossificans, m.
  ossificans progressiva, m.
  trichinous m.
myospasia
myospasm
myospasmia
myosteoma
myosthenic
myosthenometer
myostroma
myosuria
myotenositis
myotenotomy
myothermic
myotome
myotomic
myotomy
myotone
myotonia
  atrophica, m.
  congenita, m.
  dystrophica, m.
myotonic
myotonoid
myotonometer
myotonus
myotrophy
myotubule
myovascular
myringectomy
myringitis

Additional Entries

myringitis *(continued)*
 bullous m.
myringomycosis
myringorupture
myringostapediopexy
myringotome
myringotomy
myxadenitis
myxadenoma
myxangitis
myxasthenia
myxedema
 congenital m.
 heart disease, m.
 papular m.
 pituitary m.
 pretibial m.
myxedematoid
myxedematous
myxochondroma
myxochondrosarcoma
myxocystitis
myxocystoma
myxoenchondroma
myxoendothelioma
myxofibroma
myxofibrosarcoma
myxoglioma
myxoglobulosis
myxoid
 cyst, m.
 polypoid mass, m.
myxolipoma
myxoma
 virus, m.
myxomatosis
myxomatous
 degeneration of leaflet, m.
myxomembranous
 colitis, m.
myxomyoma
myxoneurosis
 intestinal m.
myxopapilloma
myxopoiesis
myxosarcoma
myxosarcomatous

Additional Entries

N

N (nitrogen)
N (number of fractions)
nabothian
 cyst, n.
 follicle, n.
 gland, n.
NAD (no appreciable disease)
NaI (sodium iodide)
nail
nailing
 hip n.
 intramedullary n.
nail patella syndrome
12N-ammonia
nanocurie (nCi)
nanogram (ng)
nanoliter (nl)
nanometer (nm)
nanophthalmos
nanosecond (ns./nsec.)
nanounit (nU.)
Na 1 radiation detector
narcoanesthesia
nares
naris
narrow
 beam, n.
 collimation, n.
 geometry, n.
 slitlike cavity, n.
narrowed intervertebral foramen
nasal
 airway obstruction, n.
 aperture, n.
 artery, n.
 bone, n.
 border, n.
 cartilage, n.

nasal *(continued)*
 cavity, n.
 concha, n.
 crest, n.
 duct, n.
 fossa, n.
 laminae, n.
 meatus, n.
 septum, n.
 sinus, n.
nasalis muscle
nasion
Nasmyth's membrane
nasoantral
nasoantritis
nasoantrostomy
nasobronchial
nasociliary
 nerve, n.
nasofrontal
 vein, n.
nasogastric (NG)
 feeding tube, n.
 intubation, n.
 suction, n.
nasograph
nasolabial
 crease, n.
 fold, n.
nasolabialis muscle
nasolacrimal
 canal, n.
 duct, n.
nasomanometer
naso-optic
naso-oral
nasopalatine
 canal, n.
 nerve, n.
 recess, n.

Additional Entries ______________________________

nasopharyngeal
electrode, n.
regurgitation, n.
nasopharyngitis
nasopharyngolaryngoscope
nasopharyngoscope
nasopharyngoscopy
nasopharynx
nasorostral
nasoscope
nasoseptitis
nasosinusitis
nasospinale
nasoturbinal
nasus
externus, n.
natatory ligament
National Council on Radiation Protection and Measurements (NCRP)
navicular
bone, n.
carpal, n.
fossa, n.
tarsal n.
Nb (niobium)
nc. (nanocurie)
NCRP (National Council on Radiation Protection and Measurements)
NCV (nerve conduction velocity)
Nb (niobium)
Nd (neodymium)
Ne (neon)
nebulizer
ultrasonic n.
neck
bladder n.
bladder n. contracture
cervix, n. of
femoral n.
neck *(continued)*
humerus, n. of
surgical n.
triangles of n.
vesical n.
necrobiotic nodule
necrometer
necroscopy
necrosis
acute tubular n.
aseptic n.
avascular n.
bone n.
central n.
cheesy n.
hepatic n.
myocardial n.
Zenker's n.
necrotic
clear cell carcinoma, n.
tumor, n.
necrotizing
enterocolitis, n.
leukoencephalopathy, n.
NED (no evidence of disease)
Nedmac, Inc.
needle inserter
negative contrast agent
negatoscope
negatron decay
Negri bodies
neighboring structure
Neill-Mooser bodies
Nelaton's
catheter, N.
line, N.
neoblastic
neodymium (Nd)
neon (Ne)
neopallium
neopathy

Additional Entries ____________________

neoplasia
neoplasm
neoplastic
  aqueduct stenosis, n.
  cells, n.
  change, n.
  lesion, n.
neothalamus
neovascularity
nephelometer
nephelometry
nephradenoma
nephric
nephridium
nephritic
nephritis
  glomerular n.
  interstitial n.
  lupus n.
  parenchymatous n.
  suppurative n.
  transfusion n.
nephritogenic
nephroabdominal
nephroangiosclerosis
nephrocalcinosis
nephrocapsectomy
nephrocardiac
nephrocele
nephrocolic
nephrocolopexy
nephrocoloptosis
nephrocystanastomosis
nephrocystitis
nephrocystosis
nephroerysipelas
nephrogastirc
nephrogenic
nephrogenous
nephrogram
  prolonged n.
nephrography
nephrohemia
nephrohypertrophy
nehoroid
nephrolith
nephrolithiasis
nephrolithotomy
nephrology
nephrolysis
nephroma
  embryonal n.
nephromalacia
nephromegaly
nephron
  lower n.
nephronophthisis
nephro-omentopexy
nephroparalysis
nephropathy
nephropexy
nephrophagiasis
nephrophthisis
nephropoietic
nephroptosis
nephropyelography
nephropyelolithotomy
nephropyeloplasty
nephropyosis
nephrorosein
nephrorrhagia
nephrorrhaphy
nephrosclerosis
  arteriolar n.
nephroscope
nephrosis
  amyloid n.
  lipid n.
  lower nephron n.
nephrosonephritis
  glomerular n.
  interstitial n.
  lupus n.
  parenchymatous n.

Additional Entries

nephrosonephritis *(cont'd)*
- suppurative n.
- transfusion n.

nephrosonography
nephrosplenopexy
nephrostoma
nephrostomy
- Cope n.
- tube, n.

nephrotic
nephrotome
nephrotomogram
nephrotomography
nephrotomy
nephrotoxic
nephrotoxicity
nephrotoxin
nephrotropic
nephrotuberculosis
nephrotyphoid
nephrotyphus
nephroureterectomy
nephroureterocystectomy
neptunium (Np)
nerve (s)
- abducent n.
- accelerator n's.
- accessory n.
- accessory n,. (spinal)
- accessory n. (vagal)
- acoustic n.
- afferent n.
- alveolar n.
- ampullar n.
- anabolic n.
- Andersch's n.
- anococcygeal n's.
- Arnold's n.
- articular n.
- auditory n.
- auricular n's.
- auricular (of vagus) n.

nerve (s) *(continued)*
- auriculotemporal n.
- autonomic n's.
- axillary n.
- Bell's n.
- Bock's n.
- buccal n.
- buccinator n.
- cardiac n.
- caroticotympanic n's.
- carotid (external) n's.
- carotid (internal) n.
- cavernous (of clitoris) n's.
- cavernous (of penis) n's.
- celiac n's.
- centrifugal n.
- centripetal n.
- cerebral n's.
- cervical n's.
- cervical, descending, n.
- cervical, transverse, n.
- chorda tympani n.
- ciliary n's.
- circumflex n.
- clunial n's.
- coccygeal n.
- cochlear n.
- cranial (II through XII) n's.
- crotaphit ic n.
- cubital n.
- cutaneous n.
- cutaneous (of abdomen) n.
- cutaneous (of arm) n.
- cutaneous (of calf) n.
- cutaneous (of foot) n.
- cutaneous (of forearm) n.
- cutaneous (of thigh) n.
- Cyon's n.

Additional Entries

nerve (s) *(continued)*
- dental inferior n.
- depressor n.
- diaphragmatic n.
- digastric n.
- digital n's.
- digital (of foot) n's.
- digital (of lateral plantar nerve, common) n's.
- digital (of lateral plantar nerve, proper) n's.
- digital (of lateral surface of great toe and of medial surface of second toe, dorsal) n's.
- digital (of medial plantar nerve, common) n's.
- digital (of medial plantar nerve, proper) n's.
- digital of median nerve, palmar, common) n's.
- digital (of median nerve, palmar, proper) n's.
- digital (of radial nerve, dorsal) n's.
- digital (of ulnar nerve, dorsal) n's.
- digital (of ulnar nerve, palmar, collateral) n's.
- digital (of ulnar nerve, palmar, common) n's.
- digital (of ulnar nerve, palmar, proper) n's.
- dorsal (of clitoris) n.
- dorsal (of penis) n.
- dorsal (of scapula) n.
- efferent n.
- eighth n.
- eleventh n.
- esodic n.
- ethmoidal anterior n.

nerve (s) *(continued)*
- ethmoidal posterior n.
- exciter n.
- excitoreflex n.
- exodic n.
- facial n.
- facial, temporal n.
- femoral n.
- fibular (common) n.
- fibular (deep) n.
- fibular (superficial) n.
- fifth n.
- first n's.
- fourth n.
- frontal n.
- furcal n.
- fusimotor n's.
- gangliated n.
- gastric n's.
- genitofemoral n.
- glossopharyngeal n.
- gluteal n.
- hemorrhoidal n's.
- Hering's n.
- hypogastric n.
- hypoglossal n.
- iliohypogastric n.
- ilioinguinal n.
- infraoccipital n.
- infraorbital n.
- infratrochlear n.
- inhibitory n.
- intercostal n's.
- intercostobrachial n's.
- intermediary n.
- intermediate n.
- interosseous (of forearm) n.
- interosseous (of leg) n.
- ischiadic n.
- Jacobson's n.

Additional Entries

nerve (s) *(continued)*
- jugular n.
- labial n's.
- lacrimal n.
- Langley's n's.
- laryngeal (inferior) n.
- laryngeal (recurrent) n.
- laryngeal (superior) n.
- lingual n.
- longitudinal of Lancisi n's.
- lumbar n's.
- lumboinguinal n.
- mandibular n.
- masseteric n.
- maxillary n.
- median n.
- medullated n.
- meningeal n.
- mental n.
- mixed n.
- motor n.
- motor (of tongue) n.
- musculocutaneous n.
- musculocutaneous (of foot) n.
- musculocutaneous (of leg) n.
- musculospiral n.
- myelinated
- mylohyoid n.
- nasociliary n.
- nasopalatine n.
- ninth n.
- nonmedullated n.
- obturator n.
- occipital (greater) n.
- occipital (internal) n.
- occipital (least) n.
- occipital (lesser) n.
- occipital (third) n.

nerve (s) *(continued)*
- oculomotor n.
- of Cotunnius, n.
- of external acoustic meatus, n.
- of Lancisi, n's.
- of Luschka, n.
- of pterygoid canal, n.
- of tensor tympani, n.
- of tensor veli palatini, n.
- of Willis, n.
- olfactory n's.
- ophthalmic n.
- optic n.
- pain n.
- palatine n.
- parasympathetic n.
- parotid n's.
- pectoral n.
- perineal n's.
- peripheral n.
- peroneal n.
- petrosal n.
- phrenic n.
- phrenicoabdominal n's.
- pilomotor n's.
- plantar n.
- pneumogastric n.
- popliteal n.
- presacral n.
- pressor n.
- pterygoid n.
- pterygopalatine n's.
- pudendal n.
- pudic n.
- radial n.
- rectal n's.
- recurrent n.
- recurrent (ophthalmic) n.
- saccular n.

Additional Entries ______________________

nerve (s) *(continued)*
sacral n's.
saphenous n.
Scarpa's n.
sciatic n.
scrotal n's.
second n.
secretory n.
sensory n.
seventh n.
sinus n.
sinu-vertebral n.
sixth n.
somatic n's.
spermatic n.
spinal n's.
splanchnic n's.
splanchnic (greater) n.
splanchnic (inferior) n.
splanchnic (lesser) n.
splanchnic (lower) n.
splanchnic (lumbar) n's.
splanchnic (pelvic) n's.
splanchnic (sacral) n's.
stapedial n.
stapedius n.
stylohyoid n.
stylopharyngeal n.
subclavian n.
subcostal n.
sublingual n.
submaxillary n's.
suboccipital n.
subscapular n's.
sudomotor n's.
supraclavicular n's.
supraorbital n.
suprascapular n.
supratrochlear n.
sural n.
sympathetic n.

nerve (s) *(continued)*
temporal (deep) n's.
temporal (subcutaneous) n's.
tenth n.
terminal n's.
third n.
thoracic n's.
thoracic (long) n.
thoracodorsal n.
tibial n.
T iedemann's n.
tonsillar n's.
transverse (of neck)
trigeminal n.
trochlear n.
trohic n.
twelfth n.
tympanic n.
ulnar n.
unmyelinated n.
utricular n.
utriculoampullar n.
vaginal n's.
vagus n.
vascular n.
vasoconstrictor n.
vasodilator n.
vasomotor n.
vasosensory n.
vertebral n.
vestibular n.
vestibulocochleear n.
vidian n.
vidian (deep) n.
Wrisberg's n.
zygomnatic n.
zygomaticofacial n.
zygomaticotemoral n.
nerve cells
nerve compression, median

Additional Entries

nerve conduction deafness
nerve conduction studies
nerve conduction time
nerve conduction velocity (NCV)
nerve decompression
nerve distribution
nerve endings
nerve entrapment
nerve fasciculi of medulla spinalis
nerve fibers of cerebral cortex
nerve root
nerve root irritation
nerve root rhizotomy
nervous system
  autonomic n.s.
  central n.s.
  parasympathetic n.s.
  peripheral n.s.
  sympathetic n.s.
nervus
  abducens n.
  accessorius n.
  acusticus n.
  alveolaris inferior n.
  alveolares superiores nn.
  ampullaris anterior n.
  ampullaris inferior n.
  ampullaris lateralis n.
  ampullaris posterior n.
  ampullaris superior n.
  anococcygei nn.
  articularis n.
  auriculares anteriores nn.
  auricularis magnus n.
  auricularis posterior n.
  auriculotemporalis n.
  axillaris n.

nervus *(continued)*
  buccalis n.
  buccinatorius n.
  canalis pterygoidei n.
  cardiacus cervicalis inferior n.
  cardiacus cervicalis medius n.
  cardiacus cervicalis superior n.
  cardiacus inferior n.
  cardiacus medius n.
  cardiacus superior n.
  cardiaci thoracici nn.
  caroticotympanici nn.
  caroticotympanicus inferior n.
  caroticotympanicus superior n.
  nervi carotici externi nn.
  caroticus internus n.
  cavernosi clitoridis nn.
  cavernosus clitoridis major n.
  cavernosi clitoridis minores nn.
  cavernosi penis nn.
  cavernosus penis major n.
  cavernosi penis minores nn.
  cerebrales nn.
  cervicales nn.
  ciliares breves nn.
  ciliares longi nn.
  clunium inferiores nn.
  clunium medii nn.
  clunium superiores nn.
  coccygeus n.
  cochleae n.
  craniales nn.

Additional Entries ____________________

nervus *(continued)*
cutaneus n.
cutaneus antebrachii lateralis n.
cutaneus antebrachii medialis n.
cutaneus antebrachii posterior n.
cutaneus antebrachii dorsalis n.
cutaneus brachii lateralis inferior n.
cutaneus brachii lateralis superior n.
cutaneus brachii medialis n.
cutaneus brachii posterior n.
cutaneus colli n.
cutaneus dorsalis intermedius n.
cutaneus dorsalis lateralis pedis n.
cutaneus dorsalis medialis n.
cutaneus femoris lateralis n.
cutaneus femoris posterior n.
cutaneus surae lateralis n.
cutaneus surae medialis n.
digitales dorsales (radialis) nn.
digitales dorsales (ulnaris) nn.
digitales dorsales pedis nn.
digitales palmares communes (mediani) nn.

nervus *(continued)*
digitales palmares communes (ulnaris) nn.
digitales palmares proprii (mediani) nn.
digitales palmares proprii (ulnaris) nn.
digitales plantares communes (plantaris lateralis) nn.
digitales plantares communes (plantaris medialis) nn.
digitales volares communes (mediani) nn.
digitales volares communes (ulnaris) nn.
digitales volares proprii (mediani) nn.
digitales volares proprii (ulnaris) nn.
dorsalis clitoridis n.
dorsalis penis n.
dorsalis scapulae n.
erigentes nn.
ethmoidalis anterior n.
ethmoidalis posterior n.
facialis n.
femoralis n.
fibularis communis n.
fibularis profundus n.
fibularis superficialis n.
frontalis n.
genitofemoralis n.
glossopharyngeus n.
gluteus inferior n.
gluteus superior n.
haemorrhoidales inferiores nn.
haemorrhoidales medii nn.

Additional Entries

nervus *(continued)*
haemorrhoidales superiores nn.
hypogastricus (dexter et sinister) n.
hypoglossus n.
iliohypogastricus n.
ilioinguinalis n.
infraorbitalis n.
infratrochlearis n.
intercostales nn.
intercostobrachiales nn.
intermedius n.
interosseus (antebrachii) anterior n.
interosseus antebrachii posterior n.
interosseus (antebrachii) dorsalis n.
interosseus (antebrachii) volaris n.
interosseus cruris n.
ischiadicus n.
jugularis n.
labiales anteriores nn.
labiales posteriores nn.
lacrimalis n.
laryngeus inferior n.
laryngeus recurrens n.
laryngeus superior n.
lingualis n.
lumbales nn.
lumboinguinalis n.
mandibularis n.
massetericus n.
masticatorius n.
maxillaris n.
meatus acustici externi n.
meatus auditorii externi n.

nervus *(continued)*
medianus n.
meningeus (medius) n.
mentalis n.
musculocutaneus n.
mylohyoideus n.
nasociliaris n.
nasopalatinus n.
obturatorius n.
occipitalis major n.
occipitalis minor n.
occipitalis tertius n.
octavus n.
oculomotorius n.
olfactorii nn.
ophthalmicus n.
opticus n.
palatini nn.
palatinus anterior n.
palatinus major n.
palatinus medius n.
palatini minores nn.
palatinus posterior n.
pectoralis lateralis n.
pectoralis medialis n.
perineales nn.
perinei nn.
peroneus communis n.
peroneus profundus n.
peroneus profundus accessorius n.
peroneus superficialis n.
petrosus major n.
petrosus minor n.
petrosus profundus n.
petrosus superficialis major n.
petrosus superficialis minor n.
phrenicus n.
phrenici accessorii nn.

Additional Entries ____________

nervus *(continued)*
plantaris lateralis n.
plantaris medialis n.
presacralis n.
pterygoideus externus n.
pterygoideus internus n.
pterygoideus lateralis n.
pterygoideus medialis n.
pterygopalatini nn.
pudendus n.
radialis n.
rectales inferiores nn.
recurrens n.
saccularis n.
sacrales nn.
saphenus n.
scrotales anteriores nn.
scrotales posteriores nn.
spermaticus externus n.
sphenopalatini nn.
spinales nn.
spinosus n.
splanchnicus imus n.
splanchnici lumbales nn.
splanchnicus major n.
splanchnicus minor n.
splanchnici pelvini nn.
splanchnici sacrales nn.
stapedius n.
subclavius n.
subcostalis n.
sublingualis n.
suboccipitalis n.
subscapularis n.
supraclaviculares nn.
supraclaviculares anteriores nn.
supraclaviculares laterales (posteriores) nn.
supraclaviculares mediales nn.
supraclaviculares medii nn.

nervus *(continued)*
supraclaviculares posteriores nn.
supraorbitalis n.
suprascapularis n.
supratrochlearis n.
suralis n.
temporales profundi nn.
temporalis profundus anterior n.
temporalis profundus posterior n.
tensoris tympani n.
tensoris veli palatini n.
tentorii n.
terminales nn.
thoracales nn.
thoracales anteriores nn.
thoracales posteriores nn.
thoracalis longus n.
thoracici nn.
thoracicus longus n.
thoracodorsalis n.
tibialis n.
transversus colli n.
trigeminus n.
trochlearis n.
tympanicus n.
ulnaris n.
utricularis n.
utriculoampullaris n.
vaginales nn.
vagus n.
vascularis n.
vertebralis n.
vesicales inferiores plexus pudendi nn.
vesicales inferiores plexus vesicalis nn.
vesicales superiores plexus vesicalis nn.
vestibuli n.

Additional Entries

nervus *(continued)*
 vestibulocochlearis n.
 zygomaticus n.
nervimotion
nervimotor
nervimuscular
nervous system
nesidioblast
nesidioblastoma
nesidioblastosis
net count rate
network
 carpal n.
 malleolar n.
Neubauer's artery
Neufeld nail
neurad
neural
 arch, n.
 canal, n.
 crest, n.
 crest tumor, n.
 folds, n.
 foramina, n.
 foraminal stenosis, n.
 groove, n.
 tube, n.
neuralgia
 facial n.
 geniculate n.
 glossopharyngeal n.
 Hunt's n.
 intercostal n.
 migrainous n.
 Morton's n.
 postherpetic n.
 trigeminal n.
neurenteric
 canal, n.
 cyst, n.
NEURET (neurad equivalent therapy)
neurilemmoma
neuritis
 acoustic n.
 brachial n.
 diabetic n.
 endemic n.
 intersititial n.
 multiple n.
 optic n.
 peripheral n.
 retrobulbar n.
 toxic n.
 traumatic n.
neuroblast
neuroblastoma
neurocanal
neurocardiac
neurocentral
neurocentrum
neurocirculatory
neurocranial
neurocranium
neuroderm
neurofibril
neurofibroma
neurofibromatosis
neurofilament
neurogangliitis
neuroganglion
neurogastirc
neurogenic
 bladder, n.
 shock, n.
neuroglia
neurogliocyte
neurogliocytoma
neuroglioma
neurogliosis
neurogram
neurolemma
neuroma
 acoustic n.
 Morton's n.
neuromalacia

Additional Entries

neuromata
neuromatosis
neuromatous
neuromechanism
neuromeningeal
neuromotor
neuromuscular
  spindles, n.
neuromyasthenia
neuromyelitis
neuromyopathic
neuromyositis
neuron (s)
  afferent n.
  efferent n.
  Golgi n.
  motor n.
  postganglionic n.
  preganglionic n.
  sensory n.
neuronal axonal dystrophy
neuronatrophy
neuronephric
neuronevus
neuronitis
neuroparalysis
neuropathic
  arthritis, n.
  joint, n.
neuropathogenesis
neuropathogenicity
neuropathy
  diabetic n.
  entrapment n.
  peripheral n.
  progressive hypertrophic interstitial n.
neuroplasm
neuroplasty
neuropore
  anterior n.
  posterior n.
neuroradiology
neuroreceptor
neuroretinitis
neuroretinopathy
neurosarcoma
neurosclerosis
neurosegmental
neurosensory
neuroskeletal
neuroskeleton
neurosonography
neurosonology
neurospasm
neurosplanchnic
neurospongium
neurotendinous
  spindles, n.
neurotome
neurotomography
neurotonometer
neurotransducer
neurotransmitter
  false n.
neurotrauma
neurotrophy
neurotropic
neurotropism
neurovascular
neutral density absorber
neutron
  activation analysis, n.
  brachytherapy, n.
  flux, n.
  induced, n.
  shielding, n.
neutrophil
  band n.
  polymorphonuclear n.
  segmented n.
  stabnuclear n.
nevoid
nevolipoma

Additional Entries

nevus
- blue n.
- compound n.
- hairy n.
- melanocytic n.
- pigmented n.
- spider n.

Newcastle disease
Newman's
- cells, N.
- dentinal sheath, N.

Newton
- guide wire, N.
- rings, N.

ng. (nanogram)
NG (nasogastric)
N gas method
Ni (nickel)
niche (s)
- multiple n.
- penetrating n.
- round wind n.
- single n.
- ulcer n.

nickel (Ni)
Nicolas-Favre disease
Niemann-Pick disease
Niemann's disease
Niewenglowski's ray
niobium (Nb)
nipple
- discharge, n.
- everted n.
- inversion, n.
- marker, n.
- retraction, n.
- shadow, n.

Nissen fundoplication
Nissl
- bodies, N.
- granules, N.

Nitabuch's layer
nitro
- MUGA, n.
- test, n.

nitrogen (N) 13 ammonia
nitrous oxide
nl. (nanoliter)
nm. (nanometer)
N-methylglucamine salts
NMG (N-methylglucamine)
NMR (nuclear magnetic resonance)
No (nobelium)
nobelium (No)
Noble's position
nodal
- arrhythmia, n.
- beat, n.
- bigeminy, n.
- bradycardia, n.
- escape, n.
- extrasystole, n.
- rhythm, n.

node (s)
- Aschoff's n.
- atrioventricular n.
- axillary n.
- Bouchard's n.
- calcified lymph n.
- cervical n.
- Durck's n's.
- Flack's n's.
- Haygarth's n's.
- Heberden's n's.
- hemal n's.
- hemolymph n's.
- Hensen's n.
- hilar n.
- inguinal n.
- jugulodigastric n.
- Keith's n.
- Keith-Flack n.
- lymph n.

Additional Entries

node (s) *(continued)*
- mediastinal n.
- Meynets n's.
- negative, n.
- obturator n.
- of Ranvier, n's.
- Osler's n's.
- pelvic n.
- positive, n.
- primitive n.
- radical inguinal n. dissection
- Ranvier n.
- Rotter's n's.
- scalene n. biopsy
- Schmorl's n.
- sentinel n.
- shotty lymph n.
- signal n.
- singer's n.
- sinoatrial n.
- sinoauricular n.
- sinus n.
- Tawara, n. of
- Troisier's n.
- Virchow's n.
- azygos n.

nodosum
- erythema n.

nodular
- density, n.
- enhancement, n.
- goiter, n.
- thyroid, n.
- tumor, n.

nodule (s)
- Albini's n.
- Aschoff's n.
- cold n.
- discrete n.
- Gandy-Gamma n.
- hot n.

nodule (s) *(continued)*
- lingular n.
- lymphatic n.
- metastatic n.
- peripheral n.
- pulmonary n.
- Schmorl's n.
- sclerosis, n.
- thyroid n.
- vocal cord n.

no evidence of disease (NED)

Nolan applicator

nominal standard dose (NSP)

nomogram

nomography

nonbarrel shaped cervix

nonbeveled needle

nonbulk disease

noncommunicating
- hydrocephalus, n.

nondisplaced
- fracture, n.

nonencapsulated

nonferrous

nonfocused block

nonfunctioning
- gallbladder, n.
- kidney, n.

nongated CT scan

nonheme

non-Hodgkin's lymphoma

nonhomogeneity

noninfarcted myocardium

nonionic
- agents, n.

nonkeratinizing

nonlooping implant

nonopaque
- stone, n.

nonosseous defect

nonossifying

Additional Entries

nonossifying *(continued)*
factor, n.
fibroma, n.
nonparallel walls
nonradiable
nonresponders
nonrotation
of the intestine, n.
non-screen film
nonspecific
ST-T wave changes, n.
urethritis, n.
nonuniformity of image
nonunion
Noonan syndrome
norepinephrine
norm
norma
basilaris, n.
frontalis, n.
lateralis, n.
occipitalis, n.
verticalis, n.
normal
convection, n.
pressure communicating hydrocephalus, n.
normoblast
acidophilic n.
basophilic n.
eosinophilic n.
polychromatic n.
normoblastic
normocapnia
normolineal
normotensive
North American Instrument Corporation
Northwest Refining Company duplicator/subtractor
Norwood snare
nose

nose *(continued)*
accessory sinuses of n.
alar cartilages of n.
arteries of n.
cartilage of septum of n.
cartilaginous frame work of n.
cavities of n.
external n.
lateral cartilages of n.
lymphatics of n.
mucous membrane of n.
muscles of n.
nerves of n.
veins of n.
nosocomial
notch
acetabular n.
angular n.
aortic n.
cardiac n.
clavicular n.
ethmoidal n.
fibular n.
gastric n.
interclavicular n.
intercondylar n. of femur
intertragic n.
jugular n.
lacrimal n.
mandibular n.
mastoid n.
maxilla, n. of
nasal n.
nasolacrimal n.
occipital bone, n. of
palatine bone, n. of
parietal n.
preoccipital n.
presternal n.
Rivinus n.

Additional Entries

notch *(continued)*
scapular n.
sciatic n.
semilunar n.
sigmoid n.
sphenoglenoid n.
sphenopalatine n.
sternum, n. of
superior thyroid n.
supraorbital n.
suprascapular n.
suprasternal n.
temporal bone, n. of
tentorial n.
thyroid n.
trigeminal n.
trochlear n.
tympanic n.
ulnar n.
umbilical n.
vertebral n.
notching
notencephalocele
notencephalus
Nothnagel's bodies
notochord
notomyelitis
novoscope
noxious gas
Np (neptunium)
ns. (nanosecond)
NSD (nominal standard dose)
nsec. (nanosecond)
N-shaped skin marker
NSR (normal sinus rhythm)
N-stage division
N1 stage
N2 stage
N3 stage
nU. (nanounit)
nucha
nuchal
ligament, n.
line, n.
rigidity, n.
Nuck's
canal, N
diverticulum, N.
nuclear
binding energy, n.
bone imaging, n.
cardiac imaging, n.
fission, n.
imaging system, n.
layer, n.
magnetic resonance (NMR), n.
membrane, n.
pulse amplifier, n.
relaxation, n.
remnants, n.
scanning, n.
spin, n.
stability, n.
structure, n.
Nuclear Associates, Inc.
Nuclear Regulatory Commission (NRC)
nucleated sheath of Schwann
nuclei
cochlear nerve, n. of
glossopharyngeal, n. of
oculomotor nerve, n. of
olivary n.
origin of motor nerves, n.
pontis, n.
trigeminal nerve, n. of
vestibular nerve, n. of
Nuclesa Cervitron II afterloader

Additional Entries ____________________

____

____

Nucletron Engineering BV
Nucletron Selectron afterloader
nucleus
- ambiguous n.
- arcuate n.
- atomic n.
- basal n.
- Bekhterev's n.
- caudate n.
- cell n.
- cochlear n.
- cuneate n.
- Darkshevich's n.
- Deiters' n.
- dentate n.
- dorsalis n.
- emboliformis n.
- facial nerve n.
- fastigii n.
- globosus n.
- gracilis n.
- Gudden, n. of
- herniated n. pulposus (HNP)
- hypoglossal n.
- hypothalamic n.
- intercalatus n.
- interpeduncular n.
- lacrimalis n.
- lenticular n.
- lentiform n.
- Luys n.
- medial longitudinal fasciculus, n. of

nucleus *(continued)*
- motor n.
- of lens, n.
- of thalamus, central n.
- of origin, n.
- of root of cerebellum, n.
- olivary n.
- paraventricular n.
- Perlia n.
- pontine n.
- pulposus, n.
- pulpy n.
- red n.
- ruber, n.
- salivatorius n.
- Schwalbe n.
- sensory n.
- subthalamic n.
- supraoptic n.
- tegmental n.
- thalamic n.
- thoracic n.
- tractus solitarius n.
- trapezoid n.
- vagus nerve n.
- vestibular n.
- Von Monakow n.

Nuel's space
Nuhn's glands
nutrient
- artery, n.
- foramen of fibula, n.

nutron/proton ratio
N-wire
nylon strands

Additional Entries

O

O (oxygen)
OAFs (off-axis factors)
oat
    cell carcinoma, o.
OB (obstetric) sonogram
O'Beirne's sphincter
obelion
Obersteiner-Redlich area
obex
object
    -film distance, o.
    image distance, o. (OID)
    -plane, o.
oblique
    cord, o.
    external o. fascia
    film, o.
    fracture, o.
    incision, o.
    ligament, o.
    line of fibula, o.
    muscle, o.
    perfusion scan, o.
    popliteal ligament, o.
    projection, o.
    ridge of clavicle, o.
    sinus of pericardium, o.
    vein, o.
    view, o.
obliquity
obliterans
    arteriosclerosis o.
obliterated
    ductus arteriosus, o.
    ductus venosus, o.
    hypogastric artery, o.
    umbilical vein, o.
obliteration
oblongata
obstetric (OB) sonogram
obstructed
    airway, o.
    lymphatic channel, o.
    thoracic duct, o.
    uropathy, o.
obstruction
    airway o.
    bile duct o.
    bladder neck o.
    bowel o.
    intestinal o.
    mechanical bowel o.
    nasal airway o.
obstructive
    airway disease, o.
    chronic o. airway disease
    chronic o. lung disease (COLD)
    chronic o. pulmonary disease (COPD)
    cardiomyopathy, o.
    hydrocephalus, o.
    nephrogram, o.
    uropathy, o.
    jaundice, o.
obturator
    artery, o.
    crest, o.
    externus muscle, o.
    fascia, o.
    foramen, o.
    groove, o.
    hernia, o.
    internus muscle, o.
    lymph node, o.
    membrane, o.
    muscle, o.
    nerve, o.
    nodal chain, o.

Additional Entries ______________________________

____

____

obturator *(continued)*
node, o.
sign, o.
tubercle, o.
vein, o.
obtuse
angle, o.
marginal, o.
occiput posterior position
occiptal
artery, o.
bone, o.
condyle, o.
crest, o.
fontanelle, o.
foramen, o.
fossae, o.
groove, o.
gyri, o.
horn, o.
lobe, o.
lymph nodes, o.
muscle, o.
nerve, o.
protuberance, o.
sinus, o.
sulcus, o.
triangle, o.
vein, o.
vertebra, o.
occipitalis
muscle, o.
occipitoanterior
occipitoaxial
ligaments, o.
occipitobasilar
occipitocalcarine
occipitocervical
occipitofacial
occipitofrontal
fasciculus, o.
oblique view, o.

occipitofrontal *(continued)*
view, o.
occipitofrontalis
muscle, o.
occipitomastoid
suture, o.
occipitomental
occipitoparietal
occipitoposterior
occipitotemporal
convolution, o.
occipitothalamic
occiput
occlude
occluding spring
occlusal position
occlusion
abnormal o.
afunctional o.
balanced o.
balloon catheter, o.
central o.
coronary o.
eccentric o.
functional o.
habitual o.
hyperfunctional o.
lateral o.
lingual o.
mesial o.
normal o.
protrusive o.
retrusive o.
traumatic o.
occlusive
arteriosclerotic peripheal o. disease
dressing, o.
occlusocervical
O'Connor's drape
occulta
spina bifida o.

Additional Entries

occupying
space o. lesion
OCG (oral cholecystogram)
ochronosis
Ochsner's muscle
OCR (off-center ratio)
ocular
adnexa, o.
bulb, o.
cup, o.
fundi, o.
humor, o.
muscle, o.
palsy, o.
pressure, o.
oculocutaneous
oculodento-osseous dysplasia
oculofacial
oculometroscope

oculomotor
nerve, o.
sulcus, o.
oculomycosis
oculopathy
oculoplastic
oculoplethysmography/carotid phonoangiography (OPG/CPA)
oculopupillary
oculospinal
oculozygomatic
Oddi's muscle
odontoblast
odontoclast
odontogenic
odontogenous
odontogram
odontograph
odontoid
fracture, o.
odontoid *(continued)*
ligaments, o.
process, o.
view, o.
odontolithiasis
odontoma
odontopathy
odontoradiography
odontoscopy
odynometer
odynophagia
OER (oxygen enhancement ratio)
OF (output factor)
off
-center, o.
-distance, o.
-focus radiation, o.
-level, o.
off-axis
CT image, o-a
factor, (OAF), o-a
off-center ratio (OCR)
Ogston's line
Oguchi's disease
Ogura system
Ohara's disease
ohm
OID (object-image distance)
oily contrast agent
Oken's canal
15 O labeled water
olecranon
bursa, o.
fossa, o.
ligament, o.
process, o.
spur, o.
oleic acid I 131
oleic acid I 125
oleoperitoneography

Additional Entries

oleothorax
olfactometer
olfactometry
olfactory
  areas, o.
  bulb, o.
  cells, o.
  fasciculus, o.
  groove, o.
  gyrus, o.
  hair, o.
  nerves, o.
  neuroblastoma, o.
  pits, o.
  projection fibers, o.
  stria, o.
  sulcus, o.
  tract, o.
  trigone, o.
  tubercle, o.
oligemia
oligemic
  lung, o.
oligodendrocyte
oligodendroglia
oligodendroglioma
oligogalactia
oligohydramnios
oligohypermenorrhea
oligomenorrhea
oligoplastic
oligopontine
  cerebellar degeneration, o.
oliguria
oliva
olivae
olivary
  body, o.
  nucleus, o.
olive-tip catheter
olivifugal
olivipetal
olivocerebellar
  fibers, o.
olivopontocerebellar degeneration
olivospinal
  fasciculus, o.
Ollier's
  disease, O.
  enchondromatosis, O.
Olshevsky roentgen-ray tube
Olympic Surgical Company
Olympus scope
OM (orbitomeatal; occipitomental)
omega
omental
  adhesive band, o.
  bursa, o.
  recess, o.
omentectomy
omentitis
omentopexy
omentoplasty
omentoportography
omentorrhaphy
omentosplenopexy
omentum
  colic o.
  gastrocolic o.
  gastrohepatic o.
  gastrosplenic o.
  greater o.
  lesser o.
  small o.
Omnipaque
Omnipaque-300
omocephalus
omoclavicular
omohyoid
  muscle, o.
omosternum

Additional Entries

omphalocele
omphaloma
omphalomesenteric
omphalophlebitis
omphalorrhagia
omphalorrhea
omphalorrhexis
oncocyte
oncocytoma
oncogene
oncogenic
oncogenous
oncolysis
oncolytic
oncometer
oncornavirus
oncotaxonomy
oncotherapy
on/in patient dosimetry
onion-scale lesion
onlay
  bone graft o.
oophoritis
oophorocystosis
oophorogenous
oophorohysterectomy
oophoroma
oophoron
oophoropathy
oophoroplasty
oophorrhagia
opacification
opacity
opaque
  calculi, o.
  foreign body, o.
  marker, o.
  medium, o.
  stone, o.
open
  beam, o.
  bladder implant, o.
open *(continued)*
  field, o.
  mouth odontoid view, o.
  needle puncture, o.
  reduction and internal
    fixation (ORIF), o.
opening
  aortic o.
  caval o.
  coronary sinus o.
  esophageal o.
  inferior vena caval o.
  pulmonary artery o.
  saphenous o.
  superior cava o.
  thoracic o.
operative
  cholangiography, o.
  venography, o.
opercula
  insula, o. of
operculum
ophthalmatrophia
ophthalmectomy
ophthalmencephalon
ophthalmic
  artery, o.
  ganglion, o.
  nerve, o.
  veins, o.
ophthalmodesmitis
ophthalmodiaphanoscope
ophthalmodiastimeter
ophthalmodonesis
ophthalmodynamometer
ophthalmodynamometry
ophthalmodynia
ophthalmoeikonometer
ophthalmograph
ophthalmomalacia
ophthalmometer
ophthalmometroscope

Additional Entries

ophthalmometry
ophthalmomycosis
ophthalmomyitis
ophthalmomyositis
ophthalmomyotomy
ophthalmoneuritis
ophthalmoneuromyelitis
ophthalmophacometer
ophthalmophlebotomy
ophthalmoplasty
ophthalmoplegia
    externa, o.
    interna, o.
    nuclear, o.
    Parinaud's o.
    partial o.
    progressive o.
    total o.
ophthalmoplegic
ophthalmorrhagia
ophthalmorrhea
ophthalmorrhexis
ophthalmoscope
    direct o.
    indirect o.
ophthalmoscopy
ophthalmostasis
ophthalmostat
ophthalmostatometer
ophthalmosteresis
ophthalmosynchysis
ophthalmothermometer
ophthalmotomy
ophthalmotonometer
ophthalmotonometry
ophthalmotrope
ophthalmotropometer
ophthalmovascular
ophthalmoxyster
opisthion
opisthionasal
opisthogenia
opisthognathism
opisthoporeia
opisthorchiasis
opisthorchosis
opisthotic
    center (of temporal bone), o.
Oppenheim's disease
opposing lateral portals
optic
    atrophy, o.
    axis, o.
    canal, o.
    chiasm, o.
    commissure, o.
    cup, o.
    disc, o.
    disk, o.
    foramen, o.
    groove, o.
    nerve, o.
    neuritis, o.
    recess, o.
    stalk, o.
    thalamus, o.
    tracts, o.
    vesicle, o.
optical
    beam-splitter optic, o.
    probe, o.
opticochiasmatic
opticociliary
opticonasion
opticopupillary
optoblast
optogram
optokinetic
optometer
optomyometer
optophone
ora
    serrata retinae, o.

Additional Entries __________

orad
Oragrafin
oral
    cavity, o.
    cholecystogram, o.
orbicular
    ligament, o.
orbiculare
orbit
    sonogram, o.
orbita
orbital
    calcification, o.
    exenteration of o. contents
    fascia, o.
    fissures, o.
    floor, o.
    floor prosthesis, o.
    gyri, o.
    margin, o.
    nerve, o.
    operculum, o.
    plates, o.
    process, o.
    pseudotumor, o.
    ridge, o.
    septum, o.
    sulcus, o.
    vein, o.
orbitography
orbitomeatal (OM)
    baseline perpendicular to film, o.
    line perpendicular to cassette, o.
orbitonasal
orbitonometer
orbitonometry
orbitosphenoid
orbitostat
orbitotemporal
orchiencephaloma
orchiepididymitis
orchiocele
orchiomyeloma
orchiopathy
orchiopexy
orchioplasty
orchioscheocele
orchioscirrhus
orchitic
orchitis
organ
    Corti o.
    effector o.
    enamel o.
    end o.
    genital o.
    Giraldes o.
    Golgi tendon o.
    Jacobson's o.
    location, o.
    mass, o.
    of Corti, o.
    of Zuckerkandl, o.
    Rosenmuller o.
    sense o.
    sensory o.
    spiral o.
    vestigial o.
    vomeronasal o.
    Weber's o.
    Zuckerkandl o.
organelle
organic benzoic acid
organoferric
organogel
organogen
organogenesis
organography
organoid

Additional Entries

organoma
organomegaly
organometallic
organon
  auditus, o.
  gustus, o.
  olfactus, o.
  spirale, o.
  visus, o.
organopathy
organopexy
organoscopy
organotropic
organ-specific compound
ORIF (open reduction and internal fixation)
orifice
  anal o.
  atrioventricular o.
  bronchial o.
  cardiac o.
  ileocolic o.
  mitral o.
  of mouth, o.
  pyloric o.
  umbilical o.
  ureteral o.
  ureteric o.
  urethral o.
  of uterus, o.
  vaginal o.
  widely patent, o.
orificulum
  externum uteri, o.
  internum uteri, o.
orocutaneous fistula
orogastric tube
orogranulocyte
orolactin-secreting microadenoma
orolingual
oromaxillary
oronasal
oropharynx
  proper, o.
Orthicon camera
orthogenesis
orthogonal film
orthoiodohippurate (131 I)
orthometer
orthomolecular
orthopedic appliance
orthopercussion
orthophony
orthopneic
orthoroentgenography
orthoscope
orthoscopy
orthostereoscope
orthotopic ureter
orthovoltage
  unit, o.
  x-ray therapy unit, o.
Os (osmium)
os (opening)
  externum uteri, o.
  uterus, external, o. of
os (pl. ossa) bone
  acromiale secondarum, o.
  basilare, o.
  breve, o.
  calcis, o.
  capitatum, o.
  centrale of corpus, o.
  centrale tarsi, o.
  cervical o.
  coccygis, o.
  costa, o.
  costae, o.
  costale, o.
  coxae, o.

Additional Entries ______________________

os (pl. ossa) bone *(cont'd)*
    cuboideum, o.
    cuneiforme primum, o.
    cuneiforme secundum, o.
    cuneiforme tertium, o.
    ethmoidale, o.
    external of uterus, o.
    frontale, o.
    hamatum, o.
    hyoideum, o.
    ilii, o.
    incae, o.
    incisivum, o.
    innominatum, o.
    internal o. of uterus
    ischii, o.
    lacrimale o.
    lunatum, o.
    magnum, o.
    multangulum, o.
    naviculare manus, o.
    naviculare pedis, o.
    occipitale, o.
    odontoideum, o.
    palatinum, o.
    parietale, o.
    pelvicum, o.
    penis, o.
    perineum, o.
    pisiforme, o.
    planum, o.
    pubis, o.
    sacrum, o.
    sphenoidale, o.
    temporale, o.
    trapezium, o.
    trapezoideum, o.
    trigonum tarsi, o.
    triquetrum, o.
    uteri, o.
    zygomaticum, o.

oscheocele
oscheohydrocele
oscheolith
oscheoma
oscillating electron
oscillating magnetic field gradient
oscillation
oscillogram
oscillograph
oscillometer
oscillometry
oscilloscope
    monitor, o.
    screen, o.
Osgood-Schlatter disease
Osler's disease
Osler's node
Osler-Weber-Rendu disease
osmesis
osmium (Os)
osmometer
osmophore
osmoreceptor
osmoscope
osmotic
    fragility, o.
    pressure, o.
    shock, o.
osphyomyelitis
ossa
    carpi, o.
    cranii, o.
    faciei, o.
    fibulare, o.
    magnus, o.
    metacarpalia, o.
    metatarsalia, o.
    nasale, o.
    pedis, o.
    sesamoidea, o.
    tarsi, o.

Additional Entries

ossa *(continued)*
tibiale, o.
osseoaponeurotic
osseocartilaginous
osseofibrous
osseomucin
osseomucoid
osseosonometer
osseosonometry
osseous
activity, o.
metastases (Mo), o.
structures, o.
ossicle (s)
auditory o.
Kerckring o.
ligament o.
mental o.
metopic o.
Riolan's o.
wormian o.
ossicula
auditus, o.
ossiculum
terminale, o.
ossification
ectopic o.
endochondral o.
intramembranous o.
osteitis
condensans generalisata, o.
condensing o.
deformans, o.
fibrosa cystica, o.
fibrosa osteoplastica, o.
fragilitans, o.
fungosa, o.
parathyroid o.
pubis, o.
sclerosing o.
osteoaneurysm
osteoarthritic
changes, o.
hypertrophic spur formation, o.
lipping, o.
osteoarthritis
osteoarthropathy
hypertrophic pulmonary o.
secondary hypertrophic o.
osteoarthrosis
osteoarticular
osteoblast
osteoblastic
osteoblastoma
osteocartilaginous
osteocele
osteocementum
osteochondral
osteochondritis
deformans juvenilis, o.
deformans juvenilis dorsi, o.
dissecans, o.
osteochondrolysis
osteochondroma
osteochondromatosis
osteochondromyxoma
osteochondropathia
osteochondropathy
osteochondrosarcoma
osteochondrosis
dissecans, o.
osteoclasia
osteoclast
osteoclastic
osteoclastoma
osteocranium
osteocystoma
osteocyte
osteodentin

Additional Entries

osteodentinoma
osteodesmosis
osteodiastasis
osteodynia
osteodysplasty
osteodystrophy
    renal o.
osteoepiphysis
osteofibrochondrosarcoma
osteofibroma
osteofibromatosis
osteogenesis
    imperfecta, o.
osteogenetic
    fibers, o.
osteogenic
    sarcoma, o.
osteogram
osteography
osteoid
osteolipochondroma
osteolipoma
osteolytic
osteoma
osteomalacia
    hepatic o.
    infantile o.
    juvenile o.
osteomatosis
osteometry
osteomiosis
osteomyelitis
    Garre's o.
    sclerosing nonsuppurative o.
osteomyelodysplasia
osteomyelography
osteopenia
osteopenic
osteoperiosteal
osteoperiostitis
osteopetrosis
osteophlebitis
osteophony
osteophyma
osteophyte
    bony o.
    bridging o.
    formation, o.
osteophytosis
osteoplaque
osteoplast
osteoplastic
osteoplasty
osteopoikilosis
osteopoikilotic
osteoporosis
    circumscripta cranii, o.
    diffuse o.
osteoporotic
osteoradionecrosis
osteorrhagia
osteorrhaphy
osteosarcoma
osteosarcomatous
osteosclerosis
    congenita, o.
    fragilis, o.
    fragilis generalisata, o.
osteosclerotic
osteoscope
osteoseptum
osteosis
osteotelangiectasia
osteothrombophlebitis
osteothrombosis
osteotome
osteotomoclasia
osteotrophy
ostia
ostial
ostium
    abdominal o.
    eustachian tube o.

Additional Entries

ostium *(continued)*
  maxillare o.
  pharyngeaal o.
  primitive urogenital o.
  primum o.
  secundum o.
otalgia
otic
  ganglion, o.
  vesicle, o.
otitic
otitis
  media, o.
otoantritis
otoblennorrhea
otocephalus
otocephaly
otocerebritis
otocleisis
otoconia
otocranium
otocyst
otoencephalitis
otoganglion
otogenous
otography
otolaryngology
otolith
otolithiasis
otomastoiditis
otomucormycosis
osomyasthenia
otomycosis
otopathy
otopharyngeal
otoplasty
otopyorrhea
ororhinolaryngology
otorhinology
otorrhagia
otorrhea
otosalpinx
otosclerosis
otoscope
otoscopy
otospongiosis
Otto disease
outer
  canthus, o.
  catheter, o.
output
  cardiac o.
  factor (OF), o.
ova
oval
  area of Flechsig, o.
  bundle, o.
  shape, o.
ovarian
  arteries, o.
  fossa, o.
  mass, o.
  plexus, o.
  tumor, o.
  veins, o.
ovariocele
ovariocentesis
ovariogenic
ovariopathy
ovariopexy
ovariorrhexis
ovariosalpingectomy
ovariotomy
ovariotubal
ovary
  polycystic o.
overflow
  incontinence, o.
overgrafting
overgrowth
overhang
  bony o.
Overhauser effect
overhead oblique view

Additional Entries

overinflation
overlap
overlapping catheter
overlying
  gas shadows, o.
  intestinal gas, o.
  mucosal thickening, o.
overriding
oviduct
oviferous
oviform
ovigenesis
oviparous
ovoid
ovula
  Naboth, o.
ovular
ovulogenous
ovum
  corona radiata of o.
  germinal spot of o.
  zona pellucida of o.
OW (oval window)
Owen's
  lines, O.
  view, O.
oxalate
  calcium o. crystals
oxalosis
oxidized cellulose
oximeter
oximetry
oxycephalic
oxycephaly
oxygen (O)
  15 labeled water, o.
oxygenated cells
oxygen enhancement ratio (OER)
oxyhemogram
oxyhemograph
oxyntic
  cells, o.
  glands, o.
oxyphil

Additional Entries

P

P (phosphorus)
Pa (protactinium)
PA (posteroanterior) projection
pacchionian
 bodies, p.
 depressions, p.
 foramen, p.
 glands, p.
 granulations, p.
pacemaker
 artificial cardiac p.
 battery, p.
 cardiac p.
 Chardack-Greatbatch p.
 cilia p.
 Cordis p.
 demand p.
 electrode, p.
 external p.
 failure, p.
 generator, p.
 Medtronic demand p.
 Nathan p.
 temporary transvenous p.
 transthoracic p.
 transvenous p.
 unipolar p. generator
 wandering p.
pachydermatocele
pachydermoperiostosis
pachygyria
pachyleptomeningitis
pachymeningopathy
pachypelviperitonitis
pachyperiosteoderma
pachyperiostitis
pachyperitonitis
pachypleuritis
pachysalpingitis
pachysalpingo-ovaritis
pachyvaginitis
pacing
 cable, p.
 catheter, p.
 electrode, p.
 impulse, p.
Pacini's corpuscles
pacinian corpuscles
pad
 abdominal p.
 fat p.
 retromolar p.
 sucking p.
Page kidney
Pagenstecher's circle
Paget's
 abscess, P.
 cell, P.
 disease, P.
pagetic
pagetoid
pagoplexia
paintbrush silhouette
pair
 annihilation, p.
 production, p.
paired
 catheter, p.
 lateral parts, p.
 lateral technique, p.
 posterior oblique, p.
Pajot hook
palatal
 process of maxilla, p.
palate
 arches of p.
 bony hard p.
 cleft p.

Additional Entries ______________________________

palate *(continued)*
  hard p.
  hook, p.
  pendulous p.
  smoker's p.
  soft p.
palatiform
palatine
  aponeurosis, p.
  artery, p.
  bone, p.
  folds, p.
  foramen, p.
  muscles, p.
  nerve, p.
  notch, p.
  process, p.
  protuberance, p.
  reflex, p.
  suture, p.
  tonsil, p.
  uvula, p.
  vein, p.
  velum, p.
palatoglossal
palatoglossus
  muscle, p.
palatognathous
palatograph
palatography
palatomaxillary
palatomyograph
palatonasal
palatopagus
palatopharyngeal
palatopharyngeus
  muscle, p.
palatoplasty
palatoplegia
palatoproximal
palatorrhaphy
palatosalpingeus
palatum
  durum, p. (hard palate)
  molle, p. (soft palate)
palencephalon
paleocerebellum
paleogenetic
paleokinetic
paleoneurology
paleopallium
paleopathology
paleostriatum
paleothalamus
palingenesis
palladium (Pd)
pallanesthesia
pallesthesia
pallesthetic
palliate
palliative
pallidofugal
pallidum
pallium
pallor
palm
palma
  manus, p.
palmar
  aponeurosis, p.
  arch, p.
  cutaneous branch of median nerve, p.
  cutaneous branch of ulnar nerve, p.
  erythema, p.
  fascia, p.
  interossei muscles, p.
  interosseous arteries, p.
  ligaments, p.
  nerves of ulnar, p.
  plexus, p.
  surface, p.
palmaris

Additional Entries

palmaris *(continued)*
    brevis muscle, p.
    longus muscle, p.
palmate folds of uterus
palpate
palpatopercussion
palpebra (pl. palpebrae)
    inferior p.
    superior p.
    tertius p.
palpebrae
palpebral
    arteries, p.
    commissures, p.
    fissure, p.
    fold, p.
    ligament, p.
    nerves, p.
    raphe, p.
    vein, p.
palpebralis
palsy
    Bell's p.
    brachial plexus p.
    bulbar p.
    cerebral p.
    Erb's p.
    facial p.
    Klumpke's p.
    Landry's p.
    ocular p.
    shaking p.
    sixth nerve p.
    Todd's p.
    ulnar p.
    wasting p.
pampiniform
    plexus, p.
pamplegia
panarteritis
panarthritis
panasthenia
panatrophy
panautonomic
panblastic
pancake coil
pancarditis
panchromatic
panchromia
Pancoast's
    syndrome, P.
    tumor, P.
pancolectomy
pancreas
    accessory duct of p.
    annular p.
    body of p.
    duct of p.
    head of p.
    lesser p.
    lymphatic vessels of p.
    neck of p.
    nerves of p.
    tail of p.
    uncinate process of p.
    ventral p.
    vessels of p.
    Willis' p.
    Winslow's p.
pancreatalgia
pancreatectomy
pancreatic
    arteries, p.
    cyst, p.
    duct, p.
    fibrosis, p.
    insufficiency, p.
    pseudocyst, p.
    veins, p.
pancreaticoduodenal
    arteries, p.
    lymph nodes, p.
    veins, p.
pancreaticoduodenostomy

Additional Entries

pancreaticoenterostomy
pancreaticogastrostomy
pancreaticojejunostomy
pancreaticolienal
 lymph nodes, p.
pancreaticosplenic
pancreatitis
 hemorrhagic, p.
pancreatoduodenectomy
pancreatoduodenostomy
pancreatoenterostomy
pancreatogenous
pancratogram
pancreatography
 endoscopic retrograde p.
pancreatoid
pancreatolipase
pancreatolith
pancreatolithectomy
pancreatolithiasis
pancreatolithotomy
pancreatopathy
pancreatotomy
pancreatotropic
pancrelipase
pancreolithotomy
pancreolysis
pancreolytic
pancreopathy
pancreotheraapy
pancystitis
pancytopenia
Pander's layer
panelectroscope
panencephalitis
 sclerosing p.
panendography
panendoscope
 Foroblique p.
panendoscopy
panesthesia
Paneth's cells
pan function
pangenesis
panhydrometer
panhypopituitarism
Panizza's plexus
panmyeloid
panmyelopathy
panmyelophthisis
panneuritis
 epidemica, p.
panniculectomy
panniculitis
 nodular nonsuppurative p.
 relapsing febrile nonsuppurative p.
panniculus (a layer of membrane)
 abdominal p.
 adiposus, p.
 carnosus, p.
panophthalmitis
panoptic
panoptosis
Panorex
panosteitis
panotitis
panproctocolectomy
Pansch's fissure
pansclerosis
panseptum
pansinusectomy
pansinusitis
pantanencephaly
pantankyloblepharon
pantochromism
pantography
Pantopaque
pantoscopic
pantothenol
pantropic
panturbinate

Additional Entries

panus
panuveitis
papaverine hydrochloride
paper chromatography
papilla (pl. papillae)
  circumvallate pp.
  conical pp.
  dental p.
  filiform pp.
  foliate pp.
  fungiform pp.
  gingival p.
  hair p.
  incisive p.
  interdental p.
  lacrimal p.
  lingual p.
  mammary p.
  of skin, p.
  of tongue, p.
  of Vater p.
  optic p.
  palatine p.
  renal p.
  sublingual p.
  tactile pp.
  urethral p.
  vallate p.
papillary
  adenocarcinoma, p.
  atrophy, p.
  carcinoma, p.
  cystadenocarcinoma, p.
  dermis, p.
  follicular metastases, p.
  layer of skin, p.
  muscle, p.
  necrosis, p.
  process, p.
  serous cystadenocarcinoma, p.
  stasis, p.
papillary *(continued)*
  thyroid carcinoma, p.
  tumor, p.
papillectomy
papilledema
papilliferous
papilliform
papillitis
  necrotizing renal p.
papilloadenocystoma
papillocarcinoma
Papillon technique
papilloma
papillomatosis
papillomatous
papillomavirus
papilloretinitis
papillosphincterotomy
papillotome
papillotomy
papular
papule
papuloerythematous
papuloid
papulopustular
papulosquamous
papulovesicular
Paquelin's cautery
para-aminohippurate
para-aortic nodes
parablast
paracardiac
paracathodic rays
paracellulose
paracenesthesia
paracentesis
  abdominal p.
paracentral
  lobule, p.
paracephalus
paracerebellar
parachordal

Additional Entries

parachute mitral valve
paracolic
    abscess, p.
    gutter, p.
paracolitis
paracolpitis
paracolpium
paracrine
paracystic
paracystitis
paracytic
paradental
paraderm
paradidymal
paradidymis
paradox
    image, p.
    Kretz, p. of
    Opie p.
    Weber's p.
paradoxical
    emboli, p.
    pulse, p.
    respiration, p.
paraesophageal
paraffin
paraffinoma
parafollicular cell syndrome
paraganglioma
paraganglion
paraglottic space
paragnosis
paragranuloma
parahepatic
parahilar
parakeratosis variegata
parallel
    grid, p.
    hole collimator, p.
    opposed field, p.
    plate, p.
    rays, p.
parallelism
parallelometer
parallel-opposed technique
parallel opposing fields
parallelism
parallel striae of Retzius
paralysis
    agitans, p.
    ascending p.
    birth p.
    bulbar p.
    central p.
    compression p.
    conjugate p.
    crossed p.
    decubitus p.
    divers' p.
    Duchenne's p.
    Erb-Duchenne p.
    facial p.
    flaccid p.
    hyperkalemic periodic p.
    hypokalemic periodic p.
    immunological p.
    infantile p.
    mixed p.
    motor p.
    progressive bulbar p.
    pseudobulbar p.
    sensory p.
    spastic p.
    tick p.
    Todd's p.
    vasomotor
paralytic
    bladder, p.
    deformity, p.
    ileus, p.
paramagnetic
    relaxation, p.
    shift, p.
paramastitis

Additional Entries

paramastoid
    process, p.
parameatal
paramedial
    sulcus, p.
paramedian
parameningococcus
parameniscitis
parameniscus
paramesial
parameter
parametritis
    posterior p.
parametrium
paramolar
paramucin
paramyelin
paramyoclonus
paramyxovirus
paraneoplastic syndrome
paranephric
    body, p.
    cyst, p.
paranephritis
    lipomatous p.
paranephroma
paranephros
paraneural
paranomia
paranormal
paranuclear
paranucleolus
paranucleus
paraoral
parapancreatic
paraparesis
parapelvic cyst
paraperitoneal
parapharyngeal lymph nodes
paraphasia
paraphasis
paraphrenitis
paraphyseal
parapineal
paraplastic
paraplegia
    ataxic p.
    cerebral p.
    flaccid p.
    senile p.
    spastic p.
paraplegic
paraplegiform
parapleuritis
paraplexus
parapneumonia
parapophysis
parapoplexy
parapraxia
paraproctitis
paraproctium
paraprostatitis
paraprotein
parapsoriasis
parapyramidal
paraqueduct
pararectal
    fossa, p.
    lymph nodes, p.
pararenal
    fat, p.
parasacral
parasalpingeal
parasalpingitis
parascapular
parasellar
parasinoidal
parasporiasis
    en plaque, p.
    lichenoides, p.
parasternal
    lymph nodes, p.
parastruma
parasympathetic

Additional Entries

parasympathetic *(continued)*
nerves, p.
nervous system, p.
parasympathomimetic
parasynovitis
parasystole
paratenon
parathormone
parathyroid
adenoma, p.
extract, p.
gland, p.
hormone, p.
insufficiency, p.
parathyroidal
parathyroidoma
parathyropathy
parathyrotoxicosis
parathyrotropic
paratoloid
paratoloidin
paratonia
paratope
paratrachoma
paratrophy
paratuberculosis
paratyphlitis
paratyphoid
paraumblical
paraungual
paraurethra
paravaginal
paravenous
paravertebral
musculature, p.
paravesical
fossa, p.
paraxial
mesoderm, p.
parencephalia
parencephalocele
parencephalon
parenchyma
brain p.
hepatic p.
lung p.
renal p.
parenchymal
active p. disease
disease, p.
infiltrate, p.
infiltration, p.
mass, p.
sarcoid, p.
scarring, p.
parent
nuclide, p.
radioisotope, p.
parepicoele
parepigastric
paresis
paresthesia
paresthetic
meralgia p.
Parham band
parietal
bone, p.
cells, p.
convolution, p.
eminence, p.
foramen, p.
lobe, p.
membrane, p.
notch, p.
operculum, p.
pleura, p.
pericardium, p.
peritoneum, p.
pleura, p.
thinning, p.
veins, p.
parietofrontal
parietography
parietomastoid

Additional Entries

parietomastoid *(continued)*
suture, p.
parieto-occipital
fissure, p.
parietosphenoid
parietosquamosal
parietotemporal
artery, p.
parietovisceral
Park's aneurysm
Parker's fluid
Parkinson's
disease, P.
facies, P.
mask, P.
sign, P.
syndrome, P.
parkinsonian
parkinsonism
pari passu (L. "at equal pace")
Paris system
paroccipital
parodontal
parodontid
parolfactory
area, p.
paromphalocele
paroniria
paronychia
paroophoritis
paroophoron
parophthalmia
parophthalmoncus
paropsis
parorchidium
parosteal
desmoid, p.
osteosarcoma, p.
parosteitis
parosteosis
parotic
parotid
duct, p.
gland, p.
lymph nodes, p.
nerve, p.
notch, p.
plexus, p.
vein, p.
parotidectomy
parotideomasseterica
fascia, p.
parotidoscirrhus
parotidosclerosis
parotitis
epidemic p.
parous
cervix, p.
introitus, p.
parovarian
cyst, p.
parovariotomy
parovaritis
paroxysm
paroxysmal
activity , p.
atrial fibrillation, p.
atrial tachycardia (PAT), p.
burst, p.
coughing spasm, p.
diffuse p. slowing
discharge, p.
nocturnal dyspnea (PND), p.
slowing, diffuse p.
tachycardia, p.
ventricular tachycardia (PVT), p.
Parrot's disease
Parry's disease
pars

Additional Entries

pars *(continued)*
centralis systematis nervosi, p.
ciliaris retinae, p.
flaccida, p.
inarticularis, p.
intermedia bulborum, p.
iridica retinae, p.
marginalis sulci cinguli, p.
plana, p.
plana corpora ciliaris, p.
squamosa, p.
tensa membranae tympani, p.
tympanica ossis temporalis, p.
Parson's disease
pars planitis
partes (pl. of pars)
genitales externae muliebres, p.
partial
absence of pericardium, p.
anomalous venous return, p.
atrioventricular canal, p.
mole, p.
scan, p.
transmission block, p.
volume effect, p.
particle
alpha p.
beta p.
bombardment, p.
decay, p.
radiation, p.
particulate
irradiation, p.
matter, p.
parumbilical
veins, p.
parvicellular
parvovirus
parvule
Paschen's bodies
Paschutin's degeneration
Passavant's
bar, P.
fold, P.
ridge, P.
passive
congestion of lung, p.
immunity, p.
range of motion, p.
Pastia's sign
patch
Dacron p.
eye p.
graft, p.
plaque disease, p.
Teflon p.
patchwork radiation therapy
patchy
area of consolidation, p.
atelectasis, p.
enhancement, p.
infiltrate, p.
patella
alta, p.
patellapexy
patellar
ligament, p.
plexus, p.
retinacula, p.
surface of femur, p.
tendon reflex, p.
tendon transposition, p.
patellofemoral
index, p.
patency
patent
blue, p.
ductus arteriosus, p.

Additional Entries ______________________

patent *(continued)*
    foramen ovale, p.
Paterson's
    bodies, P.
    syndrome, P.
Paterson-Brown-Kelly syndrome
Paterson-Kelly syndrome
Paterson-Parker
    dosimetry, P-P
    syndrome, P-P
pathfinder
pathoanatomical
pathoanatomy
pathobolism
pathoclisis
pathoformic
pathogen
pathogenesis
pathogenic
pathognomonic
pathography
pathologic
    staging, p.
pathological
    anatomy, p.
    diagnosis, p.
    fracture, p.
pathometer
pathomorphism
pathoneurosis
pathophoresis
pathophorous
pathophysiology
pathoradiography
pathoroentgenography
pathways
patrilineal
patroclinous
patrogenesis
pattern
    beta p.

pattern *(continued)*
    bowel p.
    brain wave p.
    breathing p.
    haustral p.
    intestinal gas p.
    mucosal fold p.
    spike-and-wave p.
    variable, p.
    ventricular strain p.
patulous
paucibacillary
Pauli exclusion principle
Paul-Mixter tube
Pautrier microabscess
pavilion
    ear, p. of
    oviduct, p. of
    pelvis, p. of
pavor
    diurnus, p.
    nocturnus, p.
Pavy's disease
Pawlik's triangle
Payr's clamp
Pb (lead)
PBI (protein bound iodine)
p-butyl IDA analog
pc (picocurie)
32P chromic phosphorus
Pd (palladium)
PDD (percentage depth dose)
PE (pulmonary embolism)
peak level
peakscatter factor
peak systolic/diastolic velocity ratio
peak tracking
pearl
    epithelial p.
    Eschnig's p.

Additional Entries ______________________

pearl *(continued)*
Laennec's p.
scrotal sac, p. in
Pearson position
peau d'orange
Pecquet's duct
pectinate
ligament, p.
line, p.
muscle, p.
pectineus
muscle, p.
pectiniforme septum
pectoral
fascia, p.
groove, p.
muscle, p.
nerve, p.
reflex, p.
pectoralis
major muscle, p.
minimus muscle, p.
minor muscle, p.
pectorophony
pectunculus
pectus
carinatum, p.
excavatum, p.
pedal lymphangiogram
pedal lymphangiography
pedatrophia
pedicle
clamps, p.
flap, p.
pediculosis
pediculus
pediluvium
pedionalgia
pediphalanx
peditis
pedodynamometer
pedogenesis
pedograph
pedometer
pedopathy
pedophilia
pedophilic
peduncle
cerebellar p.
cerebral p.
pineal p.
pedunculated
adenoma, p.
fibroid, p.
lesion, p.
polyp, p.
pedunculotomy
pedunculus
PEEP (positive end-expiratory pressure)
peg lateral incisor
Pel-Ebstein
disease, P.
pyrexia, P.
symptom, P.
Pelger's nuclear aanomaly
Pelger-Huet nuclear anomaly
peliosis
hepatis, p.
Pelizaeus-Merzbacher disease
pellagrosis
Pellegrini's disease
Pellegrini-Stieda disease
Pellizzi's syndrome
pelvic
angiography, p.
bone, p.
brim, p.
cavity, p.
collateral vessel, p.
colon, p.
diaphragm, p.
echogram, p.
exenteration, p.

Additional Entries ______________________

pelvic *(continued)*
floor, p.
girdle, p.
gutter, p.
inflammatory disease, p. (PID)
inlet, p.
kidney, p.
lipomatosis, p.
lymph node, p.
mass, p.
muscles, p.
node, p.
outlet, p.
plexuses, p.
pneumography, p.
portion of sympathetic system, p.
ring fracture, p.
sonogram, p.
support, p.
traction, p.
pelvicaliceal
pelvicephalography
pelvicephalometry
pelvifemoral
pelvifixation
pelvimeter
pelvimetry
pelvioileoneocystostomy
pelvioradiography
pelvioscopy
pelvirectal
pelviroentgenography
pelvis
anthropoid p.
articulations of p.
axes, p.
bifid p.
bony p.
borderline p.
boundaries of p.

pelvis *(continued)*
brim of p.
cavity of lesser p.
contracted p.
diameters of p.
frozen p.
greater p.
gynecoid p.
inferior aperture of p.
inlet of p.
lesser p.
ligaments of p.
lymph nodes of p.
major p.
minor p.
outlet of p.
portable p.
position of p.
renal p.
superior aperture of p.
pelvisacral
pelvisacrum
pelviscope
pelvisection
pelvisternum
pelviureteral
pelviureteroradiography
pelvoscopy
pelvospondylitis
pemphigoid
pemphigus
erythematosus, p.
vulgaris, p.
pencil beam algorithm
Pende's sign
pendulous
abdomen, p.
breasts, p.
pendulum tracking
penetrating
injury, p.
keratoplasty, p.

Additional Entries

penetrating *(continued)*
  niche, p.
  ulcer, p.
  wound, p.
penetration depth
penetrative power
penetrometer
penile
  implant, p.
  mini-template, p.
  prosthesis, p.
  shaft, p.
  urethra, p.
penis
  body of p.
  bulb, p.
  corona glandis p.
  corpora cavernosa of p.
  corpus cavernosum p.
  crura of p.
  deep artery of p.
  dorsal artery of p.
  dorsal veins of p.
  fascia of p.
  foreskin of p.
  fundiform ligament of p.
  glans p.
  lymphatic vessels of p.
  muscles of p.
  neck of p.
  nerves of p.
  prepuce of p.
  septum pectiniforme p.
  suspensory ligament of p.
penoscrotal
penotherapy
Penrose drain
pentad
pentagastrin
pentalogy
  Fallot, p. of
pentaploid
pentaploidy
pentetate calcium trisodium Yb 169
pentetate indium disodium In 111
pentetic acid
penumbra (that radiation just outside and adjacent to full beam) pepper-pot skull
Pepper's syndrome
peptic
  esophagitis, p.
  ulcer disease, p.
peptogenic
percent
  backscatter, p.
  resolution, p.
percentage depth dose (PDD)
percomorph
per contiguum
per continuum
percussion
  digital p.
  dullness to p.
  finger p.
  note, p.
  resonant to p.
  wave, p.
percussopunctator
percussor
percutaneous
  arteriogram, p.
  biopsy, p.
  cholangiogram, p.
  needle biopsy, p.
  needle puncture, p.
  puncture of intercricothyroid membranes, p.
  transhepatic biliary drainage (PTHBD), p.

Additional Entries

percutaneous *(continued)*
transhepatic biopsy, (PTHB), p.
transhepatic choledochoplasty (PTHC), p.
transhepatic cholangiogram/cholangiography, p. (PTC)
transhepatic stent insertion (PTHSI), p.
transhepatic stone extraction (PTHSE), p.
transluminal angioplasty, p. (PTA)
transluminal coronary angioplasty, p. (PTCA)
perfect subtraction
perfluorocarbon
perfluorochemical
perforated
appendix, p.
cathode, p.
eardrum, p.
hollow viscus, p.
viscus, p.
perforating
arteries, p.
cutaneous nerve, p.
fibers of Sharpey, p.
perforation
perforator
perfrication
perfusate
perfuse
perfusion
arterial p.
cardiac p.
defect, p.
deficit, p.
imaging, p.
lung p.

perfusion *(continued)*
pattern, p.
phase, p.
rate, p.
scan, p.
scintigraphy, p.
study, p.
ventilation p.
periacinal
periadenitis
periadventitial
periampullary
perianal
periangitis
periangioma
periaortic
adenopathy, p.
area, p.
chain, p.
lymph nodes, p.
periapex
periapical
periappendicitis
periaqueductal
periarterial
periarteritis
nodosa, p.
periarthritis
calcinosis, p.
uptake, p.
periatrial
periauricular
periaxial
periaxillary
periaxonal
periblast
peribronchial
markings, p.
thickening, p.
peribronchiolitis
peribronchitis
peribulbar

Additional Entries

peribursal
pericaliceal
pericallosal
 artery, p.
 cistern, p.
pericanalicular
pericapsular
pericardial
 area, p.
 arteries, p.
 block, p.
 cavity, p.
 constriction, p.
 cyst, p.
 effusion, p.
 fat pad, p.
 fluid, p.
 fremitus, p.
 friction rub, p.
 gas, p.
 pleura, p.
 sac, p.
 silhouette, p.
 tamponade, p.
 tear, p.
 thickening, p.
pericardiocentesis
pericardiomediastinitis
pericardiophrenic
pericardiopleural
pericarditis
 adhesive p.
 bacterial p.
 constrictive p.
pericardium
 adherent p.
 fibrous p.
 nerves of p.
 oblique sinus of p.
 parietal p.
 serous p.
 transverse sinus of p.
pericardium *(continued)*
 vessels of p.
 vestigial fold of p.
 visceral p.
pericaval region
pericecal
pericellular
pericentral
pericephalic
pericholangitis
pericholecystitis
perichondrium
perichondroma
perichord
perichordal
perichrome
pericolic
pericolitis
pericolpitis
periconchal
periconchitis
pericorneal
pericoronal
pericoronitis
pericranial
pericranium
pericyte
periderm
peridesmium
peridiverticulitis
periductal
periduodenitis
peridural
peridurogram
peridurography
periencephalitis
periencephalography
periencephalomeningitis
perienteric
perienteritis
periependymal
periepithelioma

Additional Entries

periesophageal
perifascicular
perifistular
perifocal
perifolliculitis
perigangliitis
perigastric
perigemmal
periglandular
periglial
periglottis
perigraft fluid
perihepatitis
perihernial
perihilar
    defect, p.
    fibrosis, p.
peri-insular
peri-islet
perijejunitis
perikaryon
perikeraatic
perilabyrinth
perilaryngeal
perilenticular
perilesiojnal
periligamentous
perilobar
perilymph
perimastitis
perimedullary
perimeningitis
perimeter
perimetrium
perimetrosalpingitis
    encapsulating p.
perimetry
perimyelography
perimyocarditis
perimyoendocarditis
perimyositis
perimysium
perineal
    artery, p.
    body, p.
    branch of fourth sacral nerve, p.
    fat, p.
    muscle, p.
    nerve, p.
perineocele
perineometer
perineoplasty
perineoscrotal
perineovaginal
perineovaginorectal
perineovulvar
perinephric
    abscess, p.
    fascia, p.
    fat, p.
    fluid collection, p.
perinephrium
perineum
    boundaries of p.
    central tendinous point of p.
    fascia of p.
    lymphatic vessels of p.
    muscles of p.
perincural
perineurium
perinuclear
periocular
periodontal
perioophorosalpingitis
perioral
periorbita
periorchitis
periorchium
periosteal
    bone, p.
    cyst, p.
    elevator, p.

Additional Entries

periosteal *(continued)*
reaction, p.
thickening, p.
periosteoedema
periosteoma
periosteomedullitis
periosteomyelitis
periosteophyte
periosteorrhaphy
periosteotome
periosteotomy
periosteus
periosteum
alveolar p.
periovular
peripachymeningitis
peripancreatic
peripancreatitis
peripapillary
peripartum
peripatellar
peripelvic
cyst, p.
peripenial
peripericarditis
peripharyngeal
peripherad
peripheral
arterial occlusive disease, p.
blood smear, p.
circulation, p.
cortical atrophy, p.
edema, p.
end organs, p.
fields, p.
lung field, p.
meniscal separation, p.
nervous system, p.
organs, p.
projection, p.

peripheral *(continued)*
pulmonary artery stenosis, p.
pulses, p.
rim of activity, p.
scanning, p.
tap, p.
terminations of nerves, p.
vascular disease, p.
vasodilatation, p.
vision, p.
zone, p.
epipherocentral
peripheroceptor
peripheromittor
periphery
periphlebitis
sclerosing p.
periphrastic
periphrenitis
peripleural
peripleuritis
peripneumonia
notha, p.
peripolar
periportal
periprostatic
periprostatitis
peripyema
peripylephlebitis
peripyloric
periradicular
perirectal
perirenal
air insufflation, p.
perirhinal
perirhizoclasia
perisalpingitis
perisalpingo-ovaritis
perisalpinx
periscleral
lymph space, p.

Additional Entries

perisclerium
periscope
periscopic
perisigmoiditis
perisinusitis
perispermatitis
    serosa, p.
perisplanchnic
perisplanchnitis
perisplenic
perisplenitis
perispondylic
perispondylitis
peristalsis
    mass p.
    retrograde p.
    reversed p.
peristaltic
    activity, tertiary p.
    tertiary p. activity
    waves, p.
peristoma
peristomatous
peristome
perisynovial
perisyringitis
peritendineum
peritendinitis
    adhesive p.
    calcarea, p.
    crepitans, p.
peritendinous
peritenon
peritenoneum
perithecium
perithelium
perithyroiditis
peritomy
peritoneal
    abscess, p.
    cavity, p.
    dialysis, p.

peritoneal *(continued)*
    fossae, p.
    recesses, p.
    reflection, p.
    sac, p.
    space, p.
peritoneography
peritoneomuscular
peritoneopathy
peritoneopericardial
peritoneopexy
peritoneoplasty
peritoneoscope
peritoneoscopy
peritoneotome
peritoneotomy
peritoneovenous
peritoneum
    abdominal p.
    epiploic foramen of p.
    greater sac of p.
    intestinal p.
    ligaments of p.
    lymphatic capillaries of p.
    main cavity of p.
    main horizontal disposition of p.
    main vertical disposition of p.
    mesentery p.
    omental p.
    parietal portion of p.
    vesicouterine p.
    visceral p.
peritonitis
    adhesive p.
    biliary p.
    silent p.
peritonsillar
    abscess, p.
    tag, p.

Additional Entries

peritonsillitis
peritracheal
peritrichous
peritrochanteric
perityphlic
perityphlitis
periumbilical
periungual
periureteral
periureteritis
periurethral
periurethritis
periuterine
periuvular
perivaginal
perivaginitis
perivascular
  lymph spaces, p.
perivascularity
perivasculitis
perivenous
periventricular
  leukomalacia (PVL), p.
  lucency of hydrocephalus, p.
  mass, p.
  white matter, p.
perivertebral
perivesical
perivesicular
perivesiculitis
perivisceral
perivisceritis
perivitelline
perixenitis
Perlia's nucleus
permanent
  colostomy, p.
  myocardial pacemaker, p.
  remission, p.
  sections, p.
permeative destruction
pernasal
perobrachius
perocephalus
peridactylus
peronarthrosis
peroneal
  artery, p.
  groove, p.
  muscle, p.
  nerve, p.
  retinaculum, p.
  septa, p.
  sheath, p.
  sign, p.
  tendon, p.
  vein, p.
peroneotibial
perpartum hemorrhage
perpendicular
  bisector to the plane, p.
  fasciculus, p.
  line of ulna, p.
  plate of ethmoid, p.
Perrin-Ferraton disease
Persantine
persistent positivity
pertechnetate
  imaging, p.
  ion, p.
Perthes' disease
Pertik's diverticulum
pertubation
pertussis
per vaginam
pes
  abductus, p.
  adductus, p.
  cavus, p.
  hippocampi, p.
  planus, p.
  valgus, p.

Additional Entries

pes *(continued)*
varus, p.
pessary
PET (positron emission tomography)
petechia
petechiae
petechial
hemorrhage, p.
Peters' ovum
Petit's
canal, P.
hernia, P.
triangle, P.
Petrequin's ligament
petroclinoid ligament
petromastoid
petro-occipital
fissure, p.
petropharyngeus
petrosal
ganglion, p.
nerve, p.
process, p.
sinuses, p.
petrosalpingostaphylinus
petrosphenoid
petrosphenoidal
fissure, p.
syndrome, p.
petrosquamous
sinus, p.
suture, p.
petrotympanic
fissure, p.
petrous
apex, p.
artefact, p.
bone, p.
ganglion, p.
portion, p.
pyramid, p.

petrous *(continued)*
ridge, p.
Petruschky's spinalgia
Peutz-Jeghers syndrome
Peyer's
glands, P.
patches, P.
Peyronie's disease
Peyrot's thorax
Pezzer's catheter
Pfeiffer's
disease, P.
phenomenon, P.
Pfeiffer-Gomberg method
P.FLAC (pars flaccida portion of tympanic membrane)
Pfluger's
cords, P.
tubes, P.
pg. (picogram)
phacocele
phacocyst
phacocystitis
phacoemulsification
phacoglaucoma
phacoid
phacolysis
phacomalacia
phacometer
phacopalingenesis
phacosclerosis
phacoscope
phacotherapy
phagocyte
phagocytized
phagocytoblast
phagocytolysis
phagocytose
phagocytosis
phagodynamometer
phagokaryosis

Additional Entries

phagosome
phagotherapy
phagotrophy
phakoma
phakomatosis
phalangeal
processes of Corti's rods, p.
phalangectomy
phalanges
digitorum manus, p.
digitorum pedis, p.
ungual p.
phalanx
Phalen's
maneuver, P.
sign, P.
test, P.
phallaneurysm
phallic
phalliform
phallitis
phallocrypsis
phallodynia
phalloid
phalloncus
phalloplasty
phallorrhagia
phallorrhea
phallotomy
phallus
phanerogenic
phaneroplasm
phaneroscope
phanerosis
fat p.
phantom
scattering, p.
tumor, p.
pharmacoroentgenography
pharyngeal
aponeurosis, p.

pharyngeal *(continued)*
artery, p.
bursa, p.
function study, p.
grooves, p.
membrane, p.
nerve, p.
ostium of auditory tube, p.
plexus of nerves, p.
pouches, p.
recess, p.
tonsil, p.
tubercle, p.
tumor site, p.
veins, p.
walls, p.
pharyngemphraxis
pharyngismus
pharyngitis
bacterial p.
purulent p.
streptococcal p.
viral p.
pharyngocele
pharyngoconjunctivitis
pharyngocutaneous fistula
pharyngodynia
pharyngoepiglottic
fold, p.
pharyngoesophageal
pharyngoglossus
pharyngography
pharyngokeratosis
pharyngolaryngeal
pharyngolith
pharyngomaxillary
pharyngomycosis
pharyngonasal
pharyngo-oral
pharyngopalatine
arch, p.

Additional Entries

pharyngopalatinus muscle
pharyngoparalysis
pharyngopathy
pharyngoperistole
pharyngoplasty
  Hynes p.
pharyngorhinitis
pharyngorhinoscopy
pharyngorrhagia
pharyngorrhea
pharyngosalpingitis
pharyngoscleroma
pharyngoscope
pharyngoscopy
pharyngospasm
pharyngostenosis
pharyngostoma
pharyngostomy
pharyngotherapy
pharyngotome
pharyngotonsillitis
pharyngotyphoid
pharyngoxerosis
pharynx
  aponeurosis of p.
  injected p.
  laryngeal part of p.
  mucous coat of p.
  muscles of p.
  nasal part of p.
  oral part of p.
phase
  encoding p.
  image p.
  proliferative p. endometrium
  secretory p. endometrium
  transition p.
  wash-in p.
  wash-out p.
phased
phased *(continued)*
  array scanning, p.
  array transducer, p.
phenotype
phenylephrine hydrochloride
phenylketonuria
phenolsulfonphthalein
phenylthiourea
pheochrome
pheochromoblast
pheochromoblastoma
pheochromocyte
pheochromocytoma
Philip's glands
Philips RT-50 portable radiation unit treatment gun
Philips SL 25 accelerator
Philippe-Gombault tract
Phillips catheter
philtrum
  lip, p. of
phimosis
phimotic
phlebalgia
phlebarteriectasia
phlebectasia
  laryngis, p.
phlebectopia
phlebemphraxis
phlebexairesis
phlebismus
phlebitic
phlebitis
phlebocylsis
phlebofibrosis
phlebogenous
phlebogram
phlebograph
  impedance p.
phlebography
phleboid
phlebolith

Additional Entries

phlebolithiasis
phlebomanometer
phlebometritis
phlebonarcosis
phlebopexy
phlebophlebostomy
phlebophthalmotomy
phleboplasty
phleborrhagia
phleborrhaphy
phleborrhexis
phlebosclerosis
phlebosis
phlebostasis
phlebostenosis
phlebothrombosis
phlebotome
phlegm
phlegmon
phlegmonous
phlogisticozymoid
phlogocyte
phlogocytosis
phlogogen
phlyctenule
phlyctenulosis
Phocas' disease
Pho-Con tomoscanner
phonal
phonarteriogram
phonautograph
phonendoscope
phonendoskiascope
phonoangiography
phonocardiogram
phonocardiography
phonocatheter
phonoelectrocardioscope
phonomyoclonus
phonomyogram
phonomyography
phonorenogram
phoroblast
phorocytosis
phorometer
phoroplast
phoroscope
phorotone
phosphate heart scan
phosphoroscope
phosphorus (P) P32
photic stimulation
photochemical imaging system
photochemotherapy
photochromogen
photocoagulation
photocutaneous
photodermatitis
photodermatosis
photodisintegration
photoelectric
  absorption, p.
  effect, p.
  interaction, p.
photoelectron
photoerythema
photofluorogram
photofluorography
photofluoroscope
photogastroscope
photogene
photogram
photography
photoinactivation
photokinetic
photokymograph
photoluminescence
photoma
photometer
photometry
photomicrograph
photomicroscope
photomorphogenesis

Additional Entries

photomultiplier
quantum conversion efficiency, p.
tube, p.
vacuum tube
photomyogenic
photon
beam characteristics, p.
concentration, p.
contamination, p.
deficient area, p.
deficient zone, p.
energy, p.
fluence, p.
flux density, p.
induced, p.
linear-attenuation coefficient, p.
symmetry, p.
velocity, p.
photo-onycholysis
photo-ophthalmia
photoparoxysmal
photopathy
photopeak setting
photopenic lesion
photoptometer
photoradiation
photoradiometer
photorectptor
photoretinitis
photoscan
photoscope
photostimulation
phototherapy
photronreflectometer
pH probe test
PHPV (persistent hyperplastic primary vitreous)
phrenic
ampulla, p.
arteries, p.

phrenic *(continued)*
crush, p.
ganglion, p.
lymph nodes, p.
nerve, p.
nerve canal, p.
nerve paralysis, p.
plexus of nerves, p.
vein, p.
phrenicectomized
phrenicectomy
phreniclasia
phrenicocolic
ligament, p.
phrenicocostal
sinus, p.
phrenicoexeresis
phrenicolienal
ligament, p.
phreniconeurectomy
phrenicopericardiac
ligament, p.
phrenitis
phrenocardia
phrenocolic
phrenocolopexy
phrenodynia
phrenogastric
phrenoglottic
phrenograph
phrenohepatic
phrenopathy
phrenopericarditis
phrenoplegia
phrenoptosis
phrenosplenic
phrenotropic
phronema
phrygian cap
phrynoderma
phthisis
phycochrome

Additional Entries

phycomycosis
phyllolith
physaliphore
physaliphorous
physalis
physallization
physeal
physical half-life
physicogenic
physiologic
  activity, p.
  bowing, p.
  jaundice, p.
  osteosclerosis, p.
  reflexes, p.
physiologicoanatomical
physiopathic
physocele
physocephaly
physohematometra
physohydrometra
physometra
physopyosalpinx
pia
  brain, p. of
  cord, p. of
  mater, p.
Picker Synerview
  International, P.S.
  1200 SX filtration, P.S.
  system, P.S.
Pick's disease
pickwickian syndrome
picocurie (pc.)
picogram (pg.)
picopicogram (ppg.)
picornavirus
picrosaccharometer
pictograph
Piersol's point
piesimeter
PIE (pulmonary interstitial emphysema)
  syndrome, PIE
Pierre Robin syndrome
pie-shaped dose distribution
piezocardiogram
piezometer
pigeon-breeder's disease
pigment
  bile p.
  -producing rays, p.
  respiratory p.
  skin p.
pigmented
  layer of retina, p.
  lesion, p.
  nevus, p.
  villonodular synovitis, p.
pigtail catheter
pila (pilae)
pilar
pile
  sentinel p.
piles
pileus
pili
piliform
pillar (s)
  Corti, p. of
  external abdominal ring, p. of
  fauces, p. of
  iris p.
  soft palate, p.
  tonsillar p.
pillion
pilocystic
pilomatricoma
pilonidal
  cyst, p.
pilosebaceous

Additional Entries ______________________________

Piltz-Westphal phenomenon
pilus
pimelitis
pimeloma
pimelopterygium
pimelorthopnea
pimelosis
pimeluria
pi mesons
pincushion distortion
pineal
    body, p.
    gland, p.
    recess, p.
    tumor, p.
pinealoblastoma
pinealocyte
pinealoma
    ectopic p.
pinealopathy
ping-pong fracture
pinhole
    collimator, p.
piniform
Pinkus' disease
pinna
    cartilage of p.
    ligaments of p.
pinocyte
pinocytosis
pinosome
pion
    beam, p.
pioscope
PIP (proximal interphalangeal)
PIPIDA (P-isopropylacetanilide-iminodiacetic acid) scan
piquizil hydrochloride
pirbuterol hydrochloride
piriform
    process, p.
    sinus, p.
piriformis
    muscle, p.
    fascia of p.
Pirogoff's angle
piroplasmosis
pisiform
    bone, p.
pisiuncinatus
    muscle, p.
pisohamate
    ligament, p.
pisometacarpal
    ligament, p.
p-isopropylacetanilido-iminodiacetic acid (PIPIDA)
32P isotope
pit
    anal p.
    auditory p.
    nasal p.
    stomach, p. of
    olfactory p.
Pituitrin
Pitressin
pitting cortical defect
pituitary
    adenoma, p.
    amenorrhea, p.
    apoplexy, p.
    body, p.
    dwarfism, p.
    extract, p.
    fossa, p.
    function determination, p.
    gland, p.
    growth hormone, p.
    stalk, p.

Additional Entries

pituitous
pivot
  joint, p.
  occlusal p.
pixel
  area, p.
  brightness, p.
  shifting, p.
placenta
placental
  abruption, p.
  bruit, p.
  calcification, p.
  circulation, p.
  cotyledon, p.
  cyst, p.
  forceps, p.
  fragment, p.
  imaging, p.
  insufficiency, p.
  membranes, p.
  migration, p.
  souffle, p.
placentogram
placentography
  indrect p.
Placido's disk
plafond
  tibial p.
plagiocephaly
plain
  film (PF), p.
  film angiography, p.
  radiography, p.
planar
  implant, p.
  scintigraphy, p.
Planck's constant
plane
  axial p.
  coronal p.
plane *(continued)*
  fat p.
  frontal p.
  horizontal p.
  intertubercular p.
  joint, p.
  longitudinal p.
  sagittal p.
  subcostal p.
  transpyloric p.
  transverse p.
  vertical p.
  waves, p.
planigram
planimeter
planithorax
planocellular
planoconcave
planoconvex
planocyte
planography
planta pedis
plantar
  aponeurosis, p.
  arch, p.
  arteries, p.
  aspect, p.
  calcaneal spur, p.
  cutaneous venous arch, p.
  digital veins, p.
  erythema, p.
  fascia, p.
  flexion, p.
  interosseus muscles, p.
  ligament, p.
  metatarsal arteries, p.
  nerve, p.
  reflex, p.
  spur, p.
  surface, p.

Additional Entries

plantar *(continued)*
wart, p.
plantaris
muscle, p.
plantigrade
planula
planum
nuchale, p.
occipitale, p.
planuria
plaque
atheromatous p.
calcified p.
formation, p.
Hollenhorst p.
irradiation, p.
-like linear calcification, p.
texture, p.
plasma
cell mastitis, p.
iron clearance, p.
thyroxine, p.
plasmablast
plasmacyte
plasmacytoma
radioactive strontium, p.
plasmacytosis
plasmagene
plasminogen
plasmodicidal
plasmogen
plasmoma
plasmosome
plasmotrophoblast
plasmotropic
plaster
cast, p.
of Paris cast, p.
plastic
button, p.
plastic *(continued)*
jacket, p.
sleeve, p.
stylet, p.
syringe, p.
plastidogenetic
plastosome
plate
axial p.
basal p.
bite p.
bone p.
cribriform p.
dental p.
dorsal p.
epiphyseal p.
foot p.
medullary p.
motor p.
neural p.
orbital p.
perpendicular p.
perpendicular p. of ethmoid bone
pterygoid p.
roof p.
sole p.
tarsal p.
tympanic p.
ventral p.
plateau
tibial p.
platinum (Pt)
platybasia
platycephaly
platycyte
platyglossal
platypellic
platypelloid
platysma
muscle, p.

Additional Entries ______

platyspondylysis
PLD (potentially lethal damage)
PLDL (potentially lethal damage repair)
pleocytosis
pleomorphic
pleomorphism
plessigraph
plethora
plethysmograph
plethysmographic venous study
plethysmography
 impedance p. (IPG)
 venous study p.
pleura
 cavity of p.
 cervical p.
 costal p.
 cupula of p.
 diaphragmatic p.
 lymphatic vessels of p.
 mediastinal p.
 nerves of p.
 parietal p.
 pericardial p.
 pulmonary p.
 thickened p.
 vessels of p.
 visceral p.
pleural
 based, p.
 calcification, p.
 cavity, p.
 effusion, p.
 exudate
 fremitus, p.
 friction rub, p.
 metastases, p.
 scarring, p.
 space, p.
pleural *(continued)*
 thickening, p.
pleurisy
 adhesive p.
 diaphragmatic p.
 dry p.
 fibrinous p.
 interlobular p.
 plastic p.
 purulent p.
 serous p.
 wet p.
pleuritic
 effusion, p.
pleurobronchitis
pleurocele
pleurocentesis
pleurocentrum
pleurocholecystitis
pleurocutaneous
pleurodesis
pleurodiaphragmatic adhesion
pleurodont
pleurogenous
pleurography
pleurohepatitis
pleurolith
pleuropericardial
pleuroperitoneal
 canal, p.
pleuropneumonia
pleuropulmonary
pleuroscopy
pleurotome
pleurovisceral
plexiform
 neuroma, p.
pleximeter
pleximetric
pleximetry
plexogenic

Additional Entries

plexometer
plexopathy
  lumbar p.
plexus (network of lymphatic vessels, nerves or veins)
  abdominopelvic p.
  annular p.
  aortic abdominal p.
  Auerbach's p.
  brachial p.
  cardiac p.
  carotid p.
  cavernous p.
  celiac p.
  cervical p.
  choroid p.
  coccygeal p.
  collateral p.
  corneal p.
  coronary p.
  cystic p.
  dental p.
  esophageal p.
  Exner's p.
  ganglionated p.
  gastric p.
  Heller's p.
  hemorrhoidal p.
  hepatic p.
  hypertrophy, p.
  hypogastric p.
  infraorbital p.
  internal carotid p.
  lienal p.
  lumbar p.
  lumbosacral p.
  Meissner's p.
  mesenteric p.
  myenteric p.
  nerve p.
  ovarian p.
  pampiniform p.
plexus *(continued)*
  parotid p.
  patellar p.
  pelvic p.
  pharyngeal p.
  phrenic p.
  prevertebral p.
  prostatic p.
  pterygoid p.
  pudendal p.
  pulmonary p.
  rectal p.
  renal p.
  sacral p.
  sinocarotid p.
  solar p.
  spermatic p.
  splenic p.
  submucosal p.
  subperitoneal p.
  subpleural p.
  subsartorial p.
  suprarenal p.
  sympathetic p.
  testicular p.
  thoracic p.
  tonsillar p.
  tympanic p.
  uterine p.
  uterovaginal p.
  vaginal p.
  vertebral p.
  vesical p.
  vesicoprostatic p.
pliable
plica (pl.plicae) (fold)
  fimbriata p.
  gubernatrix p.
  Hasner's p.
  Kerckring's p.
  lacrimalis p.
  semilunaris p.

Additional Entries

plica *(continued)*
- sublingualis p.
- triangularis p.
- uretericae p.
- urogenitalis p.
- vascularis p.
- ventriculares p.
- vesicalis transversa p.
- vocales p.

plicate
plication
- fundal p.
- sutures, p.

Plimmer's bodies
plombage
plug
- epithelial p.
- mucous p.
- tissue, p. of
- vaginal p.

Plummer nail
Plummer's disease
Plummer-Vinson radium applicator
Plummer-Vinson syndrome
pluriglandular
pluriocular
plurimenorrhea
pluriorificial
plurivisceral
plutonium (Pu)
PMI (point of maximal impulse)
P-31 MR spectroscopy
Pm (promethium)
PM tube
pneogaster
pneoscope
pneumal
pneumarthrogram
pneumarthrography
pneumascope
pneumatic
- cuff, p.
- tourniquet, p.

pneumatized
pneumatocele
- cranii, p.
- extracranial p.
- intracranial p.

pneumatometer
pneumatometry
pneumatoscope
pneumatosis
- coli, p.
- intestinalis, p.

pneumoalveolography
pneumoangiogram
pneumoangiography
pneumoarthrography
pneumobulbar
pneumobulbous
pneumocardial
pneumocardiograph
pneumocele
pneumocentesis
pneumocephalon
pneumocephalus
pneumocholecystitis
pneumochysis
pneumococcal
pneumocolon
pneumoconiosis
pneumocystic
pneumocystography
pneumocystosis
pneumocystomography
pneumoderma
pneumodograph
pneumoempyema
pneumoencephalitis
pneumoencephalogram
pneumoencephalographic chair

Additional Entries

pneumoencephalography
    cisternal p.
    global p.
    lumbar p.
    selective p.
pneumoencephalomyelogram
pneumoencephalomyelography
pneumoenteritis
pneumoerysipelas
pneumofasciogram
pneumogalactocele
pneumogastric
    nerve, p.
pneumogastrography
pneumogastroscopy
pneumogram
pneumograph
pneumography
    direct retroperitoneal p.
    pelvic p.
    presacral p.
pneumogynogram
pneumohemopericardium
pneumohemothorax
pneumohydrometra
pneumohydropericardium
pneumohydrothorax
pneumokidney
pneumolith
pneumomediastinogram
pneumomediastinography
pneumomediastinum
pneumomelanosis
pneumomycosis
pneumomyelography
pneumonectomy
pneumonia
    aspiration p.
    atypical p.
    bacterial p.
    bronchial p.

pneumonia *(continued)*
    broncho-p.
    caseous p.
    desquamative p.
    double p.
    hypostatic p.
    influenzal p.
    inhalation p.
    interstitial p.
    lipoid p.
    lobar p.
    Loffler p.
    miliary p.
    mycoplasmal p.
    parenchymatous p.
    pneumocystis p.
    primary atypical p.
    rheumatic p.
    round p.
    suppurative p.
    varicella p.
    viral p.
    white p.
pneumonic
    patchy p. infiltrate
    infiltrate, p.
pneumonitis
    acute interstitial p.
    aspiration p.
    granulomatous p.
    interstitial p.
    nonspecific p.
    pneumocystis p.
    radiation p.
pneumonocyte
pneumonograph
pneumonolipoidosis
pneumonolysis
pneumonomelanosis
pneumonometer
pneumonomoniliasis
pneumonopathy

Additional Entries

pneumonophthisis
pneumonopleuritis
pneumonoresection
pneumonorrhaphy
pneumopericardium
pneumoperitoneal
pneumoperitoneum
pneumoperitonitis
pneumopleuritis
pneumopleuroparietopexy
pneumoprecordium
pneumopreperitoneum
pneumopyelography
pneumopyopericardium
pneumopyothorax
pneumorachicentesis
pneumorachis
pneumoradiography
pneumoretroperitoneum
pneumoroentgenogram
pneumoroentgenography
pneumorrhagia
pneumosepticemia
pneumoserothorax
pneumosilicosis
pneumotachometer
pneumotachygraph
pneumothorax
  spontaneous p.
  tension p.
  traumatic p.
pneumotomographic chair
pneumotomography
pneumotympanum
pneumoventriculography
Po (polonium)
podarthritis
podedema
podencephalus
podocyte
pododerm
pododynamometer
podogram
podograph
poikiloblast
poikilocarynosis
poikilocyte
poikilocytosis
poikiloderma
  atrophicans vasculare, p.
  patches, p.
poikilodermatomyositis
poikiloploid
poikiloploidy
poikilosmosis
poikilotherm
poikilothermy
poikilothrombocyte
point
  auricular p.
  bleeding p.
  cardinal p.
  craniometric p.
  dose, p.
  far p.
  fixation p.
  jugal p.
  lacrimal p.
  maximum impulse, p. of (PMI)
  McBurney's p.
  near p.
  pressure p.
  source, p.
  source irradiation method, p.
  trigger p.
Poirier's glands
Poisson distribution
Poland syndrome
polarimeter
polarimetry
polariscope
polariscopy

Additional Entries

polaristrobometer
polarity
  circular p.
  elliptical p.
  plane p.
  rotatory p.
polarogram
polar
  rays, p.
  tube, p.
polarized light
pole
  cephalic p.
  fetal p.
  frontal p.
  germinal p.
  lower p. calyx
  negative p.
  occipital p.
  pelvic p.
  positive p.
  temporal p.
poliodystrophy
polioencephalitis
polioencephalomeningomyelitis
polioencephalomyelitis
polioencephalopathy
polioencephalotropic
poliomyclencephalitis
poliomyelitis
  acute p.
  anterior p.
  ascending p.
  bulbar p.
  spinal paralytic p.
poliomyelopathy
polonium (Po)
polyadenitis
polyadenoma
polyadenopathy
polyadenosis
polyadenous
polyangiitis
polyarteritis
  nodosa, p.
polyarthric
polyarthritis
  chronic villous p.
  rheumatica, p.
polyarticular
polyarticular
polyatomic
polyauxotroph
polyaxon
polyblast
polycarbonate syringe
polycarbophil
polycentric
polyceptor
polychemotherapy
polychondritis
  chronic atrophic p.
  relapsing p.
polychondropathy
polychromatocyte
polychromatophil
polychromatosis
polychromic
polyclonal
polyclonia
polycoria
polycystic
  breast, p.
  disease, p.
  kidney, p.
  liver disease, p.
  ovary, p.
  renal disease, p.
polycystoma
polycyte
polycythemia
  absolute p.
  hypertonica p.

Additional Entries

polycythemia *(continued)*
relative p.
rubra, p.
rubra vera, p.
secondary p.
stress p.
vera, p.
polydisperse nature
polydystrophy
polyelectrolyte
polyendocrinoma
polyethylene
polyganglionic
polygenic
polyglandular
polyhydramnios
polyinfection
polykaryocyte
polymastia
polymastigote
polymerize
polymetaphosphate P32
polymicrobial
polymicrolipomatosis
polymicrotome
polymorph
polymorphocellular
polymorphocyte
polymorphonuclear
leukocytes, p.
polyneuromyositis
polyneuropathy
polyneuroradiculitis
polynuclear
polyoma
polyp
adenomatous p.
cervical p.
choanal p.
colonic p.
endocervical p.
endometrial p.

polyp *(continued)*
fibrinous p.
intrauterine p.
juvenile p.
nasal p.
pedunculated p.
rectal p.
retention p.
sentinel p.
sessile p.
polypapilloma tropicum
polyparesis
polyperiostitis
hyperesthetica, p.
polyphagia
polyplegia
polypleurodiaphragmotomy
polyploid
lesion, p.
polypnea
polypoid
adenoma, p.
benign p. adenoma
cystic structure, p.
filling defect, p.
friable mass, p.
lesion, p.
tissue, p.
polyposis
polypous
polypropylene syringe
polyradiculitis
polyradiculoneuritis
polyradiculoneuropathy
polyscope
polyserositis
polysinusectomy
polysinusitis
polysomatic
polysplenia
polysyndactyly
polytendinitis

Additional Entries

polytendinobursitis
polytenosynovitis
polytome
polytomogram
polytomography
polytrophy
polyvinyl
  alcohol foam, p.
  alcohol sponge, p.
  chloride balloon, p.
Poncet's disease
Ponflick's shadow
ponograph
pons (pl. pontes)
  cerebelli, p.
  hepatis, p.
pontes
pontibrachium
pontic
ponticulus
pontine
  cerebellar p. angle
  fissure, p.
pontobulbar
pontocerebellar
pontomedullary
pontomesencephalic
pontopenducular
pontospinal fasciculus
pool contrast agent
poorly
  contoured, p.
  defined, p.
  marginated hypoechoic mass, p.
  opacified kidney, p.
popliteal
  artery, p.
  fossa, p.
  line, p.
  lymph nodes, p.
  muscle, p.
popliteal *(continued)*
  nerves, p.
  space, p.
  vein, p.
popliteus
  muscle, p.
poppet
  dysfunction, p.
  prosthetic valve, p. of
poradenolymphitis
porcelain
  gallbladder, p.
pore
  gustatory p.
porencephalia
porencephalic
  cyst, p.
porencephaly
  communicating p.
  noncommunicating p.
porocele
porokeratosis
porokeratotic
poroma
poropathy
poroplastic
porosis
porous
porphyria
  acute p.
  erythropoietic p.
  hepatic p.
  mixed p.
  variegate p.
port
  entry p.
  film, p.
  verification film, p.
porta
  hepatis, p.
portable
  chest x-ray, p.

Additional Entries

portable *(continued)*
film, p.
ionization chamber, p.
pelvis, p.
view, p.
portacaval shunt
portal
circulation, p.
cirrhosis, p.
hypertension, p.
shunt, p.
sinus, p.
systemic shunt, p.
vein, p.
vein thrombosis, p.
venous gas, p.
x-ray, p.
portio of the cervix
portocaval shunt
portoenterostomy
portography
splenic p.
port-wine hemangioma
porus
acusticus externus osseus, p.
galeni, p.
gustatorius, p.
opticus, p.
sudoriferus, p.
Posada's mycosis
Posada-Wernicke disease
positional shift
positive
beam limitation, p.
electron, p.
end-expiratory pressure, p. (PEEP)
positive contrast
agent, p.c.
encephalography, p.c.
positive contrast *(continued)*
ventriculography, p.c.
positrocephalogram
positron
decay, p.
emission tomography (PET) scan, p.
emitting source, p.
post
infective cavity, p.
irradiation, p.
stenotic dilatation, p.
postanal
postaxial
postbrachial
postbulbar
postcapillary
postcentral
sulcus, p.
postcibal
postcondylar
postcordial
postcornu
postcranial
postcubital
posteriad
posterior
alveolar artery, p.
annular ligament, p.
appositional fields, p.
basis bundle, p.
block, p.
calcaneoastragaloid ligament, p.
capsular dislocation, p.
cervical node, p.
cervical triangle, p.
circumflex numeral artery, p.
column of medulla spinalis, p.

Additional Entries

posterior *(continued)*
- common ligament, p.
- cornu of brain, p.
- cornu of medulla spinalis, p.
- costotransverse ligament, p.
- cricoarytenoid muscle, p.
- deep cervical vein, p.
- dental artery, p.
- elements, p.
- exenteration, p.
- fall-off, p.
- fossa cyst, p.
- ground bundle, p.
- humeral circumflex artery, p.
- inferior space (Morison's pouch), p.
- inferior tibiofibular ligament, p.
- interosseous artery, p.
- interosseous nerve, p.
- lip, p.
- mediastinal mass, p.
- oblique projection, p.
- oblique view, p.
- pillar of fauces, p.
- proper fasciculus, p.
- pulmonary nerves, p.
- radial carpal artery, p.
- radioulnar ligament, p.
- root of spiral nerves, p.
- sacrosciatic ligament, p.
- scapular artery, p.
- scapular nerve, p.
- scrotal nerve, p.
- segments, p.
- spinal artery, p.
- spur, p.
- superior alveolar artery, p.

posterior *(continued)*
- talotibial ligament, p.
- temporal artery, p.
- tibial artery, p.
- tibiofibular ligament, p.
- tilt, p.
- ulnar carpal artery, p.
- ulnar recurrent artery, p.
- vertebral vein, p.

posteroanterior (PA)
- penetrated view, p.
- projection, p.
- view, p.
- view with vertical beam, p.

posteroexternal

posteroinferior

posterointernal

posterolateral
- ganglionic arteries, p.

posteromedial
- ganglionic arteries, p.

posteroparietal

posterosuperior

posterotemporal

postganglionic

postglenoid

posthepatic
- lobectomy, p.

postherpetic

posthyoid

postictal

postischial

postlymphangiogram dye

postlymphangiography

postmastoid

postmature placenta

postmediastinal

postnecrotic cirrhosis

postnodular
- fissure, p.

Additional Entries

postoral
postorbital
postpalatine
postpaludal
postpharyngeal
postpituitary
postpneumonectomy radiation therapy
postpneumonic
postpyramidal
 fissure, p.
postradiation
postreduction
 films, p.
 position, p.
postrenal azotemia
postsacral
postscapular
postsphenoid
post-stress testing
postsurgical treatment-pathologic staging (pTNM)
postsylvian
post-tarsal
post-tibial
postural
 change, p.
 flattening, p.
 maneuver, p.
posture vasopressor drug
postuterine
postvoid
 residual, p.
potassium (K)
potential
 action p.
 doubling time, p. (TP)
 membrane p.
 resting p.
 sensory evoked p.
 spike p.
 visual evoked p.
potentially lethal damage (PLD)
potentially lethal damage repair (PLDR)
potassium chloride K 42
Potter-Bucky grid
Potter's syndrome
Pott's
 aneurysm, P.
 disease, P.
 fracture, P.
 Smith anastomosis, P.
pouch
 blind p.
 Douglas, p. of
 Hartmann's p.
 Morison's p.
 Prussak, p. of
 Rathke's p.
 suprapatellar p.
 vesicouterine p.
 Zenker's p.
Poupart's ligament
povidone I 125
povidone I 131
powdered tantalum
power
 law TAR method, p.
 ratio, p.
praeputium
 clitoridis, p.
 penis, p.
prenal
preaortic
 portion of duodenum, p.
preauricular
 lymph nodes, p.
 point, p.
 radiation, p.
 sulcus of ilium, p.
preaxial
precancer

Additional Entries

precancerous
precapillary
precarcinomatous
precardium
precartilage
precava
precentral
  gyre, p.
  sulcus, p.
precipitin
precipitinogen
precipitinoid
precise immobilization
precision
precocious dentition
precordial
  lead, p.
  radionuclide angiography, p.
precordium
precornu
precostal
precuneus
precursor
predetector scatter
prediverticular
preeclampsia
preganglionic
preglomerular
pregnancy
  abdominal p.
  ampullary p.
  cervical p.
  combined p.
  cornual p.
  ectopic p.
  false p.
  interstitial p.
  intraligamentary p.
  multiple p.
  mural p.
  ovarian p.

pregnancy *(continued)*
  phantom p.
  single intrauterine p.
  tubal p.
  tuboabdominal p.
  tubo-ovarian p.
pregnant
prehemiplegic
prehypophyseal
Preiser's disease
prelacrimal
prelacteal
prelaryngeal
preleukemia
preliminary
  film, p.
  view, p.
premalignant lesion
premitotic
premycotic phase
premyeloblast
prenares
prenature epiphyseal closure
preneoplastic
preoral
prep
  Betadine p.
  bowel p.
prepalatal
preparalytic
prepatellar
  bursa, p.
prepontine
  cistern, p.
prepuce
  clitoris, p. of
  penis, p. of
preputial
prepyramidal
  tract, p.
prerenal
  azotemia, p.

Additional Entries

prerenal *(continued)*
    oliguria, p.
prereticulotic parasporiasis
presacral pneumography
presbyesophagus
prescapula
presclerotic
presentation
    breech p.
    brow p.
    cephalic p.
    compound p.
    footling p.
    funis p.
    longitudinal p.
    oblique p.
    placental p.
    shoulder p.
    transverse p.
    vertex p.
presphenoid
prespondylolisthesis
pressure
    arterial p.
    blood p.
    capillary p.
    central venous p.
    cerebrospinal p.
    continuous positive p. breaathing (CPPB)
    cuff, p.
    extrinsic mass p.
    flow gradient, p.
    high p. chamber
    increased intracranial p.
    intermittent positive p. breathing (IPPB)
    intracranial p.
    intraocular p.
    mean circulatory filling p.
    negative p.

pressure *(continued)*
    osmotic p.
    overload, p.
    partial p.
    positive p.
    positive end-expiratory p.
    pulse p.
    sensation, p.
    venous p.
    wedge p.
prestyloid portion
presylvian
presystole
pretibial
    edema, p.
pretracheal
    fascia, p.
prevertebral
    artery, p.
    fascia, p.
prevesical
    facial cleft, p.
Price-Jones curve
primary
    areolae of bone, p.
    battery, p.
    dose, p.
    fibrosing alveolitis, p.
    megaloureter, p.
    radiation, p.
    rays, p.
    reticulum cell sarcoma, p.
primitive
    aorta, p.
    atrium, p.
    jugular veins, p.
    ova, p.
    sheath of nerve fiber, p.
    urogenital ostium, p.
    ventricle of heart, p.

Additional Entries

primordial dworfism
principal
pathway, p.
quantum number, p.
Pringle's disease
Priodox
prismata
adamantina, p.
prismoptometer
Pro-Banthine
probe
procarcinogen
process
accessory p.
acromial p.
alveolar p.
articular p.
axis-cylinder p.
basilar p.
Blumenbach's p.
caudate p.
ciliary p.
clinoid p.
condyloid p.
coracoid p.
coronoid p.
costal p.
descending p.
dura mater p.
ensiform p.
ethmoid p.
falciform p.
frontal p.
frontonasal p.
frontosphenoidal p.
funicular p.
glenoid p.
gblobular p.
iliac p.
inferior nasal concha p.
inflammatory p.
intrajugular p.

process *(continued)*
jugular p.
lacrimal p.
lateral nasal p.
lenticular p.
lumbar transverse p.
malar p.
mamillary p.
mandibular p.
mastoid p.
maxillary p.
muscular p.
nasal p.
odontoid p.
olecranon p.
orbital p.
palatal p.
palatine p.
papillary p.
paramastoid p.
petrosal p.
petrous p.
phalangeal p.
protoplasmic p.
pterygoid p.
pterygospinous p.
pyramidal p.
sacral p.
septal cartilage p.
sphenoidal p.
spinous p.
styloid p.
supracondylar p.
temporal p.
transverse p.
trochlear p.
trochleariform p.
uncinate p.
vaginal p.
vermiform p.
vertebral p.
vocal p.

Additional Entries

process *(continued)*
xiphoid p.
zygomatic p.
processus
styloideus, p.
proctitis
proctocolectomy
proctocolonoscopy
proctocolpoplasty
proctocystoplasty
proctocystotomy
proctogenic
proctoparalysis
proctoperineoplasty
proctopexy
proctoplasty
proctoplegia
proctoscope
proctoscopy
proctosigmoid
proctosigmoiditis
proctosigmoidopexy
proctosigmoidoscope
proctosigmoidoscopy
proctospasm
proctostasis
proctostenosis
proctostomy
proctotome
proctotomy
prodentin
production process
profundus
proglossis
proglottid
prognathism
prognathometer
progonoma
projected focal spot size
prokaryon
prokaryosis
prokaryote
prolabium
prolactin
prolactinoma
prolapse
cord, p. of
mitral valve p.
rectal p.
uterine p.
prolapsed
hemorrhoid, p.
rectum, p.
vaginal wall, p.
valve, p.
proleukocyte
proliferate
proliferation
proliferative
cycle, p.
endometrium, p.
hyperplasia, p.
phlebitis, p.
prolific
prolonged circulation time
prolymphocyte
PROM (promontory)
promastigote
promegakaryocyte
promegaloblast
promethium (Pm)
prominence
facial canal, p. of
Fallopius aqueduct, p.
gastric rugal p.
laryngeal p.
pulmonary markings, p. of
spiral p.
prominent
digital markings, p.
duct pattern, p.
promonotorium
promontory

Additional Entries

promontory *(continued)*
sacrum, p. of
tympanic cavity, p. of
promyelocyte
pronate
pronation
prone
centered to table, p.
jackknife position, p.
position, p.
view, p.
pronephric
duct, p.
pronephron
pronometer
pronormoblast
pronucleus
propantheline bromide
properitoneal
prophage
prophase
proplasmacyte
propranolol hydrochloride
proprioception
proprioceptive
proprioceptor
propriospinal
proptometer
propyliodone
prorsad
prosencephalon
prosocoele
prosoponeuralgia
prosopopagus
prosopoplegia
prosopoplegic
prosopospasm
prosoposternodymus
prostacyclin
prostaglandin E
prostate
benign hypertrophy of p.
prostate *(continued)*
gland, p.
lobes, p.
transurethral resection of p.
prostatic
benign p. hypertrophy (BPH)
catheter, p.
ducts, p.
hypertrophy, p.
plexus of nerves, p.
portion of urethra, p.
sinus, p.
utricle, p.
prostaticovesical
prostaticovesiculectomy
prostatism
vesical p.
prostatitis
prostatocystitis
prostatocystotomy
prostatodynia
prostatography
prostatolith
prostatomegaly
prostatometer
prostatomyomectomy
prostatorrhea
prostatovesiculectomy
prostatovesiculitis
prosthesis
prosthetic
patch, p.
valve thrombi, p.
prosthion
protactinium (Pa)
protein
bound iodine (PBI), p.
losing enteropathy, p.
proteolipid
proteolytic activity

Additional Entries

protoblast
protocaryon
protochondral
protochondrium
protocol
protogonocyte
protometer
proton
  beam boost, p.
  density, p.
  relaxation time, p.
protoneuron
protopathic
protoplasm
protoplast
protospasm
prototoxin
protovertebra
protraction
  mandibular p.
  maxillary p.
protruded
  intervertebral disc, p.
protrusio acetabuli
protuberance
  mental p.
  occipital p.
Prowazek's bodies
Prowazek-Greeff bodies
proximad
proximal
  convoluted tubule, p.
  insertion, p.
  interphalangeal, p. (PIP)
  tubule disorder, p.
proximate
proximobuccal
proximoceptor
proximolabial
proximolingual
prune belly
pruritic
PRUS (Prussak space)
Prussak's
  fibers, P.
  pouch, P.
psalterium
psammocarcinoma
psammoma
psammomatous calcifications
psammosarcoma
pseudarthritis
pseudarthrosis
pseudencephalus
pseudoacanthosis
  nigricans, p.
pseudoacephalus
pseudoactinomycosis
pseudoalveolar
pseudoaneurysm
pseudoankylosis
pseudoappendicitis
pseudoblock
pseudobronchiectasis
pseudobulbar
pseudocapsule
pseudocartilage
pseudocartilaginous
pseudocele
pseudocephalocele
pseudocholecystitis
pseudocholesteatoma
pseudochromosome
pseudocirrhosis
pseudoclaudication
pseudoclonus
pseudocoarctation
pseudocoele
pseudocoloboma
pseudocyst
pseudodextrocardia
pseudoencephalomalacia
pseudoendometritis
pseudoepiphysis

Additional Entries

pseudoexophthalmos
pseudofolliculitis
pseudofracture
pseudoganglion
pseudogout
pseudoglioma
pseudoglottis
pseudohypertrophic
pseudohypertrophy
pseudohypoparathyroidism
pseudoisochromatic
pseudojaundice
pseudoleukemia
pseudolipoma
pseudolithiasis
pseudomalignancy
pseudomelanosis
pseudomembranous
    angina, p.
    bronchitis, p.
    colitis, p.
    enteritis, p.
    enterocolitis, p.
    gastritis, p.
    trigonitis, p.
pseudomeningitis
pseudomicrocephalus
pseudomucin
pseudomucinous
pseudomyiasis
pseudomyxoma
pseudoneoplasm
pseudoneuroma
pseudo-obstruction
pseudo-optogram
pseudo-osteomalacia
pseudopapilla
pseudoparalysis
pseudoparaplegia
pseudoparesis
pseudopericardial
pseudoplasm
pseudoplegia
pseudopoliomyelitis
pseudopolycythemia
pseudopolyp
pseudopolyposis
pseudo-pseudo hypoparathyroidism
pseudopterygium
pseudoptosis
pseudoretinitis pigmentosa
pseudosclerosis
    spastic p.
    Strumpell-Westphal p.
pseudoscrotum
pseudospherical
pseudostratified columnar epithelium
pseudostoma
pseudostrabismus
pseudotrachoma
pseudotruncus
pseudotubercle
pseudotuberculoma
    silicoticum, p.
pseudotuberculosis
pseudotumor
pseudovacuole
pseudovalve
pseudoxanthoma elasticum
psoas
    abscess, p.
    impression, p.
    margin, p.
    muscle shadow, p.
    shadow, p.
psorenteritis
psoriasis
psoriatic
    arthritis, p.
Pt (platinum)
PTA (percutaneous transluminal angioplasty)

Additional Entries

PTC (percutaneous transhepatic cholangiography)
PTCA (percutaneous transluminal coronary angioplasty)
pterion
ossicle, p.
pterotic center of temporal bone
pterygium
colli, p.
congenital, p.
pterygoid
canal, p.
fissure, p.
fossa, p.
hamulus, p.
muscle, p.
nerve, p.
notch, p.
plate, p.
plexus of veins, p.
processes of sphenoid, p.
tubercle, p.
pterygomandibular
ligament, p.
raphe, p.
pterygomaxillary
fissure, p.
pterygopalatine
canal, p.
fossa, p.
groove, p.
nerve, p.
pterygospinous
ligament, p.
PTHB (percutaneous transhepatic biopsy)
PTHBD (percutaneous transhepatic biliary drainage)
PTHC (percutaneous transhepatic choledochoplasty)
PTHSE (percutaneous transhepatic stone extraction)
PTHSI (percutaneous transhepatic stent insertion)
pTNM (postsurgical treatment-pathological staging)
ptosis
eyelid, p. of
kidney, p. of
ptotic
ptyalocele
ptyalogenic
ptyaloith
ptyalolithiasis
Pu (plutonium)
pubic
symphysis, p.
symphysis gap, p.
tubercle, p.
pubis
angle of p.
body of p.
crest of p.
iliopectineal eminence of p.
obturator crest of p.
rami of p.
symphysis p.
xiphoid to p.
pubocapsular
ligament, p.
pubococcygeus
muscle, p.
pubofemoral
ligament, p.
puboprostatic
ligament, p.
puborectal
puborectalis
muscle, p.
pubotibial
pubovesical

Additional Entries

pubovesical *(continued)*
    ligament, p.
Puck film changer
puddle of contrast material
pudenda (sg. pudendum)
pudendal
    artery,, p.
    accessory artery, p.
    block, p.
    cleft, p.
    nerve, p.
    plexus, p.
    vein, p.
pudendum (pl. pudenda)
    muliebre, p.
pudic
    arteries, p.
pull-through tube
pulmoaortic
pulmogram
pulmometer
pulmonale
    cor p.
    P p.
pulmonary
    angiography, p.
    arterial hypertension, p.
    arteriogram, p.
    arteriography, p.
    arteriovenous communications, p.
    arteriovenous fistula, p.
    artery, p.
    artery aneurysm, p.
    artery atresia, p.
    artery hypoplasia, p.
    aspergillosis, p.
    capillary wedge pressure, p.
    chronic obstructive p. disease (COPD)
    contusion, p.

pulmonary *(continued)*
    edema, p.
    embolism, p. (PE)
    embolus, p.
    emphysema, p.
    eosinophilia, p.
    fibrosis, p.
    function studies, p.
    gangrene, p.
    hyperinflation, p.
    infiltrate, p.
    inhalation study, p.
    insufficiency, p.
    laceration, p.
    ligaments, p.
    nerves, p.
    nodule, p.
    oil emboli, p.
    oligemia, p.
    perfusion study, p.
    pleura, p.
    prominence of p. markings
    semilunar valves, p.
    sequestration, p.
    sling, p.
    stenosis, p.
    systemic flow ratio, p.
    time-activity curve, p.
    valve, p.
    vascular congestion, p.
    vascular markings, p.
    vascular redistribution, p.
    vasculitis, p.
    vein, p.
    ventilation, p.
    venous hypertension, p.
    venous obstruction, p.
    wedge pressure, p.
pulmonic
    atresia, p.

Additional Entries

pulmonic *(continued)*
insufficiency, p.
pulmonoperitoneal
pulp
calcification, p.
stone, p.
pulpa
coronale, p.
lienis, p.
splenica, p.
pulpoaxial
pulpobuccoaxial
pulpodistal
pulpolabial
pulpolingual
pulpolinguoaxial
pulpomesial
pulposus
herniated nucleus p. (HNP)
pulsating
aneurysmn, p.
arterial flow, p.
exophthalmos, p.
mass, p.
pulse (s)
bounding p.
carotid p.
dorsalis pedis p.
feeble p.
femoral p.
forming network
height analysis, p.
height analyzer, p. (window setting)
palpable p.
paradoxical p.
pedal p.
peripheral p.
pileup, p.
popliteal p.
posterior tibial p.

pulse (s) *(continued)*
radial p.
regular p.
sequence, p.
size fluctuation, p.
thready p.
tibial p.
trip-hammer p.
pulsed
digital fluorography, p.
ultrasound, p.
wave (PW) Dopper, p.
pulsimeter
pulsion diverticulum
pulvinar
punch
biopsy, p.
punctated epiphyseal dysplasia
punctiform
punctograph
punctum (pl. puncta)
caecum, p.
punctumeter
puncture
cisternal p.
lumbar p.
needle, p.
spinal p.
sternal p.
pupil (s)
Adie's p.
Argyll-Robertson p.
bounding p.
fixed p.
Hutchinson's p.
pinhole p.
tonic p.
pupillary
membrane, p.
pupillograph
pupillometer

Additional Entries

pupilloplegia
pupilloscope
pupillostatometer
Purkinje's
 cells, P.
 fibers, P.
Purtscher's disease
purulent
 arthritis, p.
puruloid
pus
pustula
pustulation
pustule
pustulosis
 vacciniformis acuta, p.
 varioliformis acuta, p.
putamen
PV (portal vein)
PVL (periventricular leukomalacia)
PW (pulsed-wave)
PW/HPRF (high-pulse repetition frequency rapid sampling)
pyelectasia
pyelectasis
pyelic
pyelitic
pyelitis
 calculous p.
 cystica, p.
 defloration p.
 encrusted p.
 glandularis, p.
 granulosa, p.
 gravidarum, p.
 hematogenous p.
 hemorrhagic p.
 suppurative p.
 urogenous p.
pyelocaliceal
pyelocaliectasis
pyelocystanastomosis
pyelocystitis
pyelocystostomosis
pyelofluoroscopy
pyelogenic cyst
pyelogram
 extretory p.
 intravenous p. (IVP)
 retrograde p.
pyelography
 antegrade p.
 drip infusion p.
 gas p.
 intramuscular p.
 intravenous p.
 retrograde p.
pyeloid metaplasia
pyeloileocutaneous
pyelointerstitial
pyelolithotomy
pyelometry
pyelonephritis
pyelonephrosis
pyelopathy
pyelophlebitis
pyeloplasty
pyeloplication
pyeloscopy
pyeloureterectasis
pyeloureterolysis
pyelovenous
pyemia
 cryptogenic p.
pyknocyte
pyknocytoma
pyknodysostosis
pyknometer
Pyle disease
pylephlebitis
pylethrombophlebitis

Additional Entries

pylethrombosis
pyloric
  antrum, p.
  artery, p.
  channel, p.
  glands, p.
  lymph nodes, p.
  orifice, p.
  stenosis, p.
  ulcer, p.
  valve, p.
  vein, p.
pyloristenosis
pyloritis
pyloroduodenitis
pylorogastrectomy
pyloromyotomy
pyloroplasty
  double p.
  Heineke-Mikulicz p.
pyloroptosis
pyloroscopy
pylorospasm
pylorus
  sphincter of p.
pyocele
pyocolpocele
pyocolpos
pyocyst
pyoderma
  gangrenosum, p.
pyogenic
  abscess, p.
  arthritis, p.
  meningitis, p.
  vertebral osteomyelitis, p.
pyohemothorax
pyolabyrinthitis
pyometrapyometritis
pyometrium
pyomyositis
pyonephritis
pyonephrolithiasis
pyonephrosis
pyonephrotic
pyopericarditis
pyopericardium
pyoperitoneum
pyoperitonitis
pyoneumocholecystitis
pyopneumocyst
pyopneumohepatitis
pyopneumopericardium
pyopneumoperitoneum
pyopneumoperitonitis
pyopneumothorax
pyorrhea
pyosalpingitis
pyosalpinx
pyosclerosis
pyosis
pyoureter
PYP (pyrophosphate) heart scan
pyramid (a/k/a pyramis)
  cerebellum, p. of
  Ferrein, p. of
  Lalouette's p.
  malpighian p.
  medulla oblongata, p. of
  renal p.
  temporal bone, p. of
  thyroid, p. of
  tympanum, p. of
  vermis, p. of
  vestibule, p. of
pyramidal
  cells, p.
  eminence, p.
  lobe, p.
  process, p.

Additional Entries

pyramidal *(continued)*
    tracts, p.
pyramidalis
    muscle, p.
    nasi muscle, p.
pyramis
    medullae oblongatae, p.
pyretogenous
pyretography
pyriform fossa
pyrogen
    free, p.
pyrometer
pyrophosphate (PYP) heart
  scan
pyroscope

Additional Entries

Q

Q angle
QF particles
QRS complex
quadrangle
quadrant
quadrantectomy
quadrate
  lobe of liver, q.
quadrigemina
quadrigeminal
  bodies, q.
  cistern, q.
quadrilateral
quadrilocular
quadripara
quadriparesis
quadriplegia
quadritubercular
quadruped
quantification
  lung scan, q.
  shunt, q.
quantum
  light, q. of
  noise, q.
  number, q.
  physics, q.
  theory, q.
quarter-intensity needle
Quatrefages' angle
Queckenstedt test
quench
Quervain's (de Quervain's) disease
Quimby
  dosimetry, Q.
  planar implant table, Q.
  style interstitial single-plane implant, Q.
  system, Q.
quinaldine blue
quinquecuspid
quinquetubercular
quintisternal

Additional Entries

R

Ra (radium)
racemose
racetrack microtron
rachigraph
rachiometer
rachiomyelitis
rachiopathy
rachitic
    bone changes, r.
    pelvic contour, r.
rad (radiation absorbed dose)
    equivalent therapy, r.
        (ret)
radarkymography
radiad
radial
    artery, r.
    bone, r.
    fibers, r.
    fossa, r.
    head, r.
    neck, r.
    nerve, r.
    notch, r.
    palsy, r.
    peculiarities of r. artery
    pulse, r.
    recurrent r. artery
    styloid, r.
    sulcus, r.
    tuberosity, r.
radiant energy (light or heat)
radiate
    ligament, r.
    sternocostal ligaments, r.
radiating fibrous septa
radiation (s)
    acoustic r.
    adaptive r.
    alpha r.
    annihilation r.

radiation (s) *(continued)*
    auditory r.
    background r.
    beta r.
    B r.
    braking r.
    burn, r.
    Cerenkov r.
    changes, r.
    corpus callosum, r. of
    corpuscular r.
    dose, r.
    dosimetry, r.
    effect, r.
    electromagnetic r.
    fibrosis, r.
    gamma r.
    gastritis, r.
    Gratiolet, r. of
    grid, r.
    heterogeneous r.
    homogeneous r.
    Huldshinsky's r.
    induced periureteral fi-
        brosis, r.
    interstitial r.
    ionizing r.
    irritative r.
    mantle technique, r.
    mitogenic r.
    monoenergetic r.
    myelopathy, r.
    occipitothalamic r.
    optic r.
    palliative r. therapy
    penetration, r.
    photochemical r.
    pneumonitis, r.
    portals, r.
    pyramidal r.
    Rollier's r.

Additional Entries ______________________________

radiation (s) *(continued)*
sensitive tumor, r.
tegmental r.
thalamic r.
thalamotemporal r.
total body r. therapy
white r.
whole brain r. therapy
y r.
Radiation Products Design, Inc.
radical
acid, r.
color, r.
free r.
radiciform
radicula
radicular
cyst, r.
radiculoganglionitis
radiculomedullary
radiculmeningomyelitis
radiculomyelopathy
radiculoneuritis
radiculneuropathy
radiculopathy
cervical r.
lumbar r.
spondylotic caudal r.
radioactive
agent, r.
balloon irradiation method, r.
colloidal gold, r.
daughter, r.
decay, r.
equilibrium, r.
gas, r.
gold, r.
half-life, r. (T 1/2)
iodine, r.
radioactive *(continued)*
iodine uptake test, r. (RAI uptake/RAIU)
isotope, r.
marker, r.
tag, r.
radioaerosol
series, r.
radiobicipital
radiocardiogram
radiocardiography
radiocarpal
angle, r.
articulation, r.
radiocarpus
radiocinematograph
radiocystitis
radioelectrocardiogram
radioelectrocardiograph
radioencephalogram
radioencephalography
radiofluoroscopic control
radiofrequency (RF)
band, r.
signal, r.
radiogenic
radiogold
radiograph
radiographic
baseline, r.
tube, r.
radiography
air contrast r.
body section r.
digital r.
double contrast r.
electron r.
mass r.
mucosal relief r.
neutron r.
panoramic r.

Additional Entries

radiography *(continued)*
  selective r.
  serial r.
  spot-film r.
radiohumeral
  joint, r.
radioimmunity
radioimmunoassay (RIA)
radioimmunodetection
radioimmunodiffusion
radioimmunoelectrophoresis
radioimmunoprecipitation
radioimmunosorbent
radioiodinated human serum albumin (RISHA)
radioiodine uptake
radioiron body distribution
radioisotope (listed alphabetically)
  bone scan, r.
  brain scan, r.
  carrier-free r.
  renal/residual urine study, r.
  renography, r.
radiolabeled
  antibodies, r.
  meal, r.
radiolead
radiolesion
radioligand
radiology
  interventional r.
  percutaneous interventional r.
radiolucency
radiolucent
  area, r.
  band, r.
  bite block, r.
  calculus, r.

radiolucent *(continued)*
  defect, r.
  ring frame, r.
radiolus
radiometallography
radiometer
radiometry
radiomictrometer
radiomuscular
radion
radionecrosis
radioneuritis
radionitrogen
radionuclide
  angiocardiography, r.
  angiogram, r.
  bone scan, r.
  brain scan, r.
  cisternography, r.
  diuretic renography, r.
  dosimetry, r.
  equilibrium angiography, r.
  imaging, r.
  liver scan, r.
  lymphangiogram, r.
  milk scan, r.
  procedure, r.
  purity, r.
  reflux studies, r.
  renal imaging, r.
  scan, r.
  ventriculography, r.
radionuclidic purity, r.
radio-osteonecrosis
radiopacity
radiopaque
  bead, r.
  clip, r.
  contrast medium, r.
  density, r.

Additional Entries ______________________

radiopaque *(continued)*
  iodized compound, r.
  marker, r.
  ruler, r.
radiopelvimetry
radiopharmaceutical
radiophotography
radiopulmonography
radioresistant
radioscleroneter
radioscope
radioscopy
radiosensitive
radiosensitizer
  infusion, r.
radiostereoscopy
radiostrontium
raadiotherapy
radiothorium
radiotracer
radiotransparent
radiotropic
radiotropism
radioulnar
  articulations, r.
  ligaments, r.
  muscles, r.
  union, r.
radio wave
radium (Ra)
  applicator, r.
  bougie, r.
  implant, r.
  needle, r. (226 Ra)
  needle extractor, r.
  needle holder, r.
  salt, r.
  seeds, r.
  sulfate, r.
  tandem, r.
  tube, r. (226 Ra)
Radium Chemical Company
radius
  fracture neck of r.
  styloid process of r.
  ulnar notch of r.
radix
  linguae, r.
  pili, r.
  pulmonis, r.
radon (Rn)
  hazard, r.
  seed implant, r. (222 Rn)
ragocyte
RAI uptake test/RAIU (radioactive iodine uptake)
Rainey's
  corpuscles, R.
  tube, R.
rami
  communicantes, r.
  conjoined, r.
  ischium, r. of
  pubis, r. of
Ramsay Hunt disease
ramus
  communicans r.
  inferior r.
  ischiopubic r.
  mandible, r. of
  nasociliary nerve, r. of
  pubic r.
  superior r.
randomization
226 Ra needle
ranine
  artery, r.
  vein, r.
Ranke's
  angle, R.
  complex, R.

Additional Entries

ranula
  pancreatic r.
Ranvier's
  crosses, R.
  nodes, R.
RAO (right anterior oblique)
raphe
  anococcygeal r.
  lateral palpebral r.
  median r.
  palate, r. of
  pharyngeal r.
  pterygomandibular r.
  scrotum, r. of
  septal r.
rapid
  alternating movements, r.
  dose falloff, r.
  eye movement, r. (REM)
  fall off of dose, r.
  flow, r.
  plasma reagin, r.
  sequence IVP, r.
  sequence changer, r.
  transit of contrast medium, r.
rarefaction
Rasmussen's aneurysm
Rathke's pouch
ratio
  arteriovenous r.
  cardiothoracic r.
  inspiratory-expiratory r.
  magnetogyric r.
Rauber's layer
Rachfuss' sling
226 Ra radioisotope needle
226 Ra radioisotope tube
ray (types listed alphabetically)
ray *(continued)*
  photon involvement, r.
Raymond's apoplexy
Raynaud's
  disease, R.
  phenomenon, R.
Rb (rubidium)
RBB (right bundle branch)
RBBB (right bundle branch block
RBE (relative biologic efficiency/effectiveness)
Re (rhenium)
reabsorption
  tubular r.
reagin
  atopic r.
real-time
  cardiac visualization, r.
  imaging, r.
  motion studies, r.
  two-dimensional real time imaging, r.
  ultrasonography, r.
recalcification
recanalization
receiver coil
receiver-operating characteristics (RDC)
receptacle
receptaculum chyli
receptor
  blurring, r.
  plane, r.
recess (s)
  cochlear r.
  costodiaphragmatic r.
  duodenal r.
  epitympanic r.
  ileocecal r.
  infundibular r.

Additional Entries ______________________

recess (s) *(continued)*
  internal ear r.
  lacrimal r.
  lateral r.
  nasopalatine r.
  omental r.
  optic r.
  paraduodenal r.
  pelvic mesocolon r.
  peritoneal r.
  pharyngeal r.
  pineal r.
  pleural r.
  pneumatoenteric r.
  retrocecal r.
  retroduodenal r.
  sphenoethmoidal r.
  Troltsch r.
recessus
  ellipticus, r.
  infundibuli, r.
  intersigmoideus, r.
  pinealis, r.
  sacciformis, r.
  sphericus, r.
  sphenoethmoidalis, r.
  spherical, r.
  suprapinealis, r.
  third ventricle, r.
Recklinghausen's disease
Reclus' disease
recirculation curve shunt
recoil electron
recrudescence
recruitment pattern
rectal
  abscess, r.
  ampulla, r.
  canal, r.
  columns of Morgagni, r.
  fistula, r.
  plug, r.
rectal *(continued)*
  prolapse, r.
  skin tag, r.
  sphincter, r.
  tear, r.
rectangular fields
recti
  diastasis r. abdominis
rectification
rectilinear
  pencil beam scanning, r.
  scanner, r.
rectoabdominal
rectocele
rectococcygeal
  muscles, r.
rectocutaneous
rectolabial
rectoromanoscope
rectoromanoscopy
rectosigmoid
rectostenosis
rerctourethroperineal fistula
rectouterine
  excavation, r.
  fold, r.
  ligament, r.
  muscle, r.
  pouch, r.
rectovaginal
  fistula, r.
  septum, r.
rectovesical
  excavation, r.
  folds, r.
  layer of pelvic fascia, r.
rectovestibular
rectovulvar
rectum
  ampulla of r.
  Houston's valves of r.
rectus sheath

Additional Entries

recumbent
- anteroposterior projection (AP), r.
- position, r.
- posteroanterior projection (PA), r.

recumbent view
recurrence time distribution
recurrent
- artery, r.
- laryngeal nerve, r.
- nerve, r.
- radial artery, r.
- tibial artery, r.
- tumor, r.
- ulnar artery, r.

recurvatum deformity
red
- blood cell-mediated deposition, r.
- Congo r.
- corpuscles, r.
- nucleus, r.
- phenol r.
- Robinson catheter, r.
- scarlet r.
- vital r.

red cell
- iron utilization, r.c.
- mass, r.c.
- sequestration, r.c.
- survival, r.c.

redistribution
- perfusion imaging, r.
- purity, r.

reduce
reducible
reduction
- closed r. of fracture
- manual r.
- open r. and internal fixation (ORIF)

redundant
- foreskin, r.
- prepuce, r.

Reese and Ellsworth system
reference
- detector, r.
- electrode, r.

reflected
- inguinal ligament, r.
- light, r.
- rays, r.
- skin flaps, r.
- sound, r.
- vesicouterine peritoneum, r.

reflection
- bladder r.
- coefficient, r.
- pleura, r. of
- peritoneal r.
- uterine r.

reflex
- abdominal r.
- accommodation r.
- Achilles tendon r.
- anal r.
- ankle r.
- auditory r.
- Babinski's r.
- biceps r.
- Brain's r.
- carotid sinus r.
- Chaddock's r.
- chain r.
- ciliary r.
- ciliospinal r.
- conditioned r.
- conjunctival r.
- corneal r.
- cough r.
- cremasteric r.
- deep r.

Additional Entries

reflex *(continued)*
deep tendon r.
digital r.
diving r.
embrace r.
gag r.
gastrocolic r.
gastroileal r.
grasp r.
Hoffmann's r.
jaw r.
jaw-jerk r.
knee r.
light r.
Magnus and de Kleijn neck r.
Mayer's r.
Mendel-Bekhterev r.
Moro r.
myotatic r.
neck righting r.
nocioceptive r.
Oppenheim's r.
orbicularis oculi r.
palatal r.
palmomental r.
patellar r.
patellar tendon r.
paths, r.
pharyngeal r.
physiologic r.
pilomotor r.
placing r.
plantar r.
proprioceptive r.
psychogalvanic r.
pupillary r.
quadriceps r.
quadrupedal extensor r.
red r.
righting r.
Rossoilimo's r.

reflex *(continued)*
spinal r.
startle r.
stepping r.
stretch r.
sucking r.
superficial r.
sympathetic dystrophy syndrome, r. (RSDS)
swallowing r.
tendon r.
tonic neck r.
triceps r.
triceps surae r.
vestibulo-ocular r.

reflux
barium, r. of
esophageal r.
esophagitis, r.
filling, r.
gastric r.
gastroesophageal r.
hepatojugular r.
intrarenal r.
mitral r.
urethrovesiculo-differential r.
vesicoureteral r.

refracted
light, r.
rays, r.

refracting media of eye

refractive edge shadowing

refracture

Refsum's disease

refusion

regime
chemotherapy r.

regional
anesthesia, r.
block, r.
colitis, r.

Additional Entries

regional *(continued)*
- enteritis, r.
- growth, r.
- ileitis, r.
- invasion, r.
- metastases, r.
- migratory osteoporosis, r.
- myocardial infarction, r.
- tidal ventilation, r.
- wall motion analysis, r.

region of interest (ROI)

Reglan

regurgitant
- refraction, r.

regurgitation
- aortic r.
- mitral r.
- tricuspid r.

Rehfuss' tube

Reichel's cloacal duct

Reichert's canal

Reichmann's disease

Reid's baseline

Reil's
- ansa, R.
- island, R.

Reisseisen's muscles

Reissner's
- fiber, R.
- membrane, R.

Reiter syndrome

relapsing polychondritis

relative biologic efficiency/effectiveness (RBE)

relaxation
- ferromagnetic r.
- isometric r.
- nuclear r.
- paramagnetic r.
- spin-lattice r.
- spin-spin r.

relaxation *(continued)*
- time, r.

relaxed
- introitus, r.
- pelvic floor, r.
- perineal body, r.

rem (roentgen equivalent man)

Remak's
- band, R.
- paralysis, R.

remnant radiation

removable implant

renal
- arteriography, r.
- artery, r.
- artery aneurysm, r.
- artery atheroma, r.
- asymmetry, r.
- backflow, r.
- calculus, r.
- calyces, r.
- capsule, r.
- cell carcinoma, r.
- colic, r.
- collecting system, r.
- columns, r.
- contour, r.
- contusion, r.
- corpuscles, r.
- cortex, r.
- cortical necrosis, r.
- cystic lesion, r.
- decortication, r.
- failure, r.
- fascia, r.
- flow study, r.
- fossa, r.
- function, r.
- hilum, r.
- imaging, r.
- implant, r.

Additional Entries

renal *(continued)*
- impression, r.
- infarct, r.
- insufficiency, r.
- lithiasis, r.
- mass, r.
- osteodystrophy, r.
- papillitis, r.
- parenchyma, r.
- parenchymal atrophy, r.
- parenchymal retention of bone scanning agents, r.
- pedicle, r.
- pelvis, r.
- plexus, r.
- pyramids, r.
- scan, r.
- sinus, r.
- sinus echo, r.
- sinus lipomatosis, r.
- size, r.
- sonogram, r.
- stenosis, r.
- tuberculosis, r.
- tubular acidosis, r.
- tubular block, r.
- tubular ectasia, r.
- tubules, r.
- vascular hypertension, r.
- vein, r.
- vein thrombosis, r.
- vessels, r.

Renaut's bodies
Rendu's tremor
Rendu-Osler-Weber disease
renin-angiotensin system
renipelvic
reniportal
renipuncture
renocortical
renocutaneous
renocystogram
renogastric
renogram
Renografin
Renografin-60
Renografin-76
renogram
- curves, r.
- 131 I-hippuran cortical renogram)

renography
renointestinal
renolithiasis
Reno-M-Dip
Reno-M-60
Reno-M-30
Renotec
renotrophic
renotropic
renopathy
Renovist II
reoxygenation
repetition time (TR)
rephasing gradient
repolarization
reproductive system
resectoscope
resectoscopy
reserpine
reservoir effect
residual
- blood pool activity, r.
- contrast material, r.
- fibrocystic r.
- post void r.

residuum
- gastric r.
- sporal r.

resistive heating
resonance
- tympanitic r.
- vesicular r.

Additional Entries

resonance *(continued)*
vocal r.
resonant
frequency, r.
percussion, r. to
radiofrequency (RF), magnetic field r.
respiration
abdominal r.
aerobic r.
anaerobic r.
artificial r.
Biot's r.
bronchovesicular r.
Cheyne-Stokes r.
cogwheel r.
electrophrenic r.
embarrassed r.
external r.
grunting r.
internal r.
Kussmaul's r.
labored r.
paradoxical r.
shallow r.
stertorous r.
suppressed r.
tissue r.
tubular r.
vesicular r.
respiratory
acidosis, r.
alkalosis, r.
apparatus, r.
arrest, r.
assistance, r.
distress, r.
embarrassment, r.
excursion, r.
failure, r.
nerve of Bell, r.
obstruction, r.
respiratory *(continued)*
standstill, r.
stridor, r.
system, r.
upper r. infection (URI)
rest exercise thallium imaging
restiform
bodies of medulla, r.
resting potential
restitutio
integrum, r.
restricted angle tomography
resurfacing procedure
ret (rad equivalent therapy)
retained
barium, r.
fecal material, r.
foreign body, r.
placental tissue, r.
products of conception, r.
secretions, r.
rete (pl. retia)
canalis hypoglossi, r.
foraminis ovalis, r.
testis, r.
retention
cyst, r.
suture, r.
urinary r.
retethelioma
retia (sg. rete)
venosa vertebrarum, r.
reticula
reticular
activating system, r.
dermis, r.
fibers of connective tissue, r.
formation, r.
lamina, r.
layer of skin, r.

Additional Entries

reticulitis
reticulocyte
reticulocytogenic
reticulocytopenia
reticulocytosis
reticuloendothelial
 marrow, r.
reticuloendothelioma
reticuloendotheliosis
reticulendothelium
reticulohistiocytoma
reticulohistiocytosis
reticuloid
reticuloma
reticulosarcoma
reticulosis
reticulothelium
reticulum
 cell sarcoma, r.
retina
 central artery of r.
 ciliary part of r.
 fovea centralis, r.
 layers of r.
 macula lutea, r.
 pars optica of r.
 pars ciliaris of r.
 pars iridica of r.
 supporting framework of r.
retinacula
 hip-joint, r. of
 patellar r.
 peroneal r.
retinaculum
 flexor r.
retinacope
retinal angioma
retinitis
 circinate r.
 disciformis, r.
 exudative r.

retinitis *(continued)*
 hemorrhagica, r.
 pigmentosa, r.
 proliferans, r.
 suppurative r.
retinoblastoma
retinochoroid
retinochoroiditis
retinograph
retinography
retinoid
retinomalacia
retinopapillitis
retinopathy
 circinate r.
 diabetic r.
 exudative r.
 hypertensive r.
 proliferative r.
retinoschisis
retinoscope
retinoscopy
retinosis
retinotopic
retinotoxic
retracted
 chest muscles, r.
 wound edges, r.
retractile mesenteritis
retraction (s)
 breast nipple r.
 eardrum r.
 scar r.
 subcostal r.
 suprasternal r.
retractor
retrad
retreatment staging (rTNM)
retroaortic node
retroareolar
 dysplasia, r.
retroauricular

Additional Entries ____________________________

retrobronchial
retrobuccal
retrobulbar
retrocalcaneal spur
retrocalcaneobursitis
retrocardiac
retrocaval ureter
retrocecal
 appendix, r.
retrocervical
retrocession
retroclavicular
retrocochlear
retrocolic
retrocollis
retrocrural
retrodental space
retroesophageal
retroflexed
retroflexion
retrogasserian
retroglandular
 sulcus of penis, r.
regrognathia
retrograde
 amnesia, r.
 arteriogram, r.
 brachial cutdown, r.
 femoral catheterization, r.
 filling, r.
 flow of barium, r.
 left ventricular route, r.
 pyelogram, r.
 pyelography, r.
 urethrogram, r.
 urogram, r.
retrography
retrogression
retrolental
retrolenticular
retrolingual
retromammary
 bursa, r.
 space, r.
retromandibular
retromastoid
retromesenteric
retromolar trigone
retronasal
retro-occipital
 fissure, r.
retro-ocular
retroparotid
retropatellar
retroperitoneal
 fat, r.
 fibrosis, r.
 fossae, r.
 pneumography, r.
 radical r. node dissection
 space, r.
retroperitoneum
retroperitonitis
retropharyngeal
 lymph nodes, r.
 space, r.
retropharyngitis
retropharynx
retroplacental
retroplasia
retropleural
retroposition
retrorectal
retrosinus
retrospondylolisthesis
retrosternal
retrosymphysial
retrotarsal
retrouterine
retroversion
retroverted
retrovesical
 septum, r.

Additional Entries

Retzius'
colored lines, R.
foramen, R.
space, R.
revascularization
Reverdin's
graft, R.
needle, R.
reverse
flow, r.
isolation, r.
reversed
butterfly pattern, r.
shunt, r.
reversible
reversion
R factor
RF (regurgitation fraction)
RF coil
Rh (rhodium)
rhabdocyte
rhabdoid
rhabdomyolysis
rhabdomyoma
rhabdomyomyxoma
rhabdomyosarcoma
rhacoma
Rh disease
rhenium (Re)
rhenium-tungsten-faced molybdenum anodes
rheoscope
rheumatoid
arthritis, r.
lung, r.
rhinal
fissure, r.
rhinalgia
rhinencephalon
rhinenchysis
rhinesthesia
rhinoanemometer
rhinoantritis
rhinobyon
rhinocephaly
rhinocheiloplasty
rhinocoele
rhinodacryolith
rhinogenous
rhinolaryngitis
rhinolith
rhinolithiasis
rhinomanometer
rhinomanometry
rhinometer
rhinonecrosis
rhinopathy
rhinopharyngitis
rhinopharyngocele
rhinopharyngolith
rhinopharynx
rhinophycomycosis
rhinophyma
rhinoplasty
rhinopneumonitis
rhinorrhea
rhinosalpingitis
rhinoscleroma
rhinoscope
rhinoscopy
rhinostenosis
rhinotracheitis
rhizoblast
rhizodontropy
rhizoid
rhizoplast
rhodium (Rh)
rhodium-106
rhodopsin
rhombencephalon
rhombic
grooves, r.

Additional Entries

rhombic *(continued)*
  lip,r .
rhombocoele
rhomboid
  fossa, r.
  impression, r.
  ligament, r.
rhomboideus
  major muscles, r.
  minor muscle, r.
  occipitalis muscle, r.
rhythm
  atrioventricular .r
  auriculoventricular r.
  bigeminal r.
  cardiac r.
  circadian r.
  escape r.
  gallop r.
  idioventricular r.
  nodal r.
  regular sinus r.
  strip, r.
  theta r.
  ventricular r.
RIA (radioimmunoassay)
rib (s)
  asternal r.
  cage intact, r.
  cervical r.
  false r.
  floating r.
  infarct, r.
  notching, r.
  slipping r.
  true r.
  vertebrochondral r.
  vertebrosternal r.
ribbon ribs
Ribe's ganglion
Richet's aneurysm
Richter's hernia
Richter-Monro line
ridge
  dental r.
  dermal r.
  epipericardial r.
  ganglion r.
  genital r.
  healing r.
  interureteric r.
  mammary r.
  mesonephric r.
  oblique r.
  Passavant's r.
  supracondylar r.
  suprarenal r.
  synaptic r.
  trapezoid r.
  urethral r.
  urogenital r.
ridging
Ridley's sinus
Riedel's lobe
Rieder's cell
Riegel's pulse
Riehl's melanosis
Riesman's pneumonia
Rieux's hernia
RIF-1 fibrosarcoma
Riga-Fede disease
right
  angled wedge, r.
  anterior oblique position, r. (RAO)
  anterior oblique view, r.
  aortic arch, r.
  atrial angiography, r.
  atrium, r.
  auricle, r.
  auricular appendix, r.
  coronary artery, r.
  coronary plexus, r.
  coronary veins, r.

Additional Entries

right *(continued)*
- ductus, r.
- gastroepiploic lymph nodes, r.
- heart catheterization, r.
- heart failure, r.
- iliac fossa, r.
- lateral view, r.
- lower lobe, r. (RLL)
- posterior oblique position, r. (RPO)
- posterior oblique view, r.
- recumbent lateral projection, r.
- shoulder girdle, r.
- sided collecting structures, r.
- sided lesions, r.
- -to-left shunt, r.
- ventricle, r.
- ventricular infarction, r.
- ventriculography, r.

rigid
- bronchoscope, r.
- esophagoscopy, r.
- segment, r.
- stomach, r.

Riley-Day syndrome

rim

rima
- glottidis, r.
- mouth, r. of
- palpebrarm, r.
- pudendal, r.
- vestibuli, r.

ring (s)
- abdominal r.
- Bandl's r.
- Cannon's r.
- ciliary r.

ring (s) *(continued)*
- conjunctival r.
- constriction r.
- deep inguinal r.
- enhancement, r.
- external inguinal r.
- fibrous r.
- forceps, r.
- hymenal r.
- internal inguinal r.
- Kayser-Fleischer r.
- retraction r.
- Schwalbe's r.
- shaped, r.
- superficial inguinal r.
- third cartilaginous r.
- tracheal r.
- tympanic r.
- umbilical r.
- vascular r.

Ring-McLean catheter

ring fracture

ring-wall lesion

Riolan's
- arc, R.
- anastomosis, R.

ripple reduction

RISHA (radioiodinated human serum albumin)

risorius muscle

Ritter's disease

Rivinus's
- ducts, R.
- notch, R.

RL (right lateral)

RLL (right lower lobe)

RM 50 (racetrack microtron)

R-meter

R/minute

Rn (radon)

222 Rn radioisotope seed

Additional Entries

Robert's
ligament, R.
pelvis, R.
Robertson's pupil
Robinson catheter
Robinson's circle
Robson's
point, R.
position, R.
ROC (receiver-operating characteristics)
rocker-bottom syndrome
rod (s)
box device, r.
Corti r.
intermedullary r.
olfactor r.
retinal r.
Rush r.
rod bipolars of retina
rod granules of retina
roentgen-equivalent-man (rem)
roentgenkymography
roentgenocardiogram
roentgenocinematography
roentgenogram
roentgenography
roentgenolucent
roentgenomcter
rocntgenometry
roentgenoscope
roentgenoscopy
roentgenotherapy
roentgen
radiation, r.
rays, r.
Roger's disease
Rogers' sphygmomanometer
Rohl's marginal corpuscles
ROI (region of interest)
Rokitansky's
Aschoff sinus, R.
disease, R.
diverticulum, R.
Rolando
fissure of R.
substantia gelatinosa of R.
tubercle of R.
Rolf-circle
Roller's nucleus
Rollet's chancre
Rollet's stroma
Rollier's radiation
Romanovsky's stained smear
Romberg's disease
Romberg's
sign, R.
station, R.
root
anterior r.
aortic r.
decompression, nerve r.
dorsal r.
lung r.
mesentery, r. of
nerve r.
penis r.
posterior r.
resorption, r.
sclerosis, r.
sensory r.
sheath, r.
sheath cyst, r.
sleeve, r.
spinal nerve r.
teeth, r. of
tongue, r. of
transverse mesocolon, r. of
ventral r.

Additional Entries ______

rosary beading
Rosch-Thurmond catheterization set
rose bengal scintigraphy (I 131)
rose bengal sodium I 125
Rosenmuller's
 body, R.
 fossa, R.
 lymph node, R.
 organ, R.
Rosenthal's
 canal, R.
 vein, R.
Rosch catheter
Rose position
Ross's bodies
Rossbach's disease
Rostan's asthma
rostrad
rostral
rostrum
 corpus callosum, r.
 sphenoidal r.
ROT (right occipitotransverse)
rotary
 scoliosis, r. joint
 subluxation, r.
 thoracolumbar scoliosis, r. joint
rotating
 chair, r.
 frame, r.
 gantry system, r.
rotation
 advancement flap, r.
 apex, r. of
 speed, r.
 technique, r.
 therapy, r.
 vertebral r.
rotational
 electron beam dosimetry, r.
 field, r.
 technique, r.
 movement, r.
rotator
 cuff injury, r.
 cuff tear, r.
 muscles, r.
rotatory scoliosis
Roth's disease
Roth's spots
Roth-Bernhardt disease
rotoscoliosis
Rouget's
 bulb, R.
 cells, R.
Rougnon-Heberden disease
round
 atelectasis, r.
 back, r.
 metal marker, r.
 pneumonia, r.
round ligament
 hip joint, r.l. of
 liver, r.l. of
 uterus, r.l. of
Rous sarcoma
Roussy-Levy disease
Rouviere, nodes of
Royal Flush catheter
RPF (renal plasma flow)
RPO (right posterior oblique)
RSDS (reflex sympathetic dystrophy syndrome)
rTNM (retreatment staging)
Ru (ruthenium)
rubber
 catheter, r.
 jaws, r.

Additional Entries

Rubenstein-Taybi syndrome
rubidium (Ru)
rubidium chloride Rb 86
rubrospinal
  fasciculus, r.
rudimentary
  horn, r.
  uterus, r.
Ruffini's corpuscles
ruga (pl. rugae)
rugal
  coarsening, r.
  folds, r.
  pattern, r.
  prominence, r.
rugoscopy
rugous
rugosity
Rummo's disease
rump
runoff
  arteriofemoral r.
  arterial r.
rupture
  Achilles tendon r.
  membranes, r. of artificial
rupture *(continued)*
  premature r. of membranes
  prolonged r. of membranes
ruptured
  aneurysm, r.
  bullae, r.
  esophagus, r.
  ectopic, r.
  intervertebral disc, r.
  organ, r.
  pneumatosis coli, r.
  tracheobronchial tree, r.
  viscus, r.
Rusconi's anus
Russell's bodies
Russell-Silver dwarfism
ruthenium-106
rutherford unit
Ruysch's tube
RVH (right ventricular hypertrophy)
RWHM (full width at half maximum)
Rye modification
Ryle's tube

Additional Entries

S

S (sulfur)
SAC (spinal accessory chain)
sac
  air s.
  alveolar s.
  amniotic s.
  aortic s.
  conjunctival s.
  conjunctival cul-de-sac
  cul-de-sac
  dental s.
  Douglas cul-de-sac
  dural s.
  fluid-filled s.
  free fluid in cul-de-sac
  intrauterine gestational s.
  lacrimal s.
  lesser s.
  peritoneal s.
  thecal s.
  umbilical s.
saccharascope
saccular
  outpouching, s.
sacculated
sacculation
  colon, s. of
saccule
  laryngeal s.
  ear, s. of
  vestibule, s. of
sacculi
sacculocochlear
sacculus
saccus
  lacrimalis, s.
  vaginalis, s.
Sachs' disease
sacrad
sacral
  artery, s.
  canal, s.
  cornua, s.
  crest, s.
  foramina, s.
  groove, s.
  hiatus puncture method, s.
  lymph nodes, s.
  nerves, s.
  nucleus, s.
  parasympathetic nerves, s.
  plexus, s.
  prominence, s.
  spine, s.
  sympathetics, s.
  tuberosity, s.
  veins, s.
sacralization
sacrococcygeal
  ligaments, s.
sacrococcyx
sacrocoxitis
sacrogenital
  folds, s.
sacroiliac
  articulation, s.
  joint, s.
  ligaments, s.
  notch, s.
sacrolisthesis
sacrolumbar
sacroperineal
sacroposterior
sacropromontory
sacrosciatic
  ligaments, s.
sacrospinal

Additional Entries ______________________________

____

____

sacrospinalis
    muscles, s.
sacrotransverse
sacrotuberous ligaments
sacrouterine
sacrovertebral
    angle, s.
    joint, s.
sacrum
    ala of s.
    apex, s.
    articulations of s.
    auricular surface of s.
    base of s.
SAD (source-to-axis distance)
    linear accelerator, SAD
saddle
    block anesthesia, s.
    deformity of nose, s.
    joint, s.
Saenger's macula
sagittal
    fontanelle, s.
    fossa, s.
    plane, s.
    projection, s.
    sinus, s.
    sulcus, s.
    suture, s.
sala's cells
saline
    formaldehyde gel, s.
    infusion pressure-flow study, s.
salivary
    duct, s.
    fistula, s.
    glands, s.
    parotid gland, s.
    sublingual glands, s.
    submaxillary glands, s.

salivary *(continued)*
    view, s.
salpingion
salpingocele
salpingography
salpingolithiasis
salpingolysis
salpingo-oophorocele
salpingo-oothecitis
salpingo-oothecocele
salpingopalatine
    fold, s.
salpingoperitonitis
salpingopexy
salpingopharyngeal
    fold, s.
salpingopharyngeus
    muscle, s.
salpingoscopy
salpingostomatomy
salpingostomatoplasty
salpingostomy
salpingotomy
salpinx
Salter's
    fracture, S.
    incremental lines, S.
    I,II,III,IV,V,VI fracture, S.
Salter-Harris Type II fracture
salt loading
salvage surgery
Salzmann's nodular corneal dystrophy
samarium (Sm)
Sampson's cyst
sandbag
Sanders' disease
Sandstrom's glands
sandwich technique
Sandwith's bald tongue
Sanfilippo syndrome

Additional Entries

sanguinopurulent
sanguirenal
saniopurulent
sanioserous
Santorini's
  cartilages, S.
  duct, S.
saphenous
  greater s. system
  high s. vein ligation
  lesser s. system
  nerves, s.
  opening, s.
  system, s.
  veins, s.
  vein graft, s.
  vein ligation, s.
Sappey's fibers
SAR (scatter-to-air ratio)
sarcoblast
sarcocarcinoma
sarcocele
sarcocyst
sarcocyte
sarcogenic
sarcoglia
sarcohydrocele
sarcoid
sarcoidosis
sarcolemma
sarcoma
  Abernethy's s.
  adipose s.
  alveolar soft part s.
  ameloblastic s.
  botryoid s.
  botryoides, s.
  chicken s.
  chloromatous s.
  chondroblastic s.
  colli uteri hydropicum papillare, s.

sarcoma *(continued)*
  deciduocellular s.
  embryonal s.
  endometrial stromal s.
  Ewing's s.
  fascial s.
  fibroblastic s.
  fowel s.
  giant cell s.
  granulocytic s.
  Hodgkin's s.
  idiopathic multiple pigmented hemorrhagic s.
  Jensen's s.
  Kaposi's s.
  Kupffer cell s.
  leukocytic s.
  lymphatic s.
  melanotic s.
  mixed cell s.
  multiple idiopathic hemorrhagic s.
  osteoblastic s.
  osteogenic s.
  osteoid s.
  osteolytic s.
  parosteal s.
  polymorphous s.
  reticulocytic s.
  reticuloendothelial s.
  reticulum cell s.
  retrothelial s.
  Rous s.
  serocystic s.
  synovial s.
  telangiectatic s.
sarcomata
sarcomatoid
sarcomatosis
sarcomatous
sarcomphalocele
sarcoplasm

Additional Entries

sarcoplast
sarcosis
sarcotubule
sarcous
sartorius
    muscle, s.
satellite
    collimator, s.
    lesion, s.
    nodule, s.
    peak, s.
    platform, s.
    skin nodule (s), s.
satellitosis
Sattler's layer
saturation-recovery
saucer-shaped pressure defect
Saunders' disease
Saynac rays
Sayre's apparatus
Sb (antimony)
Sc (scandium)
scala
    media, s.
    tympani, s.
    vestibuli, s.
scale
    false color s.
    gray s.
scalene
    fat pad, s.
    lymph node, s.
    node biopsy, s.
    tubercle, s.
scalloped cortex
scalp
    avulsion, s.
    defect, s.
    gyrate s.
scan
    axial s.
    bone s.

scan *(continued)*
    CAT (computerized axial tomography) s.
    CT (computerized tomography) s.
    flow s.
    gallium s.
    liver-spleen s.
    medronate s.
    MUGA (multiple gated acquisition) s.
    PIPIDA s.
    stacked s.
    thallium s.
    ventillation perfusion (VQ) s.
    VQ (ventilation perfusion) s.
Scanditronix RM50 accelerator
Scanditronix M 22 accelerator
scandium (Sc)
scanner (scanners under alpha listing)
    emission computerized tomographic s.
    GE 9800 high resolution CT s.
    high field strength s.
    total body s.
scanning
    device, s.
    electron microscopy s.
    mode, s.
    radioisotope s.
scanography
scapha
scaphocephaly
scaphoid
    abdomen, s.
    bone, s.

Additional Entries ____________________

____

____

scaphoid *(continued)*
  fossa, s.
  scapula, s.
scaphoiditis
scapula
  acromion of s.
  coracoid process of s.
  glenoid cavity of s.
  scaphoid s.
  semilunar notch of s.
  spine of s.
scapular
  arteries, s.
  circumflex artery, s.
  nerve, s.
  notch, s.
scapuloanterior
scapuloclavicular
  articulation, s.
scapulodynia
scapulohumeral
scapuloposterior
scapus
  pili, s.
scar
  bolus, s.
  carcinoma, s.
  hypertrophied s.
  massive s. tissue
  operative s.
  retraction, s.
  revision, s.
scarification
Scarpa's
  fascia, S.
  foramina, S.
  ganglion, S.
  nerve, S.
  sheath, S.
  triangle, S.
scatter
  maximum ratio, s. (SMR)

scatter *(continued)*
  radiation, s.
  to air ratio, s. (SAR)
  to primary ratio, s.
scattered
  diverticula, s.
  dose, s.
  photon, s.
  radiation, s.
  radiation contrast, s.
  radiation quality, s.
  rays, s.
scattergram
scattering
  broad beam, s.
  foils, s.
Schacher's ganglion
Schachowa's spiral tubes
Schatzki's ring
Schaumann's bodies
Scheie syndrome
schematic diagram
Scheuermann's disease
Schiefferdecker's disk
Schiff's biliary cycle
Schilder's disease
Schiller's test
Schilling test
Schimmelbusch's disease
schindylesis
Schiotz tonometer
schistothorax
schizencephalic
schizencephaly
schizogenous
Schlatter's disease
Schlatter-Osgood disease
Schlemm's canal
Schmidt's fibrinoplastin
Schmincke tumor
Schmorl's
  bacillus, S.
  disease, S.

Additional Entries

Schmorl's *(continued)*
node, S.
nodule, S.
Schnabel's caverns
schneiderian membrane
Schoemaker's line
Scholz's disease
Schonlein's disease
Schonlein-Henoch disease
Schonlein-Henoch purpura
Schottmuller's disease
Schreger's
bands, S.
lines, S.
Schridde's disease
Schroeder's
disease, S.
syndrome, S.
Schron's granule
Schron-Much granules
Schuffner's dots
Schuller's
disease, S.
method, S.
position, S.
view, S.
Schuller-Christian disease
Schultze's
cells, S.
fold, S.
sign, S.
test, S.
Schultz's micrococcus
Schumann rays
Schwalbe's
corpuscles, S.
nucleus, S.
schwannoma
Schwann's
cell, S.
sheath, S.
Schwartz introducer
Schweigger-Seidel sheath
sciatic
artery, s.
foramen, s.
nerve, s.
nerve distribution, s.
notch, s.
veins, s.
scimitar
sign, s.
syndrome, s.
scintigraphic
appearance, s.
features, s.
pattern, s.
study, s.
scintigraphy
67 Ga s.
I 131 rose bengal s.
scintillation
camera, s.
crystal detector, s.
detector, s.
scintiphoto
scintiphotograph
scintiscan
scintiscanner
scirrhoid
scirrhoma
scirrhophthalmia
scirrhous
sclera
buckling of s.
scleradenitis
sclerae
scleral
sclerencephaly
sclerenchyma
sclerenchymatous
scleriasis
scleroblastema
sclerochoroiditis
scleroconjunctival

Additional Entries

sclerocorneal
junction, s.
scleroderma
circumscribed s.
systemic s.
sclerodermatous
sclerokeratitis
sclerokeratosis
scleroma
scleromalacia
scleromyxedema
sclero-oophoritis
sclerophthalmia
sclerosarcoma
sclerosing
adenosis, s.
cholangitis, s.
hemangioma, s.
panencephalitis, s.
sclerosis
Alzheimer's s.
amyotrophic lateral s.
multiple s.
primary lateral s.
progressive systemic s.
sclerostenosis
sclerotic
area, s.
keratitis, s.
mastoiditis, s.
metaphyseal bands, s.
thickening, s.
sclerotome
sclerotomy
anterior s.
posterior s.
sclerous
scoliosis
concavity to left/right, s. with
dextro s.
kyphosis and s.

scoliosis *(continued)*
levo s.
lumbar s.
rotary s.
thoracic s.
thoracolumbar s.
scotogram
scotoma
annular s.
central s.
colar s.
mental s.
negative s.
peripheral s.
physiologic s.
positive s.
relative s.
ring s.
scintillating s.
scotomagraph
scotomata
scotometer
scotoscopy
scout
film, s.
image, s.
view, s.
screenage function
screen-film sensitivity
screening mammography
Scribner arteriovenous shunt
scrotal
mass, s.
ultrasound, s.
scrotocele
scrotoplasty
scrotum
dartos tunic of s.
integument of s.
raphe of s.
scybalous
stool, s.

Additional Entries

scybalum
scyphoid
scytoblastema
Se (selenium)
sebaceous
  cyst, s.
  gland, s.
Sebileau's bands
sebolith
seborrhea
seborrheic
  dermatitis, s.
  keratosis, s.
sebum
  cutaneum, s.
sec (second)
secant integral
Sechenoff's center
second (sec)
  cervical vertebra, s. (C2)
  cuneiform bone, s.
  metacarpal bone, s.
  metatarsal bone, s.
  nerve, s.
  order subtraction, s.
  portion of duodenum, s.
secondary
  areolae of bone, s.
  barrier, s.
  dentin, s.
  rays, s.
  sensory fasciculus, s.
  spermatocytes, s.
  tympanic membrane, s.
  wave, s.
secretion (s)
  aspiration of s.
  gastric s.
  respiratory s.
  retained s. in the stomach
  tenacious mucoid s.

secretion (s) *(continued)*
  wax-like s.
section
  axial s.
  coronal s.
  cross s.
  frozen s.
  paraffin s.
  permanent s.
  sagittal s.
  transverse s.
sector scanning
secular equilibrium
seed
  array, s.
  125 I s.
  radon s. implantation
Seessel's pouch
segment (s)
  basal s.
  lower uterine s.
  medullary s.
  spinal s.
segmenta
segmental
  atelectasis, s.
  bronchi, s.
  colon resection, s.
  defect, s.
  infiltrate, s.
  loss, s.
  perfusion defect, s.
segmentation
segmented
  cells, s.
  forms, s.
  lesion, s.
  neutrophils, s.
Seidel's scotoma
Seidelin bodies
seismocardiogram
seismocardiography

Additional Entries

seizure pattern
Seldinger
    catheter, S.
    double-wall femoral arterial puncture technique, S.
    method, S.
    puncture needle, S.
    technique, S.
selective
    adrenal venography, s.
    angiography, s.
    angiocardiography, s.
    arteriography, s.
    azygos vein injection, s.
    energy absorption, s.
    irradiation, s.
    renal angiography, s.
    venography, s.
Selectron afterloading system
selenium (Se)
    75m s.
selenomethionine Se 75
self-retaining catheter
self-sealing
    decomposition, s.
    valve, s.
sella (pl. sellae)
    dorsum, s.
    enlarged s.
    small s.
    truncated s.
    turbuclum s.
    turcica, s.
sellae
sellar polytomograph
Selter's disease
semiaxial position (a/k/a Titterington's position)
semicanal
semicartilaginous
semicircular
semicircular *(continued)*
    canal, s.
    duct, s.
semiconductor detector
semierect position
semiflexion
semifluctuating
semilithotomy position
semilogarithmic
    coordinates, s.
    graph paper, s.
    plots, s.
semilunar
    artery, s.
    bone, s.
    cartilage, s.
    fibrocartilages of knee, s.
    fold of colon, s.
    ganglion of abdomen, s.
    ganglion of trigeminal nerve, s.
    notch of ulna, s.
    valves, s.
semimembranosis muscle
semimembranous
seminal
    duct, s.
    vesicles, s.
    vesiculography, s.
seminiferous
    tubules, s.
seminoma
semiprone position (a/k/a Sims' position)
semireclining position
semirecumbent position
semisupine position
semitendinosus muscle
semitendinous
semitransparent beam-splitting mirror

Additional Entries

semiupright position
Sengstaken-Blakemore multi-lumen tube
sense
    color s.
    decreased position s.
    kinesthetic s.
    light s.
    muscle s.
    posture s.
    pressure s.
    stereognostic s.
sensitive
    critical organs, s.
    organs, s.
sensitivity
sensitizer enhancement ratio (SER)
sensitometric
    curve, s.
    measurement, s.
sensor
sensoriglandular
sensorimuscular
sensorineural
sensorivascular
sensory
    abnormality, s.
    ataxia, s.
    changes, s.
    deficit, s.
    ganglia of nerves, s.
    neural deafness, s.
    pathways, s.
    receptor, s.
sentinel
    loop, s.
    nodes, s.
    polyp, s.
separation
    acromioclavicular s.
    fracture site, s. at
septal
    aortic s. defect
    cartilage, s.
    interatrial s. defect
    interventricular s. defect
    penetration, s.
    raphe, s.
    ventral s. defect
    ventricular s. defect
septate
    bladder, s.
    uterus, s.
septic
    arthritis, s.
    infarction, s.
septicemia
septo-otic dysplasia
septula
    testis, s. of
septum
    aortic s.
    atrioventricular s.
    canalis musculoturbarii, s.
    cartilaginous s.
    crural s.
    deviated nasal s.
    femorale, s.
    inferius of heart, s.
    interalveolar s.
    interatrial s.
    interdental s.
    intermedium, s.
    interventricular s.
    lucidum, s.
    mobile nasi, s.
    nasal s.
    orbital s.
    pellucid s.
    pellucidum, s.
    primum, s.
    rectovaginal s.

Additional Entries ____________________

septum *(continued)*
rectovesical s.
secundum, s.
spurium, s.
subarachnoid, s.
tongue, s.
transversum, s.
urorectal s.
ventricular s.
ventriculorum, s.
sequela (pl. sequelae)
sequence
rapid s. intravneous pyelogram (IVP)
sequential
plane imaging, s.
point imaging, s.
sequestra
sequestrectomy
SER (sensitizer enhancement ratio)
serial
film changer, s.
film radiography, s.
imaging, s.
series
gallbladder s.
GB (gallbladder) s.
GI (gastrointestinal) s.
upper gastrointestinal s.
serioscopy
serocolitis
serofluid
serogastria
serolemma
seroma
seromembranous
seromucus
seromuscular
seronegative
seroperitoneum
seropneumothorax
seropurulent
serosa
serosal
fibroids, s.
fold, s.
layer, s.
metastases, s.
serosanguinous
seroscopy
serosynovial
serosynovitis
serous
coat, s.
cystadenocarcinoma, s.
effusion, s.
fluid, s.
glands, s.
membrane, s.
otitis media, s.
papillary s. cystadenocarcinoma
serpiginous
serrata
ora, s.
Serres' angle
Sertoli's cell
sesamoid
bone, s.
cartilage, s.
fracture, s.
sesamoiditis
sessile
lesion, s.
polyp, s.
Setchenow's centers
setting a window
seven-pinhole
collimator system, s-p
longitudinal tomography, s-p
seventh nerve
Sever's disease

Additional Entries

Sezary syndrome
SFA (superficial femoral artery)
shadow (s)
  confluent s.
  nipple s.
  overlying gas s.
shadowing artifacts
shaft
  calcification, s.
  femur, shaft of.
  fibula, shaft of
  humerus, s. of
  penile s.
  tibial s.
  ulnar s.
Sharpey's fibers
Shaver's disease
sheath
  arteries, s. of
  carotid s.
  connective tissue s.
  crural s.
  cyst, s.
  cystoscope s.
  dentinal s.
  dilatation, s.
  dural s.
  femoral s.
  flexor tendon s.
  Henle's s.
  medullary s.
  myelin s.
  optic nerve s.
  rectus s.
  rectus abdominis muscle s.
  root s.
  Schwann, s. of
  synovial s.
  tendon s.
  tumor, s.
Sheehan's syndrome
sheet of lead rubber
shelf
  rectal s.
shelling out of lesion
shelling out procedure
shell location
shelving
  edge of Poupart's ligament, s.
Shenton's line
Shepard formula
Shepherd's fracture
Sherwood Medical
Shick test
shield
shielding block
Shimadzu Ralston afterloader
shim coil
shimming
shin
  bone, s.
Shiner's radiopaque tube
shine-through
shock
  lung, s.
  nephrogram, s.
Shope papilloma
short
  border, s.
  calcaneocuboid ligament, s.
  gastric veins, s.
  half-life positron, s.
  plantar ligament, s.
  saphenous nerve, s.
  saphenous vein, s.
  treatment distance, s.
shotty
  consistency, s.
  lymph nodes, s.
  nodes, s.

Additional Entries

shoulder
    blade, s.
    girdle, s.
    hand syndrome, s.
    harness, s.
    joint, s.
Shrapnell's membrane
shunt
    arteriovenous s.
    cardiovascular s.
    Blalock-Taussig s.
    blockage, s.
    Cimino arteriovenous s.
    complication, s.
    evaluation, s.
    formation, s.
    Javid's s.
    left-to-right s.
    LeVeen s.
    pentose s.
    portacaval s.
    quantification, s.
    recirculation curve, s.
    Scribner arteriovenous s.
    Silastic ventriculoperitoneal s.
    Teflon s. tube
    Torkildsen s.
    venous s.
    ventriculoatrial s.
    ventriculocaval s.
    ventriculocisternal s.
    ventriculoperitoneal s.
    ventriculopleural s.
    Waterston s.
shrinking of tumor
shrunk
shunt quantification
shutter correction
Si (silicon)
SI (sacroiliac joint)
sialadenitis
sialadenography
sialadenosis
sialoadenectomy
sialoadenotomy
sialoangiectasis
sialoangiitis
sialoangiography
sialocele
sialodochoplasty
sialogram
sialography
sialoma
Sibson's
    aponeurosis, S.
    fascia, S.
sickle cell anemia
SID (source-image distance)
side-mounted periscope
sideroblast
siderocyte
siderofibrosis
siderophore molecule
sideroscope
sidewinder catheter
Siegle's otoscope
Siemens Elema Cisal I injector
Siemens Elema Cisal II injector
Siemens Elema Cisal AB injector
Siemens Mevatron KD accelerator
Siemerling's nucleus
sievert
    integral, S.
    method, S.
sight
    organ of s.
sigmoid
    arteries, s.

Additional Entries

sigmoid *(continued)*
  cavity, s.
  colon, s.
  colostomy, s.
  diverticulosis, s.
  flexure, s.
  loop colostomy, s.
  mesocolon, s.
  notch, s.
  sinus, s.
  sulcus, s.
sigmoidoproctostomy
sigmoidoscope
sigmoidoscopy
sigmoidosigmoidostomy
sigmoidostomy
sigmoidovesical
Sigmund's glands
signal
  averaging, s.
  filtration, s.
  intensity, s.
  to noise ratio, s. (SNR)
silastic beads
silastic ventriculoperitoneal shunt
silent thyroiditis
silhouette sign
silicon (Si)
silicon elastomer
silicosis
silicotuberculosis
silver (Ag)
  fork deformity, s.
  halide crystals, s.
  iodide, s. (AgI)
  rod, s.
Silverman needle
Simmonds' disease
Simmons 1 catheter
Simmons 2 catheter
Simmons 3 catheter
Simmons 5/7 French catheter
Simon afterloading tube
Simon's position (a/k/a Edebohls' position)
Simon-Heyman capsules
simple
  bone cyst, s.
  cyst, s.
  thyroiditis, s.
  trauma, s.
simple
  compression fracture, s.
  cyst, s.
  fracture, s.
  tumor removal (STR), s.
simplex
  herpes virus s.
Simpson
  catheter, S.
  electric arc light, S.
  splint, S.
Sims' position (a/k/a semi-prone position)
simulation
simulator
simultaneous iterative reconstruction technique (SIRT)
sine qua non
single
  annihilation escape peak, s.
  breadth imaging, s.
  breath inhalation image, s.
  contrast, s.
  crystal gamma camera, s.
  dose, s.
  emulsion film, s.
  exposure, s.
  field isodose curve, s.
  film, s.

Additional Entries ______________________

single *(continued)*
foil system, s.
gutter guide, s.
hit damage, s.
hit killing, s.
hole collimator, s.
hole spinning top, s.
homolateral field, s.
lumen catheter, s.
niche, s.
patient visit equivalent (SPVE) treatment, s.
phase, s.
phase alternating voltage line, s.
phase operation, s.
photon absorptiometry, s.
photon emission computed tomography (SPECT), s.
photon emission tomography, s.
photon tomography, s.
piece applicator, s.
plane, s.
plane electrodes, s.
slice projection, s.
ventricle, s.
vessel clot, s.
sinistrocardia
sinistrocerebral
sinistrocular
sinistropedal
sinistrotorsion
sinoatrial
block, s.
bundle, s.
node, s.
sinoauricular
heart block, s.
node, s.
sinobronchitis
sinodural plate
Sinografin
sinography
sinopulmonary
sinoventricular
sinovertebral nerves
sinus (es)
air s.
anal s.
aortic s.
basilar s.
branchial s.
carotid s.
cavernous s.
cervicalis s.
circular s.
coccygeal s.
confluence of s.
coronary s.
costomediastinal s.
cortical s.
dura mater s.
epididymis s.
ethmoid s.
external jugular vein s.
frontal s.
intercavernous s.
lactiferous s.
laryngeal s.
lateral s.
longitudinal s.
maxillary s.
medullary s.
Morgagni s.
oblique s.
occipital s.
oral s.
nose, s. of
paranasal s.
pericardial s.
petrosal s.

Additional Entries

sinus (es) *(continued)*
petrosquamous s.
phrenicocostal s.
pilonidal s.
piriform s.
pocularis s.
prostatic s.
pyriformis s.
rectal s.
renal s.
rhomboidalis s.
Rokitansky-Aschoff s.
sagittal s.
sclerae s.
septum s.
sigmoid s.
sphenoidal s.
sphenoparietal s.
straight s.
tentorial s.
thyroglossal s.
tonsillaris s.
transverse s.
tract, s.
urogenital s.
Valsalva s.
venarum cavarum, s.
venosus s.
sinusitis
sinusoid
Minot, s. of
myocardial s.
sinuventricular
Sipple syndrome
Sippy dilator
SIRT (simultaneous iterative reconstruction technique)
site identification
situ
carcinoma in s.
situs
ambiguous, s.

situs *(continued)*
indeterminate, s.
inversus, s.
mixed, s.
solitus, s.
sitz bath
six-cavity accelerating structure
six-pulse
sixth nerve
Sjogren's syndrome
skeletal
abnormalities, s.
absorptiometry, s.
angiomatosis, s.
appendicular s.
axial, s.
deformity, s.
imaging, s.
metastases, s.
muscle activity, s.
survey, s.
tracer, s.
traction, s.
skeletization
skeletogenous
skeletography
skeleton
appendicular s.
axial s.
fetal s.
Skene's
ducts, S.
glands, S.
skenoscope
skiagraph
skiameter
Skillern's fracture
skin
appendages of s.
arteries of s.
cleavage lines, s.

Additional Entries

skin *(continued)*
corium, s.
cutis vera s.
dimpling of s.
epidermis, s.
flap, s.
fold, s.
furrows of s.
gap, s.
graft, s.
hemorrhoidal s. tags
Langer's lines of s.
loss, s.
lymphatic capillaries of s.
metastases, s.
nerves of s.
nodules, s.
papillary layer of s.
rake, s.
reticular layer of s.
retraction, s.
scrapings, s.
sparing, s.
stratum corneum, s.
stratum mucosum, s.
tags, s.
thickening, s.
true s.
skinny needle
skip
areas, s.
lesion, s.
metastases, s.
skull
cap, s.
exterior of s.
fossa of s.
interior of s.
trauma, s.
upper surface of base of s.
skyline view
slant
brain fields,, s.
hole collimator, s.
SLDR (sublethal damage repair)
sleep
deprived EEG (electroencephalogram), s.
EEG (electroencephalogram), s.
slice
body pictures, s. of
fracture, s.
orientation, s.
profile, s.
selection, s.
thickness, s.
sliding
hiatal hernia, s.
flap, s.
technique, s.
slightly oblique brow-up cross-table lateral position
sling
levator s.
Rauchfuss' s.
Velpeau s.
slipped
capital femoral epiphysis, s.
epiphysis, s.
meniscus, s.
slit
diaphragm, s.
dorsal s.
lamp biomicroscopy, s.
lamp examination, s.
ventral s.
slough
sloughed mucosa
sloughing

Additional Entries

sloughing *(continued)*
skin s.
sludge
Sm (samarium)
SMA (superior mesenteric artery)
small
bore butterfly needle, s.
bore needle, s.
bowel series, s.
caliber needle, s.
cardiac vein, s.
foam pad, s.
heart of Adison's disease, s.
hila, s.
intestine, s.
irregular opacity, s.
jejunum of s. intestine
localizing cone, s.
lymphatic nodules of s. intestine
Meckel's diverticulum of s. intestine
mucous membrane of s. intestine
muscular coat of s. intestine
nerves of s. intestine
occipital nerve, s.
Peyer's patches of s. intestine
rounded opacity, s.
saphenous vein, s.
sciatic nerve, s.
serous coat of s. intestine
submucous coat of s. intestine
valvulae conniventes of s. intestine
villi of s. intestine

small *(continued)*
wings of sphenoid, s.
smaller
cardiac veins, s.
occipital nerve, s.
Smithers Medical Products
Smith's
disease, S.
fracture, S.
Smith-Petersen nail
SML (superior malleolar ligament)
smooth
muscle, s.
liver edges, s.
wall, s.
SMR (scatter-maximum ratio)
SMV (submentovertex) view
Sn (tin)
snowstorm shadow
sodium (Na)
acetrizoate, s.
arsenate (As 74)
benzoate, s.
bicarbonate, s.
biphosphate, s.
cellulose phosphate, s.
chlorate, s.
chloride (Na 22)
chromate (Cr 51)
dehydrocholate, s.
diatrizoate, s.
fluoride, s. (18F)
glutamate, s.
iodide, s. (Na 1) (I 125; I 131)
ipodate, s.
molybdate (Mo 99)
nitroprusside, s.
pertechnetate, s. (Tc99m)

Additional Entries

sodium (Na) *(continued)*
- phosphate, s. (32P)
- rays, s.
- salt, s.
- succinate, s.
- sulfate, s. (S35)
- thiamylal, s.

soft
- applicator, s.
- copper seeds, s.
- lesion, s.
- palate, s.
- tissue, s.
- tissue emphysema, s.
- tissue mass, s.
- tissue technique, s.

solar plexus

sole
- foot, s. of
- muscles of s.

solenoidal coil

solenoma

soleus muscle

solid
- bony union, s.
- organ, s.
- state dosimetry, s.
- stool, s.
- support column chromatography, s.

solitary
- abnormality, s.
- bone cyst, s.
- cells of medulla spinalis, s.
- coin lesion, s.
- cold lesion, s.
- hepatic cyst, s.
- lesion, s.
- myeloma, s.
- nodule, s.
- palpable nodule, s.

solitary *(continued)*
- simple cyst, s.

soluble indigo blue

Solutrast

somatic
- fibers, s.
- layer, s.

somaticovisceral

somatoceptor

somatodidymuse

somatogram

somatome

somatomegaly

somatometry

somatopathy

sompatoplasm

somatopleural

somatoscopy

somatotropic

somatotrope

somatotrophic

somatotropic

somersault with rotating chair

somnocinematograph

Sones technique

sonic liver mass

sonogram

sonography

sonologist

sonolucency

sonolucent
- liver mass, s.
- mass, s.
- superior pole, s.

Soret band

Sottas disease

souffle
- cardiac s.
- placental s.
- umbilical s.

sound wave

Additional Entries

source
  axis distance, s. to (SAD)
  calibration, s.
  collimator distance, s.
  construction, s.
  fiberoptic light s.
  image distance, s. (SID)
  skin distance, s. to (SSD)
  surface technique, s.
Souttar tube
space (s)
  Blessig's s.
  Bogros's s.
  Bowman's s.
  Burns' s.
  Colles' s.
  consuming mass, s.
  corneal s.
  Cotunnius' s.
  Crookes s.
  Czermak's s.
  dead s.
  disc s.
  Disse's s.
  Douglas' s.
  episcleral s.
  extradural s.
  Faraday's dark s.
  of Fontana, s's.
  foraminal s.
  globular s's of Czermak
  haversian s.
  Henke's s.
  His's perivascular s.
  Holzknecht's s.
  intercostal s.
  interglobular s.
  interpleural s.
  intervertebral disc s.
  intrathecal s.

space (s) *(continued)*
  joint s.
  Kiernan's s's.
  Kiesselbach's s.
  Kretschmann's s.
  Larrey's s's.
  Lesgraft's s.
  Magendie's s's.
  Malacarne's s.
  Marie's quadrilateral s.
  Meckel's s.
  Mohrenheim's s.
  Nance's leeway s.
  Nuel's s's.
  Obersteiner-Redlich s.
  occupying lesion, s.
  parapharyngeal s.
  Parona's s.
  perichoroidal s.
  pleural s.
  Poiseuille's s.
  popliteal s.
  preputial s.
  prevesical s.
  proximal s.
  proximate s.
  Prussak's s.
  retropharyngeal s.
  retropubic s.
  Retzius s.
  Robin's s's.
  Schwalbe's s's.
  subarachnoid s.
  subdural s.
  suprasternal s.
  Tarin's s.
  Tenon's s.
  thenar s.
  Traube's semilunar s.
  Troltsch's s's.
  vesicovaginal s.
  Virchow-Robin s's.

Additional Entries ______________________________

____

____

space (s) *(continued)*
Westberg's s.
Zang's s.
spade field
Spallone's analysis
spasm
spatia zonularia
spatial
distortion, s.
filtration, s.
resolution, s.
uniformity, s.
spatium
spear
specialized blocking procedure
specificity
special
contrast medium, s.
mode, s.
nonroutine projection, s.
specific
activity, s.
ionization, s.
specimen
pathological s.
tube with black rubber cork, s.
SPECT (single photon emission computed tomography)
spectral broadening
spectrofluorometer
spectrograph
spectrometer
spectrophotofluorometer
spectrophotometer
spectroscope
spectroscopy
spectrum
Spee's curve
Spence, tail of
Spencer Wells facies
Spengler's fragments
spermatic
artery, s.
canal, s.
cord, s.
fascia, s.
nerve, s.
plexus, s.
vein, s.
spermatoblast
spermatocele
spermatocyst
sphaceloderma
S-phase
sphenobasilar
sphenocephaly
sphenoethmoid
sphenoethmoidal
recess, s.
suture, s.
sphenofrontal
suture, s.
sphenoid
bone, s.
body, s.
fontanelle, s.
pterygoid process of s.
sinus, s.
wing of s.
sphenoidal
air sinuses, s.
conchae, s.
crest, s.
process, s.
rostrum, s.
spine, s.
structures, s.
turbinated processes, s.
sphenomandibular
ligament, s.
sphenomaxillary

Additional Entries

sphenomaxillary *(continued)*
fissure, s.
fossa, s.
suture, s.
spheno-occipital
spheno-orbital
sphenopalatine
artery, s.
foramen, s.
ganglion, s.
nerves, s.
notch, s.
sphenoparietal
sinus, s.
suture, s.
sphenosquamous
suture, s.
sphenotemporal
suture, s.
sphenoturbinal
sphenovomerine
sphenozygomatic
spherical
ball, s.
shape, s.
tumor, s.
spherocyte
spherocytosis
spheroid
shaped, s.
spherule (s)
of Fulci, s.
rod s.
spidery collecting system
sphincter
anal s.
ani, s.
ani externus muscle, s.
cardiac s.
gastroesophageal s.
incompetent esophageal s.
sphincter *(continued)*
internus muscle, s. of
muscle of pylorus, s.
muscle of urethra, s.
muscle of urinary bladder, s.
Oddi, s. of
pharyngoesophageal s.
pupillae muscle, s. of
pyloric s.
rectal s.
recti muscle s.
stenosis, s.
urethrae membranaceae muscle, s.
vaginae muscle, s. of
vesicae, s.
sphincteroscope
sphincterotome
sphingolipid
sphingolipidosis
sphymobologram
sphygmobolometer
sphygmocardiogram
sphygmocardioscope
sphygmochronograph
sphygmodynamometer
sphygmogram
sphygmograph
sphygmography
sphygmometer
sphygmometrograph
sphygmometroscope
sphygmo-oscillometer
sphygmoplethysmograph
sphygmoscope
Bishop's s.
sphygmotonograph
spider
angioma, s.
cell, s.
nevi, s.

Additional Entries

spider web meninx (meninx-
  lining)
Spieghel's line
spigelian lobe of liver
spillage of tumor
spin
  coupling, s.
  density, s.
  down state, s.
  echo imaging, s.
  echo pulse image, s.
  lattice relaxation, s.
  spin, s.
  spin relaxation, s.
spina
  angularis, s.
  bifida cystica, s.
  bifida occulta, s.
  helicis, s.
  scapulae, s.
spinal
  accessory nerve, s.
  afferent fibers of s.
    nerves
  arteries, s.
  autonomic fibers of s.
    nerves
  bifida cystica, s.
  bulb, s.
  canal, s.
  column, s.
  connections with sympa-
    thetic s. nerves
  cord, s.
  cord block, s.
  cord compression, s.
  cord concussion, s.
  cord decompression, s.
  cord dysfunction, s.
  dysraphism, s. (defective
    fusion)
  fibers of s. nerves
spinal *(continued)*
  fusion, s.
  ganglia, s.
  lemniscus, s.
  manometer, s.
  meningitis, s.
  muscular atrophy, s.
  nerves, s.
  parasympathetic fibers of
    s. nerves
  points of emergence of
    s. nerves
  puncture, s.
  reflex paths, s.
  roots of s. nerves
  segments, s.
  somatic efferent fibers of
    s. nerves
  stenosis, s.
  subarachnoid block, s.
  sympathetic fibers of s.
    nerves
spindle
  aortic s.
  cataract, s.
  cell, s.
  neuromuscular s.
  neurotendinous s.
  shaped, s.
spindling
activity, s.
  pattern, s.
spine
  alar s.
  anterior maxillary s.
  anterior superior iliac s.
  cervical s.
  dorsal s.
  ethmoidal s.
  field, s.
  frontal bone s.
  iliac s.

Additional Entries

spine *(continued)*
ischial s.
lumbar s.
lumbosacral s.
maxillary s.
mental s.
nasal s.
neural s.
palatine s.
pubic s.
scapular s.
sphenoidal s.
suprameatal s.
thoracic s.
tibial s.
trochlear s.
spinifugal
spinipetal
spinobulbar
spinocellular
spinocerebellar
degeneration, s.
spinocostalis
spinoglenoid
ligament, s.
spinogram
spino-olivary fasciculus
spin orientations
spinotectal fasciculus
spinothalamic tract
spinous
foramen, s.
process, s.
spin-spin relaxation
spinthariscope
spintherometer
spin-warp imaging
spiny projection
spiradenoma
spiral
artery, s.
canal, s.

spiral *(continued)*
fracture, s.
ganglion, s.
ligament, s.
line, s.
organo of Corti, s.
thread, s.
tip catheter, s.
spiroid
spirometer
spirometry
bronchoscopic s.
Spitzka's nucleus
Spitzka-Lissauer tract
splanchnic
block, s.
fibers, s.
nerve, s.
splanchnoblast
splanchnocele
splanchnocranium
splanchnography
splanchnolith
splanchnopleural
splanchnoptosis
splanchnosclerosis
splanchnoscopy
splanchnoskeleton
splaying
spleen
accessory s.
contour, s.
hilus of s.
imaging, s.
malpighian bodies of s.
supernumerary s.
trabeculae of s.
splenadenoma
splenatrophy
splenial center of ossification
splenic
anoxia, s.

Additional Entries

splenic *(continued)*
arteriography, s.
artery, s.
artery thrombosis, s.
calcification, s.
capsule, s.
cells, s.
cyst, s.
flexure of colon, s.
irradiation, s.
localization, s.
lymph nodes, s.
plexus, s.
pulp, s.
vein, s.
vein thrombosis, s.
splenium
corporis callosi, s. of
splenoblast
splenocele
splenocolic
splenocyte
splenogram
splenohepatomegaly
splenoid
splenoma
splenomedullary
splenomegaly
splenometry
splenomyelogenous
splenomyelomalacia
splenopancreatic
splenopathy
splenophrenic
splenopneumonia
splenoportography
splenorenal
splenosis
split
course external irradiation, s.
course irradiation, s.
split *(continued)*
course radiation, s.
splitting
zero-field s.
spoke wheel
spondylarthritis
anklylopoietica, s.
spondylitis
ankylosing s.
hypertrophic s.
rheumatoid s.
spondylocostal dysostosis
spondyloepiphyseal dysplasia congenita
spondylolisthesis
spondylolysis
spondylomalacia
spondylometaphyseal dysplasia
spondylopathy
spondylosis
narrow vertebral canal, s. with
ridge, s. with
spondylotic
spondylous
sponge
holding forceps, s.
stick, s.
spongiform
spongioblast
spongioblastoma
multiforme, s.
unipolare, s.
spongiocyte
spongioid
spongioplasm
spongiosis
spontaneous
closure, s.
pneumothorax, s.
reflux, s.

Additional Entries

sporoblast
sporocyst
sporoduct
sporogenous
sporophore
sporophyte
sporoplasm
spot
  Bitot's s.
  blind s.
  cafe-au-lait s.
  film, s.
  hat s.
  Koplik's s.
  liver s.
  Mariotte's s.
  mongolian s.
  radiation, s.
  Soemmering's s.
  view, s.
Sprengel deformity
spring
  guide holder, s.
  guide wire, s.
  ligament, s.
sprue (a/k/a catarrhal dysentery)
spur
  bone s.
  calcaneal s.
  degenerative s.
  formation, s.
  heel s.
  Morand's s.
  plantar s.
  posterior s.
  retrocalcaneal s.
spurring
  degenerative s.
  hypertrophic s.
SPVE (single patient visit equivalent treatment)
squama (pl. squamae)
  frontal s.
  occipital s.
  temporal s.
squamate
squamocellular
squamocolumnar
  junction, s.
squamofrontal
squamomastoid
squamo-occipital
squamoparietal
squamopetrosal
squamosa
squamosal
squamosoparietal
squamosphenoid
squamotemporal
squamous
  cell carcinoma, s.
  epithelial cells, s.
  epithelium, s.
  metaplasia, s.
Sr (strontium)
Sr/Y applicator (90Sr/90Y applicator)
Sr 85 ion
Sr 90 isotope (plaque)
Sr 90 surface dose rage
SSD (source-to-skin) distance
S-shaped
stab
  cell, s.
  incision, s.
  wound, s.
stable fracture
stacked scans
Staderini's nucleus
Stage I, II, III, IV
staghorn
  calculus, s.
Stahr gland

Additional Entries ______________________

____

____

stainless steel
afterloading needle (open end), s.s.
afterloading stylet (closed end), s.s.
syringe, s.s.
stalk
optic s.
pituitary s.
Stallard applicator
standard
blocks, s.
deviation, s.
fluoroscopic system, s.
low-dose myelogram, s.
radiographic system, s.
target volume, s.
standing wave
stannous (Sn)
chloride, s.
pyrophosphate, s.
sulfur colloid, s.
stapedial
nerve, s.
tendon, s.
stapedioplasty
stapediotenotomy
stapediovestibular
stapedius
muscle, s.
nerve, s.
tendon, s.
stapes
annular ligament of s.
fixation of s.
footplate, s.
staphyloangina
staphyloderma
staphyloma
staphylomatous
staphylopharyngorrhaphy
staphyloplasty
staphyltome
Starck
cardioesophageal dilator, S.
dilator, S.
star pattern
stasis
changes, s.
cirrhosis, s.
intestinal s.
ulcer, s.
urinary s.
venous s.
static
ataxia, s.
B-mode ultrasonography, s.
image, s.
tremor, s.
view, s.
stationary
field, s.
grid, s.
statoacoustic
nerve, s.
statocyst
statolith
statometer
steady state
steatitis
steatocele
steatocystoma
steatoma
steatomatosis
steatonecrosis
steatopygous
steatorrhea
steatosis
cardiaca, s.
Steell's murmur
steep
dose-response curve, s.

Additional Entries

steep *(continued)*
- right posterior oblique position, s.

steeple sign
steerable
- basket catheter, s.
- biopsy brush, s.
- catheter system, s.

steered focused ultrasound system
Steiner's tumors
Stein-Leventhal syndrome
Steinmann's pin
stella
stellate
- fracture, s.
- ganglion, s.
- ligament, s.
- scar, s.
- tear, s.
- veins of kidney, s.

stem
- brain s.

stenosing
- tendinitis, s.
- tenosynovitis, s.

stenosis
- aortic s.
- calcific aortic s.
- cervical s.
- coronary sinus ostium, s. of
- esophageal s.
- idiopathic hypertrophic subaortic s.
- IHSS (idiopathic hypertrophic subaortic) s.
- meatal s.
- mitral s.
- pulmonary s.
- pyloric s.
- subaortic s.

stenosis *(continued)*
- supraclinoid carotid s.
- tracheal s.
- tricuspid s.
- urethral meatal s.
- valvular s.

stenothorax
stenotic
Stensen's
- canal, S.
- duct, S.
- foramen, S.
- veins, S.

stent
- antegrade ureteral s.
- biliary s.
- tie-over s.
- ureteral s.

Stenver's view
step
- down heating, s.
- up transformer, s.
- wedge, s.
- wedge block, s.

stepped spinal cord block
stephanion
- skull, s. of

stercoroma
stercorous
stereoanesthesia
stereoblastula
stereocilium
stereocinefluorography
stereogram
stereometer
stereo-ophthalmoscope
stereophorometer
stereophoroscope
stereophotography
stereophotomicrograph
stereoplasm
steropsis

Additional Entries

stereoradiography
stereoroentgenography
stereoroentgenometry
stereosalpingography
stereoscope
stereoscopic
  film, s.
  view, s.
stereoshift film
stereotactic
  biopsy, s.
  technique, s.
stereotaxy
stereo view
sternad
sternal
  angle, s.
  border, s.
  depression, s.
  end of clavicle, s.
  foramen, s.
  intercostal retractions, s.
  notch, s.
  plate, s.
  ribs, s.
  splitting incision, s.
  wire sutures, s.
Sternberg's disease
Sternberg-Reed cells
sternoclavicular
  articulations, s.
  joint, s.
sternoclavicularis
  muscle, s.
sternocleidomastoid
  artery, s.
  muscle, s.
  vein, s.
sternocostal
  articulations, s.
  ligaments, s.
  surface of heart, s.
sternogoniometer
sternohyoid
  muscle, s.
sternoid
sternomanubrial area
sternomastoid
  artery, s.
  muscle, s.
sternopericardial
  ligaments, s.
sternoscapular
sternoschisis
sternothyroid
  muscle, s.
sternotracheal
sternovertebral
sternoxiphopagus
Stern's position
sternum
  articulations of s.
  cleft s.
  ensiform s.
  gladiolus s.
  manubrium s.
  xiphoid s.
steroid
  induced avascular necrosis, s.
  therapy, s.
stethendoscope
stethogoniometer
stethograph
stethokyrtograph
stethometer
stethomyositis
stethoparalysis
Stewart-Hamilton equation
Sticker's disease
Stieda's diesease
stigmatometer
stigmatoscope
Still's disease

Additional Entries

stillicidium
lacrimarum, s.
narium, s.
urinae, s.
Stilling's canal
stimulating hormone
increase, s.h.
suppression, s.h.
stimulation
areal s.
audio-visual-tactile s.
carotid sinus s.
nonspecific s.
paradoxical s.
paraspecific s.
photic s.
punctual s.
transcutaneous nerve s.
stimulator
transcutaneous electrical nerve s.
TENS (transcutaneous electrical nerve) s.
stipple
cell, s.
stippled epiphyses
stippling
basophilic, s.
sTNM (surgical evaluative staging)
Stoerk's blennorrhea
Stokes' disease
Stokes-Adams disease
stoma
ostomy s.
stomach
bed, s.
body of s.
curvatures of s.
duodenopyloric constriction of s.
fundus of s.

stomach *(continued)*
glands of s.
greater curvature of s.
lesser curvature of s.
pyloric antrum of s.
pyloric glands of s.
pyloric orifice of s.
pylorus of s.
rugal folds of s.
rugal pattern of s.
valve, s.
serous coat of s.
stomal
stomata
stomatitis
aphthous s.
herpetic s.
necrotizing ulcerative s.
stomatocyte
stomatocytosis
stomatogastric
stomatoglossitis
stomatognathic
stomatography
stomatomalacia
stomatomycosis
stomatonecrosis
stomatopathy
stomatoplasty
stomatorrhagia
stomatoscope
stomodeum
stone
basket, s.
biliary s.
calyceal s.
extraction, s.
impacted s.
kidney s.
nonopaque s.
opaque s.
partially opaque, s.

Additional Entries ____________

stone *(continued)*
radiolucent s.
staghorn s.
unusual manifestation of s.
ureteral s.
stopcock
stopper
storage pools
stored mask mode
storiform
fibrous histiocytoma, s.
Storm van Leeuwen chamber
Storz ureteroscope
STR (simple tumor removal)
strabismometer
strabismus
straddling atrioventricular valves
straight
anterior oblique position, s.
back syndrome, s.
blockage border, s.
brow-up cross-table lateral position, s.
strand
strangulated
hernia, s.
strangulation
intestinal s.
Strasburger's cell plate
strata
stratified
stratiform fibrocartilage
stratigram
stratum
compactum, s.
corneum, s.
germinativum, s.
granulosum cerebelli, s.
intermedium, s.

stratum *(continued)*
lemnisci, s.
lucidum hippocampi, s.
opticum, s.
spongiosum, s.
zonale, s.
strawberry
hemangioma, s.
straw-colored
streptokinase
stress
cystogram, s.
fracture, s.
incontinence, s.
induced ischemia, s.
MUGA, s.
reaction, s.
redistribution, s.
stressors
stria (pl. striae)
longitudinal s.
striate
arteries, s.
veins, s.
striated
muscle, s.
pelvis, s.
reticulum, s.
stricture
anal s.
anastomotic s.
annular s.
cicatricial s.
esophageal s.
false s.
urethral s.
stringy
vitreous floaters, s.
striocellular
striocerebellar
striomuscular
strip

Additional Entries

strip *(continued)*
  boost, s.
  chart, s.
stripe
  Hensen, s. of
  sign, s.
striped muscle
stripping tool
stroma
  iris, s. of
  kidney, s. of
  ovary, s. of
stromal
  distortion, s.
  hyperplasia, s.
  invasion, s.
  opacity, s.
strontium (Sr)
  90 applicator, s.
  chloride Sr 85, s.
  ion, s. (Sr 85 ion)
  isotope, s.
  nitrate, s.
  90 Sr surface dose rate, s.
  yttrium applicator, s. (90 Sr/90Y applicator)
structural
  anomaly, s.
  lesion, s.
structure (s)
  anatomic s.
  low-contrast s.
  model, s.
  osseous s.
struma ovarii
Strumpell's disease
Strumpell-Leichtenstern disease
Strumpell-Marie disease
Strumpell-Westphal pseudosclerosis
struvite
study
  flow s.
  pressure s.
  redistribution s.
stump
  amputation s.
  appendiceal s.
  bronchial s.
  cervical s.
Sturge's disease
Sturge-Weber disease
stylatic implant catheter
stylet
styloglossus
  muscle, s.
stylohyal part of styloid process
stylohyoid
  ligament, s.
  nerve, s.
stylohyoideus
  muscle, s.
styloid
  bone, s.
  process, s.
stylomandibular
  ligament, s.
stylomastoid
  artery, s.
  foramen, s.
stylomaxillary
  ligament, s.
stylomyloid
stylopharyngeus
  muscle, s.
stylostaphyline
stylosteophyte
S.TYMP. (sinus tympani)
styrofoam beads
subabdominal
subabdominoperitoneal

Additional Entries

subacetabular
subacute thyroiditis
subadventitial fibroplasia
subaortic
    idiopathic hypertrophic s. stenosis (IHSS)
subapical
subarachnoid
    block, s.
    cavity, s.
    cisternae, s.
    hemorrhage, s.
    myelography, s.
    sclerosis, s.
    septum, s.
    space, s.
subarcuate
    fossa, s.
subareolar
subarticular
    cyst, s.
    erosions, s.
    sclerosis, s.
subastragalar
subatloidean
subaural
subaurale
subcallosal gyrus
subcapsular
    afferent lymphatic vessels, s.
    cataract, s.
subcardinal veins
subcarinal
    adenopathy, s.
subchondral
subclavian
    artery, s.
    catheter, s.
    steal syndrome, s.
    triangle, s.
    vein, s.
subcortical
subcostal
    arteries, s.
    zone, s.
subcutaneous
    connective tissue, s.
    emphysema, s.
    extravasation of blood, s.
    fat layer, s.
    inguinal ring, s.
    plane, s.
    tissue, s.
    tunnel, s.
subcuticular
subdiaphragmatic
    free s. air
    hernia, s.
    region, s.
subdigastric lymph nodes
subdural
    abscess, s.
    cavity, s.
    cyst, s.
    extravasation, s.
    hematoma, s.
    hemorrhage, s.
    instillation, s.
    needle, s.
    space, s.
subendocardial
    infarction, s.
    ischemia, s.
subepithelial plexus
subependymal
    nodule, s.
    siderosis, s.
subfrontal gyre
subgaleal
subgallate
subgemmal
subglossitis

Additional Entries

subhepatic
subicteric
subinguinal lymph nodes
subinvolution
  uterus, s. of
subjacent
subjugal
sublesional
sublethal damage repair (SDR)
sublingual
  artery, s.
  fold, s.
  gland, s.
sublobe
sublobular
  veins, s.
subluxate
subluxation
submammary
submandibular
  duct, s.
  lymph nodes, s.
  salivary gland, s.
submaxillary
  artery, s.
  duct,. s.
  ganglion, s.
  gland, s.
  triangle, s.
submedial
submental
  vertex position, s.
  vertex view, s. (SMV)
submentovertical position
submerged tooth
submucosa
subnasale
subnatant
subneural
subnucleus
suboccipital
suboccipital *(continued)*
  muscles, s.
  triangle, s.
suboptimal
subparietal
  sulcus, s.
subperiosteal
  ossification, s.
subperiosteally
  rib s. resected
subperitoneal
  connective tissue, s.
subphrenic
  abscess, s.
  collection, s.
subpial
subpleural
  mediastinal plexus, s.
subpreputial
subpubic
  ligament, s.
subpulmonary
  effusion, s.
  fluid, s.
subpyramidal
subsartorial plexus
subscapular
  angle, s.
  artery, s.
  fascia, s.
  fossa, s.
  nerves, s.
subscleral
subsclerotic
subsegmental bibasilar atelectasis
subserous
  fascia, s.
substantia (pl. substantiae)
  adamantina dentis, s.
  alba, s.
  eburnea dentis, s.

Additional Entries __________

substantia *(continued)*
- ferruginea, s.
- nigra, s.
- propriacorneae, s.

substernal
- goiter, s.
- thyroid, s.

substernomastoid
substrate
substratum
substructure
subsulcus
subsylvian
subtalar
- joint, s.

subtemporal
subtenial
subtentorial
subthalamic tegmental region
subthalamus
subtraction
- digital s. angiogram (DSA)
- direct x-ray s.
- electronic s.
- photographic s.

subtractor
subtrochanteric
subtrochlear
subungual
suburethral
subvaginal
subvalvular stenosis
subvertebral
suction tube
Sudan stain
sudanophilia (staining readily with Sudan stain)
sudanophilic degeneration
Sudeck's
- atrophy, S.
- disease, S.

sudogram
sudoriferous glands
sulci
- brain, s. of

sulcus (pl. sulci)
- alveolabial s.
- anterior longitudinal s.
- calcaneal s.
- carpal s.
- central s.
- centralis cerebri, s.
- cerbral s.
- cingulate s.
- circular s.
- circularis s.
- coronary s.
- frontal s.
- gingival s.
- infraorbital s.
- intermedius s.
- intraparietal s.
- lacrimal s.
- lateral cerebral s.
- lunate s.
- malleolar s.
- medial frontal s.
- medial s.
- mentolabial s.
- Munro s.
- nasolabial s.
- nasolacrimal s.
- occipital s.
- occulomotor s.
- olfactory s.
- orbital s.
- palatine s.
- paracolic s.
- paramedial s.
- parieto-occipital s.
- postcentral s.
- posterior median s.
- preauricular s.

Additional Entries

sulcus (pl. sulci) *(continued)*
precentral s.
pulmonary s.
radial s.
retroglandular s.
sagittalis s.
sclerae s.
scleral s.
sigmoid s.
spirales s.
subparietal s.
tali s.
temporal s.
terminal s.
tympanic s.
vomerovaginal s.
sulfa crystals
sulfhydryl-containing compound
sulfobromophthalein sodium
sulfur (S)
sulfur colloid
sulfuric acid
sunburst appearance
Sundt shunt
sunken
acetabulum, s.
supercilia
superciliary
arches, s.
superconducting magnet
superficial
abrasion, s.
atrophy, s.
bleeders, s.
cervical artery, s.
epigastric artery, s.
external pudendal artery, s.
fascia, s.
femoral artery, s. (SFA)
iliac circumflex artery, s.

superficial *(continued)*
long plantar ligament, s.
orthovoltage beam, s.
palmar arch, s.
perineal artery, s.
peroneal nerve, s.
spreading, s.
stopper, s.
sylvian vein, s.
temporal artery, s.
transverse ligament, s.
unit, s.
volar artery, s.
x-ray, s.
Super-Flab
superflexion
superfrontal
gyre, s.
superimposed
angiogram, s.
bowel gas, s.
scout film, s.
superimposition
superior
articular arteries, s.
calcaneocuboid ligament, s.
cerebellar peduncles, s.
constrictor muscle, s.
dental nerve, s.
diverging spine field, s.
epigastric artery, s.
intercostal artery, s.
lingualis muscle, s.
longitudinal sinus, s.
maxillary nerve, s.
mediastinum, s.
medullary velum, s.
mesenteric arteriography, s.
nasal concha, s.
nuchal line, s.

Additional Entries

superior *(continued)*
oblique muscle, s.
orbital fissure, s.
pancreaticoduodenal artery, s.
petrosal sinus, s.
profunda artery, s.
pulmonary artery, s.
sagittal sinus, s.
segment, s.
semicircular canal, s.
stopper, s.
tarsal plate, s.
thoracic artery, s.
thyroid artery, s.
tibiofibular articulation, s.
tympanic artery, s.
ulnar collateral artery, s.
vena cava, s.
vesical artery, s.
vocal cords, s.
supernumerary
cervical ribs, s.
digits, s.
spleen, s.
super scan
appearance, s.s.
pattern, s.s.
supersphenoid
superstructure
Super-Stuff
supernumerary
bone, s.
kidney, s.
tooth, s.
superoinferior view
supervascularization
supervoltage
radiation, s.
roentgenography, s.
supine
supine *(continued)*
decubitus view, s.
external oblique projection, s.
film, s.
frontal anteroposterior projection, s.
internal oblique projection, s.
oblique position, s.
oblique view, s.
position, s.
view, s.
supporting
cells of Hensen, s.
cells of Sertoli, s.
frame-work of retina, s.
suppurative
appendicitis, s.
encephalitis, s.
hepatitis, s.
hidradenitis, s.
phlebitis, s.
tonsillitis, s.
supra-acromial
nerves, s.
supra-anal
supra-auricular
supra-axillary
suprabuccal
supracallosal
gyrus, s.
supracardiac
supracervical
suprachoroid
supraciliary
supraclavicular
branches, s.
bruit, s.
fossa, s.
lymph nodes, s.
supraclinoid carotid stenosis

Additional Entries ____________________

____

____

supracondylar
  fracture, s.
  process, s.
supracostal
supracostalis muscle
supracranial
supradiaphragmatic
supraepicondylar
supraepitrochlear
supraglenoid
  tuberosity, s.
supraglottic larynx
suprahepatic
  space, s.
suprahyoid
  aponeurosis, s.
  artery, s.
  muscles, s.
  triangle, s.
suprainguinal
supraintestinal
supralumbar
supramalleolar
supramammary
supramandibular
supramarginal
  gyrus, s.
supramastoid
  crest, s.
suprameatal
  spine, s.
  triangle, s.
supramediastinal mantle
supramental
supramesocolic region
supranasal
supranuclear
supraoccipital
supraocular
supraorbital
  artery, s.
  foramen, s.

supraorbital *(continued)*
  margin, s.
  nerve, s.
  notch, s.
  vein, s.
suprapatellar
  bursa, s.
  effusion, s.
  pouch, s.
suprapelvic
suprarenal
  arteries, s.
  glands, s.
  plexus, s.
  veins, s.
suprarenoma
suprascapular
  artery, s.
  ligament, s.
  nerve, s.
  notch, s.
suprascleral
suprasellar
  mass, s.
supraseptal
supraspinal
  ligament, s.
supraspinatous
  fascia, s.
  fossa, s.
  muscle, s.
supraspinous
  ligament, s.
  muscle, s.
suprastapedial
suprasternal
  nerves, s.
  notch, s.
  space, s.
suprastructure
suprasylvian
supratemporal

Additional Entries

suprathoracic
supratonsillar
    fossa, s.
supratrochlear
    foramen, s.
    nerve, s.
supratympanic
supraumbilical
supravascular stenosing ring of left atrium
supraventricular
    arrhythmia, s.
    premature s. contractions
    tachycardia, s.
sural
    arteries, s.
    cutaneous nerve, s.
    nerve, s.
surface
    anatomy, s.
    application, s.
    articular s.
    coils, s.
    dorsal s.
    dose, s.
    lateral s.
    occlusion s.
    palmar s.
    plantar s.
surgical
    artifact, s.
    emphysema, s.
    survical evaluative staging (sTNM), s.
    neck, s.
surgicopathologic staging
Surgi-Lift stretcher
suspension intracavitary irradiation method
suspensory
    ligament, s.
suspensory *(continued)*
    muscle of duodenum, s.
sustentacular
    fibers of Muller, s.
sustentaculum
    lienis, s.
    tali, s.
Sutton's
    disease, S.
    nevus, S.
sutura
    dentata, s.
    harmonia, s.
    limbosa, s.
    notha, s.
    serrata, s.
    squamosa, s.
    vera, s.
sutural
    bones, s.
    diastasis, s.
    ligament, s.
suture
    coronal s.
    frontal s.
    frontoethmoidal s.
    frontozygomatic s.
    lambdoidal s.
    metopic s.
    occipitomastoid s.
    parietomastoid s.
    petro-occipital s.
    petrosquamous s.
    sagittal s.
    sphenoethmoidal s.
    sphenofrontal s.
    sphenoparietal s.
    sphenopetrosal s.
    sphenosquamosal s.
    sphenozygomatic s.
    squamosal s.
    squamosomastoid s.

Additional Entries

suture *(continued)*
- zygomaticofrontal s.
- zygomaticotemporal s.

Suzanne's gland
SVR (stroke volume ratio)
swallow
- barium s.

swallowing function study
Swan-Ganz catheter
swayback
sweat glands
Swediaur's disease
sweep
- duodenal bulb and s.

Swift's disease
swimmer's view
swish-and-swallow
Swyer-James
- hyperlucent lung, S-J
- syndrome, S-J

Syed/Neblett prostate template
Sylvest's disease
sylvian
- aqueduct, s.
- artery, s.
- cistern, s.
- cortex, s.
- fissure, s.
- fossa, s.
- line, s.
- triangle, s.
- point, s.
- vein, s.

Sylvius
- angle of S.
- aqueduct of S.
- valve of S.

Symington's body
Symmers' disease
symmetrical
symmetry
sympathectomy
sympathetic
- activity, s.
- block, s.
- chain, s.
- fibers, s.
- nerves, s.
- nervous system, s.
- plexuses, s.
- system, s.
- trunks, s.

sympatheticoparalytic
sympathetoblast
sympathicoblast
sympathicoblastoma
symphalangism
symphoricarpus
symphyocephalus
symphyseal
symphysis
- mandible, s. of
- pubis s.
- sacrococcygea, s. of

symphytum
synarthrosis
synchondrosis
- neurocentral s.

synchronia
synchronism
synchronous
syncytial
- layer, s.

syncytiotrophoblast
syndactyly
syndesmochorial
syndesmography
syndesmoma
syndesmo-odontoid
syndesmopexy
syndesmophyte
syndesmoplasty
syndesmorrhaphy

Additional Entries

syndesmosis
    tibiofibularis, s.
syndrome
    blue toe s.
    carpal tunnel s.
    cubital tunnel s.
    empty sella s.
synechia
synechiae
synechotome
synencephalocele
synencephaly
syneresis
synergistic action
syngenesioplastic
syngenesis
synophthalmia
synoptoscope
synostosis
synovectomy
synovia
synovial
    bursa, s.
    capsule, s.
    cyst, s.
    fluid, s.
    fluid analysis, s.
    fold, s.
    herniation, s.
    joint, s.
    membrane, s.
    sheath, s.
    tumor, s.
synovioblast
synoviocyte
synovioma
synoviosarcoma
synoviparous
synovitis
    dry s.
    purulent s.
    serous s.

synovitis *(continued)*
    sicca s.
    simple s.
    tendinous s.
    villonodular s.
synovium
synpneumonic
synreflexia
syntenosis
synteresis
synthescope
synthesis
synthesize
synthetic graft
syntropic
syntropy
syphilis
syphilitic aortitis
syringoadenoma
syringobulbia
syringocarcinoma
syringocele
syringocystadenoma
    papilliferum, s.
syringocystoma
syringoencephalomyelia
syringoid
syringoma
syringomeningocele
syringomyelia
    traumatic s.
syringomyelitis
syringomyelocele
syringotome
system
    atrioventricular conduction s.
    autonomic nervous s.
    calyceal s.
    canalicular s.
    cardiovascular s.
    circulatory s.

Additional Entries

system *(continued)*
collecting s.
external jugular s.
gastrointestinal s.
genitourinary s.
greater saphenous s.
hepatic ductal s.
immune s.
internal carotid s.
lesser saphenous s.
lower collecting s.
lymphatic s.
peripheral circulatory s.
peripheral nervous s.
renal collecting s.
respiratory s.
reticular activating s.
reticuloendothelial s.
skeletal s.
sympathetic nervous s.
upper collecting s.
urogenital s.
ventricular s.

systemic
absorption, s.
blood flow, s.
cardiac output, s.
chemotherapy, s.
circulation, s.
iron overload, s.
lupus erythematosis, s.
veins, s.

systole
atrial s.
auricular s.

systolic
apical murmur, s.
blood pressure, s.
click, s.
ejection murmur, s.
ejection rate, s.
gradient, s.
heave, s.
hypertension, s.
murmur, s.

Additional Entries

T

T (tesla)
T1 longitudinal or spin lattice relaxation time constant
T1 values
T1 weighted coronal image
T1 weighted image
T1 weighted sagittal image
T 1/2 (radioactive half-life)
T 1/2 B (tumor biological half-life)
T 1–201 (thallous chloride)
T2 image contrast
T2 transverse or spin-spin relaxation time constant
T2 values
T2 weighted image
T3 (thyroxine)
T4 (triiodothyronine)
Ta (tantalum)
    182 Ta isotope, wire
tabes dorsalis
table Bucky
tabletop absorption
tachyarrhythmia
tachycardia
    atrial t.
    ectopic t.
    junctional t.
    nodal t.
    paroxysmal t.
    paroxysmal atrial t. (PAT)
    paroxysmal ventricular t. (PVT)
    reflex t.
    sinus t.
    supraventricular t.
    ventricular t.
tachycardic
tachygastria
tachypnea
tachyrhythmia
taenia (pl. taeniae)
    coli, t.
    pontis, t.
    semicircularis, t.
    thalami, t.
    ventriculi quar
tag
    hemorrhoidal skin t.
    rectal skin t.
    tonsilar t.
tagliacotian rhinoplasty
tail
    gut, t.
    pancreas, t. of
Taillefer's valve
Takayashu arteritis
talar
tali
taliped
talipedic
talipes
    calcaneovalgus, t.
    calcaneovarus, t.
    calcaneus, t.
    cavovalgus, t.
    cavus, t.
    equinovalgus, t.
    equinovarus, t.
    equinus, t.
    planovalgus, t.
    valgus, t.
    varus, t.
talipomanus
Talma's disease
talocalcaneal
    articulation, t.
talocalcaneonavicular
    articulation, t.

Additional Entries ______________________________

talocrural
 articulation, t.
talofibular
 ligament, t.
talonavicular
 joint, t.
talotibial
 ligament, t.
talus
Tamm-Horsfall proteinuria
tamponade
 cardiac t.
tandem
 needle technique, t.
tangential
 beam, t.
 field, t.
 posteroanterior projection, t.
 view, t.
Tangier disease
tantalum (Ta)
 182 Ta Ta isotope, wire, t.
 182 Ta ophthalmic applicator, t.
taper-point surgical needle
tapetum
TAR (tissue-air ratio)
target
 background ratio, t. to
 cell, t.
 depth, t.
 film, t. to
 material, t.
 object distance, t.
 skin distance, t.
 tabletop distance, t.
 volume, t.
 volume localization, t.
Tarlov cyst
tarsal
tarsal *(continued)*
 artery, t.
 bone, t.
 gland, t.
 plate, t.
tarsi of eyelids
tarsoepiphyseal
tarsomegaly
tarsometatarsal
 articulations, t.
tarso-orbital
tarsophalangeal
tarsophyma
tarsoplasty
tarsorrhaphy
tarsotarsal
tarsotibial
tarsus
 bony t.
 inferior t.
 superior t.
 synovial membranes of t.
taste
 buds, t.
 fibers, t.
 nerves of t.
 organ of t.
Tawara's node
Tay's disease
Tay-Sachs disease
Tb (terbium)
TB
 patch test, TB
 smear, TB
T-bar
TBG (thyroxine-binding globulin)
TBI (total body irradiation)
TBPA (thyroxine-binding prealbumin)
Tc (technetium)
Tc 99m

Additional Entries ______________

Tc 99m *(continued)*
aggregated albumin, Tc 99m
albumin colloid, Tc 99m
albumin macroaggregated, Tc 99m
albumin microspheres, Tc 99m
antimony trisulfide colloid, Tc 99m
diethylene-triamine pentaacetic acid (DTPA), Tc 99m
diisopropylacetanilideiminodiacetic acid (DISIDA), Tc 99m
dimercaptosuccinic acid (DMSA), Tc 99m
dimethylacetanilide-iminodiacetic acid (HIDA), Tc 99m
diphosphonate, Tc 99m
DISIDA, Tc 99m (diisopropylacetanilideiminodiacetic acid or Tc 99m sulfur colloid)
disofenin, Tc 99m
DMSA, Tc 99m (dimercaptosuccinic acid)
DTPA (diethylene-triamine pentaacetic acid)
DTPA aerosol lung imaging
DTPA brain scanning
DTPA radioisotope, Tc 99m (diethylene-triamine pentaacetic acid)
DTPA renal imaging
etidronate, Tc 99m
ferpentetate, Tc 99m
GHP, Tc 99m (glucoheptonate)

Tc 99m *(continued)*
gluceptate, Tc 99m
glucoheptonate (GHP), Tc 99m
HDP, Tc 99m (hydroxydiphosphonate)
HIDA, Tc 99m (dimethylacetanilide-iminodiacetic acid)
HIDA liver scintigraphy, Tc 99m
hydroxydiphosphonate (HDP), Tc 99m
labeled A.C., Tc 99m
labeled stannous methylene diphosphonate, Tc 99m
lidofenin, Tc 99m
MAA, Tc 99m
MAA radioisotope, Tc 99m (macroaggregated albumin)
macroaggregated albumin (MAA), Tc 99m
MDP, Tc 99m (methylene diphosphonate)
mebrofenin, Tc 99m
medronate disodium, Tc 99m
methylene diphosphonate, Tc 99m
oxidronate, Tc 99m
pentetate, Tc 99m
pentetic acid, Tc 99m
PIPIDA, Tc 99m (P-isopropylacetanilide iminodiacetic acid)
P-isopropylacetanilide iminodiacetic acid (PIPIDA), Tc 99m
polyphosphate PYP (pyrophosphate), Tc 99m

Additional Entries

Tc 99m *(continued)*
PYP, Tc 99m (pyrophosphate)
pyridoxylidene glutamate, Tc 99m
pyrophosphate (PYP), Tc 99m
sodium pertechnetate, Tc 99m
stannous pyrophosphate, Tc 99m
stannous phytate, Tc 99m
succimer, Tc 99m
sulfur colloid, Tc 99m
tagged to phosphate, Tc 99m
thyroid scan, Tc 99m
trimetaphosphate, Tc 99m
T-cell
TCP (tumor control probability)
TD (tolerance dose/tumor doubling time)
TDF (time-dose-factor)
Te (tellurium)
TE (echo time)
TE/T2 ratio
technetium (Tc) (see under Tc 99m above)
Technicare Corporation
tectospinal
fasciculus, t.
Teff 1/2 (tumor effective half-life)
Teflon
Angiocath catheter, T.
ball, T.
button, T.
catheter, T.
coated needle, T.
Teflon *(continued)*
graft, T.
needle, T.
patch, T.
prosthesis, T.
shunt tube, T.
tegmen
tympani, t.
tegmental part of pons
tegmentum
tela (pl. telae) (any weblike tissue)
elastica, t.
telangiectasia
telangiectasis
spider t.
telangiitis
telangion
telangiosis
telecardiogram
telecardiography
telecardiophone
Telecobalt
telecord
telecurietherapy
telefluoroscopy
telectrocardiograph
telencephalon
teleneuron
Telepaque
teleradiography
teleradium
teleroentgenogram
teleroentgentherapy
telescope
Holinger t.
right-angle t.
telescopic mirror
telescoping catheter
telesthetoscope
teletherapy machine
tellurium (Te)

Additional Entries

TEM Cathetron afterloader
template
  applicator, t.
  table, t.
temporal
  arteries, t.
  arteritis, t.
  bone, t.
  electrode, t.
  facial nerve, t.
  fascia, t.
  fossa, t.
  gyri, t.
  headache, t.
  hemianopia, t.
  lines, t.
  lobe of brain, t.
  muscle, t.
  nerve, t.
  operculum, t.
  process, t.
temporalis
  muscle, t.
temporoauricular
temporofacial
temporofrontal
temporohyoid
temporomalar
  nerve, t.
temporomandibular
  articulation, t.
  joint, t.
temporomandibular joint syndrome (TMJ)
temporomaxillary
  vein, t.
temporo-occipital
temporoparietal
  muscle, t.
temporopontile
temporospatial
temporosphenoid
temporozygomatic
  suture, t.
tenacious
  mucoid secretions, t.
tenacity
  cellular t.
tendinitis
  stenosing t.
tendinoplasty
tendinous
  arch, t.
  inscriptions of rectus abdominis muscle, t.
  levator ani muscle, t.
tendo
  Achilles, t.
  calcaneus, t.
  oculi, t.
tendon (s)
  Achilles t.
  adductor t. release
  advancement, t.
  calcaneal t.
  common t.
  conjoined t.
  coronary t's.
  cricoesophageal t.
  deep t. reflexes (DTR)
  hamstring t.
  heel t.
  kangaroo t.
  lengthening, t.
  membranaceous t.
  of diaphragm, central t.
  of diaphragm, cordiform t.
  of diaphragm, intermediate t.
  of Hector, t.
  of perineum, central t.
  of Zinn, t.
  patellar t.

Additional Entries

tendon (s) *(continued)*
- pulled t.
- quadriceps t.
- riders' t.
- sheath, t.
- slipped t.
- transfer, t.
- transposition, t.
- trefoil t.

tendonitis
tendoplasty
tendovaginal
tendovaginitis
tendril fibers
tenesmus
tennis racquet catheter
tenodesis
tenodynia
tenolysis
tenomyoplasty
temomyotomy
Tenon's
- capsule, T.
- fascia, T.
- membrane, T.
- space, T.

tenonectomy
tenonitis
tenonometer
tenontodynia
tenontography
tenontophyma
tenontothecitis
tenophyte
tenoplasty
tenorrhaphy
tenostosis
tenosynovectomy
tenosynovitis
- adhesive t.
- stenosing t.
- villonodular t.

tenotomy
- curb t.
- graduated t.

TENS (transcutaneous electrical nerve stimulator)
tensiometer
tension
- arterial t.
- extraocular t.
- intraocular t.
- lines, t.
- muscle t. artifact
- ocular t.
- oxygen t.
- pneumothorax, t.
- surface t.
- wall, t.

tenth nerve
tenth value layer
tentorial sinus
tentorium
- cerebelli, t.

tentum
teratoblastoma
teratocarcinogenesis
teratocarcinoma
teratogen
teratogenesis
teratogenic
teratoid tumor
teratoma
- adult t.
- benign cystic t.
- malignant t.
- mature t.
- trophoblastic malignant t.

terbium (Tb)
teres
- major muscle, t.
- minor muscle, t.
- notch of ligamentum t.

Additional Entries ____________________

terminal
 crest, t.
 exponential region, t.
 ileal loop, t.
 ileitis, t.
 ileum, t.
 sulcus, t.
 vein, t.
 ventricle, t.
tertiary
 contractions, t.
 peristaltic activity, t.
 wall t.
 wave, t.
tesla (T)
testes
testicle
testicular
 lesion, t.
 torsion, t.
testiculoma
testis (pl. testes)
 appendages of t.
 appendix of t.
 coverings of t.
 descent of t.
 lobules of t.
 tunica albuginea t.
tethered cord
tetrablastic
tetrabrachius
tetrabromophthalein sodium
tetrad
 Fallot's t.
tetradactyly
tetralogy
 of Fallot, T.
tetranophthalmos
tetraparesis
tetraplegia
texture
 matrix t.
TGF (therapeutic gain factor)
TGG (time-controlled gain)
Th (thorium)
thalamectomy
thalamocoele
thalamocortical
thalamolenticular
thalamomamillary
thalamotegmental
thalamus
 optic t.
thalassemia
 major, t.
 trait, t.
thallium (Tl)
 chloride (Tl-201)
 rest exercise imaging, t.
 scan, t.
 stress redistribution perfusion imaging, t.
 stress test, t.
 201 (Tl-201) radioisotope, t.
 T1–201 thallous chloride
thanatophoric dwarfism
Thaysen's disease
thebesian
 valve, t.
 veins, t.
thebesius
 foramina of t.
 valve off t.
 veins of t.
theca (pl. thecae)
thecal
 luteal cyst, t.
 sac, t.
thecoma
thecitis
thecomatosis
thecostegnosis

Additional Entries

Theile's glands
Theiler's disease
thenad
thenar
    atrophy, t.
    eminence, t.
    facial cleft, t.
    facial compartment, t.
    muscles, t.
    space, t.
therapeutic
    embolization, t.
    failure, t.
    gain factor, t. (TGF)
    ratio, t. (TR)
therapy
    aversion t.
    immunosuppressive t.
    localization, t.
    radiation t.
TheraSeed implant
Theratron 780 cobalt 60 machine
thermacogenesis
thermaerotherapy
thermal
    equillibrium, t.
    injury, t.
    plastic, t.
thermistor-plethysmography
thermocautery
thermocoagulation
thermocouple
thermodiffusion
thermodilution
thermoelectric
thermoflex mold
thermogenesis
thermogenous
thermogram
    liquid crystal t.
thermograph
thermograph *(continued)*
    continuous scan t.
thermography
thermogravimeter
thermohyperalgesia
thermolamp
thermolaryngoscope
thermoluminescence (TL)
thermoluminescent dosimeter (TLD)
thermomastography
thermometer
thermonuclear
thermoplastic catheter
thermoscope
thermosteresis
thermotaxis
thermotolerance
thermotonometer
Thermotron-8 systen
thermotropism
Thessalus of Tralles
theta
    activity, t.
    frequency, t.
    wave, t.
thick x-ray target
thickened
    cortex, t.
    folds, t.
    gastric folds, t.
    placenta, t.
    rugae, t.
    small bowel folds, t.
thickening
    apical pleural t.
    bladder wall, t. of
    breast t.
    diffuse t.
    focal t.
thigh
    bone, t.

Additional Entries ______________________

thimble
chamber, t.
ionization chamber, t.
thin
liver block, t.
lung block, t.
needle, t.
placenta, t.
skull, t.
wall, t.
walled mass, t.
x-ray target, t.
thiol depletor
thiopentone
thiophosphate
third
cartilaginous ring, t.
cranial nerve, t.
cuneiform bone, t.
degree atrioventricular block, t.
degree cystocele, t.
degree heart block, t.
degree burn, t.
degree rectocele, t.
degree uterine prolapse, t.
healing by t. intention
metacarpal bone, t.
metatarsal bone, t.
nerve, t.
trimester, t.
trochanter, t.
ventricle, t.
Thiry's fistula
Thoma's ampulla
Thoma-Zeiss cell
Thomsen's
disease, T.
phenomenon, T.
thoracentesis
thoracic
thoracic *(continued)*
aneurysm, t.
aorta, t.
arteries, t.
axis, t.
cage, t.
cardiac nerves, t.
cavity, t.
duct, t.
esophagus, t.
inlet, t.
nerves, t.
nodes, t.
outlet, t.
outlet decompression, t.
portion of gangliated cord, t.
scoliosis, t.
spine, t.
venography, t.
vertebrae, t.
vertebral body, t.
thoracoacromial
artery, t.
thoracobronchotomy
thoracodorsal
artery, t.
nerve, t.
thoracoepigastric
system, t.
vein, t.
thoracolumbar
sympathetics, t.
thoracopathy
thoracopneumograph
thoracoscope
thoracostenosis
thoracostomy
thoracotomy
post t. changes
tube, t.
thorax

Additional Entries

thorax *(continued)*
barrel-shaped t.
bony t.
symmetrical t.
Thorel's bundle
thoriagram (photo made with thorium)
thorium (Th) 232
Thorotrast
induced reticuloendothelial blockage, T.
threatened abortion
three-dimensional
Fourier transformation, t-d
view, t-d
volume imaging, t-d
three-field
arrangement, t-f
box technique, t-f
technique, t-f
treatment beam geometry, t-d
x-ray beam dosimetry, t-d
three-phase
bone scanning, t-p
bone scintigraphy, t-p
three-way stopcock
threshold dose
thromboangiitis
obliterans, t.
thromboarteritis
thrombocyst
thrombocyte
thrombocytopenia
idiopathic t.
thrombocytopoiesis
thrombocytopoietic
thrombocytosis
thromboembolism
thromboendarterectomy
thromboendarteritis
thromboendocarditis
thrombogenesis
thrombogenic
thrombolymphangitis
thrombolysis
thrombophlebitis
migratory deep vein t.
superficial t.
suppurative t.
thrombopoiesis
thrombopoietic
thrombopoietin
thrombosinusitis
thrombosis
deep veinous t.
venous t.
thrombotic
occlusion, t.
thrombus
formation, t.
mural t.
occluding t.
through-and-through technique
thulium (Tm)
thumb
thymectomy
thymic
dysplasia, t.
hypertrophy, t.
lobule, t.
nodules, t.
thymidine
labeling index, t. (TLI)
thymitis
thymocyte
thymogenic
thymoma
thymopathy
thymopoietin

Additional Entries

thymoprivous
thymus
  gland, t.
thyroadenitis
thyroarytenoid
  ligament, t.
  muscle, t.
thyrocardiac
thyrocarditis
thyrocele
thyrocervical
  trunk, t.
thyroepiglottic
  ligament, t.
  muscle, t.
thyrofissure
thyrogenous
thyroglobulin assay
thyroglossal
  cyst, t.
  duct, t.
thyrohyoid
  ligament, t.
  membrane, t.
  muscle, t.
thyroid
  aberrant t.
  accessory t.
  acini, t.
  acropachy, t.
  adenoma, t.
  ala, t.
  arteries, t.
  axis, t.
  bed, t.
  body, t.
  cartilage, t.
  deficiency, t.
  eye disease, t.
  extract, t.
  foramen, t.
  gland, t.
thyroid *(continued)*
  insufficiency, t.
  intrathoracic t.
  isthmus, t.
  lingual t.
  lobe of t.
  needle biopsy, t.
  notch, t.
  probe, t.
  retrosternal t.
  scintigram, t.
  scintiscan, t.
  sonogram, t.
  stimulating hormone, t. (TSH)
  substernal t.
  radioiodine uptake, t.
  uptake, t.
  veins, t.
thyroidism
thyroiditis
  creeping t.
  de Quervain t.
  giant cell t.
  granulomatous t.
  Hashimoto's t.
  lymphocytic t.
  painless t.
  silent t.
  simple t.
  subacute t.
thyromegaly
thyromimetic
thyropathy
thyropenia
thyroptosis
thyrotome
thyrotomy
thyrotoxic
  goiter, t.
  heart disease, t.
thyrotoxicosis

Additional Entries

thyrotoxicosis *(continued)*
factitia, t.
medicamentosa, t.
thyrotropic
thyrotropin (thyroid stimulating hormone TSH)
receptors, t.
releasing hormone, t. (TRH)
thyroxine (T4)
binding globulin, t. (TBG)
binding prealbumin, t. (TBPA)
I 125, t.
I 131, t.
Ti (titanium)
TIA (transient ischemic attack)
tibia
saber t.
saber-shaped t.
valga t.
vara t.
tibial
artery, t.
bowing, t.
collateral ligament, t.
condyle, t.
crest, t.
epiphysis, t.
muscle, t.
nerve, t.
plafond, t.
plateau, t.
shaft, t.
spine, t.
surfaces of femur, t.
torsion, t.
tubercle, t.
tuberosity, t.
vein, t.
tibialis
anterior muscle, t.
anticus muscle, t.
posterior muscle, t.
tibiofibular
articulation, t.
joint, t.
ligament, t.
mortise, t.
syndesmosis, t.
tibionavicular
ligament, t.
tibiotarsal
articulation, t.
tidal
air, t.
volume, t.
Tiedemann's nerve
tie-on needle
tie-over stent
tie sternum
Tillaux's disease
tilted, foot down
tilting radiographic table
time controlled gain (TCG)
time-course uptake
time-dose-fraction (TDF) equivalent
time interval difference imaging
time interval difference mode
time-modulated pseudorandom coded aperture collimator
timer accuracy
tinea
capitis, t.
pedis, t.
tinged
fluid, blood t.
sputum, blood t.
stools, blood t.

Additional Entries

tinnitus
tip
- aspirating t.
- spleen t.
- whistle t. catheter

tissue
- adenoid t.
- adipose t.
- adventitial t.
- air ratio, t. (TAR)
- areolar t.
- cancellous t.
- cartilaginous t.
- cicatricial t.
- clearance, t.
- compensation, t.
- compensator, t.
- concentration, t.
- connective t.
- devitalized t.
- diagnosis, t.
- elastic t.
- endothelial t.
- epithelial t.
- erectile t.
- equivalent bolus, t.
- fibrous t.
- forceps, t.
- glandular t.
- heterogeneity, t.
- inhomogeneities, t.
- interstitial t.
- loose connective t.
- lymphoid t.
- massive scar t.
- maximum ratio, t. (TMR)
- mucous t.
- muscular t.
- myeloid t.
- nerve t.

tissue *(continued)*
- osseous t.
- phantom ratio, t. (TPR)
- reticular t.
- scar t.
- skeletal t.
- slice, t.
- soft t.
- soft t. calcification
- soft t. damage
- soft t. density
- soft t. injury
- soft t. swelling
- subcutaneous t.
- voxels, t.

titanium (Ti)
- clips, t.
- rays, t.

Titterington position (a/k/a semiaxial position)
Tl (thallium)
Tl-201
- imaging, t.
- kinetics, t.
- myocardial scan, t.
- scintigraphy, t.
- stress testing, t.
- washout half-time, t.

TL (thermoluminescence)
TLD (thermoluminescent dosimeter)
TLI (thymidine labeling index)
Tm (thulium)
TMR (tissue-maximum ratio)
TNM system (tumor, node metastases grading)
tocograph
tocometer
TOD (target-object distance)
Todd bodies

Additional Entries

Todd's palsy
toe
    hammer t.
toenail
toggle action
tolazoline hydrochloride
tolbutamide sodium
tolerance dose
tolpovidone I 131
toluidine blue
Tomes' fibers
Tommaselli's disease
Tomocat
tomogram
tomograph
tomography
    cardiac transaxial t.
    computed t.
    CAT (computerized axial) t.
    CATT (computerized axial transverse t.)
    computerized axial transverse t. (CATT)
    computerized axial t. (CAT)
    ECAT (emission computer assisted t.)
    emission computer assisted, t. (ECAT)
    frontal t.
    nephro t.
    restricted angle t.
    single photon emission t.
    transaxial emission t.
    ultrasonic t.
    positron emission transaxial t.
tomographic
    view, t.
tomoscintigraphy
tone
    loss of muscle t.
    rectal sphincter t.
    uterine muscle t.
tongue
    depressor, t.
    dorsum of t.
    fissured t.
    frenulum of t.
    glands of t.
    hairy t.
    mucous membrane of t.
    papillae of t.
    root of t.
    septum of t.
tonicity
tonoclonic
    spasm, t.
tonofibril
tonofilaments
tonograph
tonography
tonometer
    Schiotz t.
tonometry
    applanation t.
    digital t.
tonoscope
tonotopic
Toomey syringe
Tooth's disease
Topinard's angle
topoanesthesia
topographically
topography
toposcopic catheter
topper sponges
top spin
Torcon NB catheter
Torkildsen shunt
Tornwaldt's bursa

Additional Entries

torque
torsade de pointes (arrhythmia)
torsion
 negative t.
 positive t.
 testicular t.
torsionometer
torsiversion
torsoclusion
torticollis
tortipelvis
tortua
tortuosity
tortuous
 aorta, t.
 varicosities, t.
 vessels, t.
toruloma
torus
 auditory tube, t. of
 fracture, t.
 uretericus, t.
 uterinus, t.
total
 anomalous venous anomaly, t.
 body irradiation, t. (TBI)
 body photon radiation, t.
 body scan, t.
 filtration, t.
 lymphoid irradiation, t.
 nodal irradiation, t.
 skin irradiation, t.
 uterine length, t.
totipotency
touch fibers
Towne-Chamberlain position
Towne projection
Towne view
toxic
 adenoma, t.
 convulsion, t.
 diffuse goiter, t.
 dilatation, t.
 goiter, t.
 megacolon, t.
 multinodular goiter, t.
 nodular goiter, t.
 uninodular goiter, t.
toxoplasmosis
Toynbee's otoscope
TPN (total parenteral nutrition)
TPR (tissue-phantom ratio)
TR (repetition time)
trabecula (pl. trabeculae)
 carneae, t.
 penis, t. of
 spleen, t. of
 testis, t. of
trabeculation
 coarse bladder t.
 trigone, t. of
tracer
 accumulation, t.
 material, t.
 radioactive t.
trachea
 birfurcation of t.
 carina, t. of
 midline, t.
 shifted to right, t.
tracheal
 artery, t.
 bifurcation nodes, t.
 catheter, t.
 compression, t.
 diverticulosis, t.
tracheoaerocele
tracheobronchial
 lavage, t.

Additional Entries

tracheobronchial *(continued)*
    lymph nodes, t.
    toilet, t.
    tree, t.
tracheobronchitis
tracheobronchomegaly
tracheobronchoscopy
tracheocele
tracheoesophageal
    fistula, t.
tracheofissure
tracheogenic
tracheolaryngeal
tracheolaryngotomy
tracheomalacia
tracheomegaly
tracheopathia osteoplastica
tracheopharyngeal
tracheoplasty
tracheorrhagia
tracheostenosis
tracheostoma
tracheostomy
    button, t.
    cuff, t.
    stoma, t.
    tube, t.
tracheotome
traachcotomy
trachoma
    glands, t.
    inclusion conjunctivitis t.
trachomatous
tracing
    electrocardiogram t.
    electroencephalogram t.
    fetal heart monitor t.
track
    length, t.
    width, t.
tract (s)
    alimentary t.

tract (s) *(continued)*
    anterior basis bundle t.
    ascending t.
    Bekhterev's t.
    biliary t.
    Bruce's t.
    bulbar t.
    bulbospinal t.
    Burdach's t.
    cerebellar t.
    cerebellorubral t.
    cerebellorubrospinal t.
    cerebellospinal t.
    cerebellothalamic t.
    cerebrospinal t., lateral
    cornucommissural t.
    corticobulbar t.
    corticocerebellar t's.
    corticohypothalamic t.
    corticonuclear t.
    corticopontine t's.
    corticorubral t.
    corticospinal t.
    corticothalamic t.
    crossed t., marginal
    Deiters' t.
    descending t.
    digestive t.
    direct spinocerebellar t.
    dorsal peripheral band t.
    dorsolateral t.
    extracorticospinal t.
    extrapyramidal t.
    Flechsig's t.
    foraminous spiral t.
    frontopontine t.
    gastrointestinal t.
    geniculocalcarine t.
    genitourinary t.
    Goll's t.
    Gowers' t.
    habenular t's.

Additional Entries ______________________________

tract (s) *(continued)*
- habenulopenduncular t.
- Helweg's t.
- illiopubic t.
- iliotibial t.
- intermediolateral t.
- internuncial t.
- intersegmental t.
- intestinal t.
- lateral basis bundle t.
- Lissauer's t.
- Lowenthal's t.
- Maissiat's t.
- mamillopeduncular t.
- mamillotegmental t.
- mamillothalamic t.
- Marchi's t.
- Monakow's t.
- motor t.
- occipitopontine t.
- of auditory nerve, t.
- of bulb, t.
- of cranial nerves, t.
- of Flechsig, t.
- of medulla oblongata, t.
- of Meynert, t.
- of Philippe-Gombault, t.
- of Schultze, t.
- of spinal cord, t.
- of thymus, t.
- of trigeminal nerve, t.
- of trigeminal nerve, t.
- of trigeminal nerve, t.
- of Vicq d'Azyr, t.
- olfactory t.
- olivocerebellar t.
- olivospinal t.
- optic t.
- parietopontine t.
- predorsal t.
- prepyramidal t.
- projection t.

tract (s) *(continued)*
- pyramidal t.
- pyramidoanterior t.
- pyramidolateral t.
- respiratory t.
- reticulospinal t.
- rubroreticular t.
- rubrospinal t.
- Schultze's t.
- semilunar t.
- sensory t.
- septomarginal t.
- spinocerebellar t.
- spinocervicothalamic t.
- spino-olivary t.
- spinotectal t.
- spinothalamic t.
- spiral t.
- Spitzka's t.
- Spitzka-Lissauer t.
- strionigral t.
- sulcomarginal t.
- supraopticohypophyseal t.
- tectobulbar t.
- tectocerebellar t.
- tectospinal t.
- tegmental t.
- tegmentospinal t.
- temporopontile t.
- temporopontine t.
- thalamocortical t.
- thalamo-occipital t.
- thalamo-olivary t.
- transverse t.
- triangular t.
- trigeminothalamic t.
- tuberohypophyseal t.
- urinary t.
- uveal t.
- vestibulocerebellar t.
- vestibulospinal t.

Additional Entries

traction diverticulum
tragus
transabdominal
transaortic
transappendageal
transatrial
transaxial
    emission computed tomography, t.
    single photon emission tomographic images, t.
    slice, t.
    tomography, t.
transaxillary needle
transbasal
transcalvarial
transcatheter
transcervical
transcondyloid
transcortical
transcricothyroid
transducer
    applicator, t.
transduodenal cholangiography
transdural
transection
transepidermal
transepithelial
transferrin
transfixing
transformation constant
transformer
transfrontal
transglottic cancer
transhepatic cholangiogram
transient
    bladder herniation, t.
    equilibrium, t.
transillumination
transischiac
transit
transit *(continued)*
    time, t.
transition
    cell, t.
    phase, t.
transitional
    carcinoma, t.
    cell carcinoma, t.
    epithelial cells, t.
    epithelium, t.
    zone, t.
translateral
translate-rotate procedure
translucent
translumbar
    aortography, t.
    approach, t.
transluminal angioplasty
transmission target
transmitted light
transmural
    infarction, t.
    ischemia, t.
    perforation, t.
transocular
transorbital
transparent
    template, t.
transpectoral pathway
transperineal
    metallic guide, t.
    needle biopsy, t.
transperitoneal
transplant
    autogenous t.
    bone marrow t.
    homogenous t.
    organ t.
    tissue t.
transpleural
transposition
    great arteries, t. of

Additional Entries ______________________________

transposition *(continued)*
great vessels, t. of
patellar tendon, t. of
transpubic
transpyloric plane
transsegmental
transseptal
needle, t.
route, t.
transsphenoidal microsurgery
transthoracic
angiography, t.
biopsy, t.
lateral view, t.
transudate
peritoneal t.
transurethral
resection of bladder tumor, t. (TUR)
resection of prostate, t. (TURP)
transvenous
epicardial pacemaker, t.
transventricular
transversa colli artery
transversalis
artery, t.
fascia, t.
muscle, t.
transverse
acetabular ligament, t.
aorta, t.
axis, t.
carpal ligament, t.
cervical artery, t.
cervical nerve, t.
colon, t.
colostomy, t.
crural ligament, t.
diameter, t.
digital subtraction, t.
facial artery, t.

transverse *(continued)*
facial vein, t.
fibers, t.
fissure, t.
folds, t.
lie, t.
ligament, t.
lingualis muscle, t.
magnetization, t.
mesocolon, t.
occipital sulcus, t.
plane, t.
portion, t.
process, t.
scapular artery, t.
sinus, t.
temporal tyri, t.
transvesical
Trantas' dots
trapeziometacarpal
trapezium
trapezius muscle
trapezoid
body, t.
bone, t.
ligament, t.
nucleus, t.
ridge, t.
trapezoidal block
Traube's
body, T.
curves, T.
Traube-Hering curves
trauma
traumatic
amputation, t.
bowing fracture, t.
coagulopathy, t.
periostitis, t.
pneumothorax, t.
rupture of leaflet, t.
traveling wave

Additional Entries

Treacher Collins syndrome
Treacher Collins Franceschetti syndrome
treatment
- aids, t.
- portals, t.

tree
- biliary t.
- bronchial t.
- tracheobronchial t.

Treitz
- arch, T.
- ligament of T.

tremogram
Trendelenburg
- cannula, T.
- position, T.

trephine
trepidation
T3 resin uptake
Treves fold
TRH (thyrotropin-releasing hormone)
triad
- portal t.
- syndrome, t.

triangle (s)
- Alsberg t.
- Assezat t.
- Beclard t.
- Bolton t.
- Bonwill t.
- Bryant's t.
- Burger's scalene t.
- Calot t.
- carotid t.
- cervical t.
- Codman t.
- costohepatic t.
- digastric t.
- Dunham t's.
- Einthoven t.

triangle (s) *(continued)*
- Farabeuf t.
- femoral t.
- Garland t.
- Gerhardt t.
- Gombault-Philippe t.
- Grocco t.
- Grynfeltt t.
- habenular t.
- Henke t.
- Hesselbach t.
- hypoglossal t.
- inguinal t.
- Jackson safety t.
- Kanavel t.
- Koranyi-Grocco t.
- Labbe t.
- Langenbeck t.
- Lesgaft t.
- Lesser t.
- Lieutaud t.
- Livingston t.
- lumbar t.
- Macewen t.
- Malgaigne t.
- mesenteric t.
- Minor t.
- muscular t.
- neck t.
- occipital t.
- Pawlik t.
- pectineal t.
- Petit t.
- Pinaud t.
- Pirogoff t.
- pubourethral t.
- Rauchfuss' t.
- Reil t.
- sacral t.
- Scarpa's t.
- sternocostal t.
- subclavian t.

Additional Entries

triangle (s) *(continued)*
submaxillary t.
submental t.
suboccipital t.
supraclavicular t.
suprahyoid t.
suprameatal t.
Trautmann t.
Tweed t.
vagal t.
von Weber t.
Ward t.
Wernicke t.
trapping
air, t. of
triangular
articular disk, t.
bandage, t.
bone, t.
fascia, t.
fold, t.
ligament, t.
muscle, t.
trichoepithelioma
trichoesthesiometer
trichoglossia
trichomegaly
trichopathy
trichoscopy
tricuspid
atresia, t.
insufficiency, t.
malformation, t.
ring, t.
stenosis, t.
valve, t.
valve incompetency, t.
tricyclic
tridermic
tridermoma
trifacial
nerve, t.
trifid
trigastric
trigeminal
ciliary ganglion, t.
mandibular division, t.
maxillary division, t.
neuralgia, t.
ophthalmic division, t.
otic ganglion, t.
semilunar ganglion, t.
sphenopalatine ganglion, t.
submaxillary ganglion, t.
trigeminy
trigger finger
trigone
hypertrophy of t.
bladder, t. of
trigonitis
trigonocephaly
triiodothyronine (T3)
trilateral
trilobar prostatic enlargement
trilogy
Fallot, t. of
trimalleolar
trimanual
trineural
trinucleate
tripartite
triphalangeal
triphasic
triple
line, t.
lumen catheter, t.
voiding, t.
tripod position
trisomy 13, 18, 21
tritiated
thymidine, t. (3HTdR)
water, t.
tritium

Additional Entries

trivalve
trocar
trochanter
greater t.
lesser t.
third t.
trochanteric
bursa, t.
fossa, t.
trochlea
humerus, t. of
trochlear
fovea, t.
nerve, t.
process, t.
spine, t.
trochocephaly
trochoid
joint, t.
Trolard
anastomotic vein, T.
plexus, T.
trolley-type couch
Troltsch
corpuscles, T.
recess, T.
trophoblast
trophocyte
trophoneurosis
trophoplasm
trophoplast
trophospongium
tropochrome
trough level
TR/T1 ratio
Trousseau's syndrome
TRS (tumor-reductive surgery)
TruCut needle biopsy
true
aneurysm, t.
angle, t.
true *(continued)*
aphasia, t.
cords, t.
labor, t.
lateral position, t.
lateral projection, t.
mantle field, t.
pelvis, t.
positive, t.
skin, t.
vocal cords, t.
truncal
truncated sella
truncus
arteriosus, t.
costocervicalis, t.
sympathicus, t.
thyreocervicalis, t.
trunk
brachiocephalic t.
celiac t.
costocervical t.
length, t.
pulmonary t.
sympathetic t.
thyrocervical t.
vagal t.
TSH (thyroid stimulating hormone: thyrotropin) receptors
T-shaped uterus
TSK Surecut modified Menghini needle
TTT (tensor tympani tendon)
T-tube
cholangiogram, T-t
tuba
auditiva, t.
uterina, t.
tubal
abortion, t.
air cells, t.

Additional Entries

tubal *(continued)*
- block, t.
- fulguration, t.
- insufflation, t.
- ligation, t.
- occlusion, t.
- pregnancy, t.
- sterilization, t.

tubes (listed alphabetically)

tuber
- cinereum, t.
- frontale, t.
- parietale, t.

tubercle
- adductor t.
- anterior t.
- articular t.
- atlas, t. of
- auricular t. of Darwin
- carotid t.
- coccygeal t.
- conoid t.
- cuneate t.
- cuneiform t.
- dorsal radial t.
- epiglottis t.
- femur t.
- fracile t.
- greater t.
- humerus, t. of
- infraglenoid t.
- intercondylar t.
- intervenous t.
- jugular t.
- labial t.
- lacrimal t.
- lesser t.
- Lower, t. of
- marginal t.
- mental t.
- obturator t.
- olfactory t.

tubercle *(continued)*
- peroneal t.
- pharyngeal t.
- posteriot t.
- postglenoid t.
- pubic t.
- pterygoid t.
- quadrate t.
- rib, t. of
- Rolando, t. of
- scalene t.
- supraglenoid t.
- tibial t.

tube-film image

tubercular

tuberculocele

tuberculoderm

tuberculofibroid

tuberculoid

tuberculoma

tuberculomyces

tuberculosis
- disseminated t.
- genital t.
- miliary t.
- pulmonary t.
- warty t.

tuberculous
- adenitis, t.
- cavitation, t.
- meningitis, t.

tuberosity
- coracoid t.
- costal t.
- cuboid, t. of
- deltoid t.
- fifth metatarsal bone, t. of
- gluteal t.
- greater t.
- humerus, t. of
- iliac t.

Additional Entries

tuberosity *(continued)*
  infraglenoid t.
  ischial t.
  lesser t.
  maxillary t.
  navicular bone, t. of
  palatine bone, t. of
  radial t.
  sacral t.
  supraglenoid t.
  tibial t.
  ulna t.
tuberous
  sclerosis, t.
tubiferous
tuboabdominal
tubo-ovarian mass
tuboperitoneal
tubotympanum
tubouterine
tubovaginal
tubular
  accumulation, t.
  acidosis, t.
  acute t. necrosis
  carcinoma, t.
  defect, t.
  dysfunction, t.
  hypoplasia of aorta, t.
  interstitial disease, t.
  necrosis, t.
  renal t. acidosis
  respiration, t.
tubule (s)
  collecting t's.
  Henle's t's.
  renal t's.
  seminiferous t's.
  testicular t.
tubulocyst
tubulus (pl. tubuli)
  renal t.
Tudden's tract
tuft
  erosion, t.
  ungual t.
TUL (total uterine length)
tumor
  activity, t.
  bearing area, t.
  benign t.
  biological half-life (T 1/2 b)
  biopsy, t.
  cluster of t. cells
  control probability, t. (TCP)
  depth, t.
  dose, t.
  doubling time, t. (TD)
  effective half-life (Teff 1/2)
  encapsulated t.
  foci, t.
  Ewing's t.
  false t.
  formation, t.
  giant cell t.
  granular cell t.
  gross t.
  heterologous t.
  homologous t.
  Hurthle cell t.
  infiltration, t.
  inoperable t.
  invasion, t.
  islet cell t.
  lobulated t. mass
  localization, t.
  malignant t.
  mast cell t.
  melanotic t.
  metastatic t.
  mixed t.

Additional Entries

tumor *(continued)*
papillary t.
physical half-life (T 1/2 p)
primary t.
reductive surgery, t. (TRS)
residual t.
response, t.
satellite t. nodules
site, t.
tolerance, t.
volume, t.
Wilson's t.
tumoricidal dose
tumoritis
tungsten (W)
anode, t.
shielding, t.
target, t.
tunic
dartos t.
fibrous t.
tunnel
carpal t.
carpal t. decompression
carpal t. release
carpal t. syndrome
Corti, t. of
flap, t.
graft, t.
table, t.
view, t.
Tuohy-Borst introducer
turbid
fluid, t.
turbinate
inferior t.
middle t.
nasal t.
superior t.
turbinated
turbinated *(continued)*
bone, t.
processes, t.
turcica
sella t.
Turck
bundle, T.
zone, T.
Turcot syndrome
turgescence
turgid
Turk cell
Turner
intraparietal sulcus of T.
sulcus, T.
syndrome, T.
tooth, T.
Tuttle
pH probe test, T.
proctoscope, T
TVL (tenth value layer)
twelfth nerve
twelve-pulse
Twinning's view
two-dimensional
echocardiography, t-d
study, t-d (real-time)
view, t-d
two fixed coaxial lateral fields
two fixed technique
two frame gated imaging
two phase
two-plane
two-way catheter
tympanic
antrum, t.
artery, t.
canaliculus, t.
cavity, t.
lip, t.
membrane, t.

Additional Entries

tympanic *(continued)*
  nerve, t.
  plexus, t.
  ring, t.
  sulcus, t.
tympanitic
tympanocentesis
tympanoeustachian
tympanogenic
tympanogram
tympanohyal
  part of temporal bone, t.
tympanolabyrinthopexy
tympanomalleal
tympanomandibular
tympanomastoid
  cavity, t.
  fissure, t.
tympanomastoiditis
tympanomeatal
  flap, t.
tympanometry
tympanoplasty
tympanosclerosis
tympanosquamosal
tympanostapedial
tympanotemporal
tympanum
Tyndall light
Tyndall phenomenon
typhlitis
typhlocolitis
typhlolithiasis
typhlomegaly
typhus
  nodule, t.
typoscope
tyroma
tyromatosis
tyropanoate sodium
tyrosine
tyrosinemia
Tyrrell fascia
Tyrrell hook
Tyson crypts
Tzanck
  cell, T.
  smear, T.
T zone

Additional Entries

U

U (uranium)
Uhl anomaly
ulcer
  active u.
  antral u.
  crater, u.
  Curling's u.
  decubitus u.
  gastric u.
  niche, u.
  penetrating u.
  peptic u.
  perforated u.
  prepyloric u.
  regimen, u.
  stasis u.
  stress u.
  varicose u.
  venereal u.
ulcerate
ulcerated
  plaque, u.
  tumor, u.
ulcerative
  colitis, u.
ulcerogangrenous
ulcerogenic
ulcerogranuloma
ulceromembranous
ulcerous
ulna
  bone, u.
ulnad
ulnar
  artery, u.
  collateral artery, u.
  deviation, u.
  recurrent artery, u.
  nerve, u.
  notch of radius, u.

ulnar *(continued)*
  palsy, u.
  pulse, u.
  reflex, u.
  styloid bone, u.
  vein, u.
ulocarcinoma
uloglossitis
ulorrhagia
ulorrhea
ultimobranchial bodies
ultradolichocephalic
ultrafilter
ultrafiltration
ultragaseous
ultramicron
ultramicroscope
ultrasonic
  echorenography, u.
  nebulizer, u.
ultrasonogram
ultrasonography
  A-mode u.
  B-mode u.
  B-scan u.
  computerized reconstruction u.
  Doppler u.
  gray-scale u.
  guided procedure for diagnosis, u.
  guided procedure for therapy, u.
  real-time u.
  special nonroutine projection u.
ultrasonometry
ultrasound
  abdominal scanning, u.
  breast u.

Additional Entries ______

ultrasound *(continued)*
cardiovascular u.
continuous wave u.
Doppler u.
high-frequency u.
imaging, u.
pelvic u.
pulsed u.
real-time u.
ultraviolet rays
ultra x-ray
umbilical
artery, u.
catheter, u.
circulation, u.
cord, u.
folds, u.
fossa, u.
hernia, u.
notch, u.
pathway, u.
souffle, u.
tape, u.
vein, u.
venography, u.
vesicle, u.
zone, u.
umbilicus
symphysis to u.
umbo (a round projection)
tympanic membrane, u. of
umbrascopy
unciform
bone, u.
uncovertebral
unctuous
uncus
Underwood's disease
undescended testes
undulation (wavelike motion)
unfolded aorta
ungual
phalanx, u.
tuft, u.
ungues
uniarticular
uniaxial
unibasal
unicameral
unicellular
unicentral
unicuspid
unifocal
uniform echo pattern
uniform failure
unigeminal
unigerminal
uniglandular
unilaminar
unilateral
facet dislocation, u.
hyperlucent lung, u.
hypoplasia, u.
mass effect, u.
parametrial portal, u.
translucency, u.
wedge pair field, u.
unilobar
unilocular
cyst, u.
structure, u.
union
bony u.
delayed u.
fibrous u.
Union Miniere Company
uniparous
Unipoint Industries
unipolar
lead, u.
pacemaker generator, u.
United States Catheter and Instrument Corporation

Additional Entries

unmodified x-ray beam
unopacified
unrest
  peristaltic un.
Unverricht's disease
upper airway obstruction
upper gastrointestinal (GI) series
upright
  chest cassette holder, u.
  film, u.
  frontoposterior projection, u.
  view, u.
uptake
  decreased u.
  diminished u.
  heterogenous u.
  high u.
  increased u.
  probe, u.
  radioiodine u.
  radioisotope u. studies
  rate, u.
urachovesical
urachus
uranium (U)
  nuclei, u.
  series, u.
uratoma
Urbach-Oppenheim disease
uremic pericarditis
ureter
ureteral
  meatus, u.
  necrosis, u.
  orifice, u.
  reflux, u.
  septa, u.
  stent, u.
  structure, u.
ureteralgia
ureterectasis
ureterectomy
ureteric
  notching, u.
  stricture, u.
ureteritis
  cystica, u.
ureterocele
  ectopic u.
  simple u.
ureterocelectomy
ureterocervical
ureterocolic fistula
ureterocystoscope
ureterocystostomy
ureterodialysis
ureteroduodenal
ureteroenteric
  fistula, u.
ureterogram
ureterography
ureteroileostomy
ureterointestinal
ureterolith
ureterolithiasis
ureteropelvic
  junction, u. (UPJ)
  junction obstruction, u.
ureterophlegma
ureteropyelitis
ureteropyelography
ureteropyelonephritis
ureterorectal
ureterorectoneostomy
ureterorenoscope
ureterorrhagia
ureterosigmoidostomy
ureterostenoma
ureterostenosis
ureterostoma
ureterostomy
ureterotomy

Additional Entries

ureterotrigonoenterostomy
ureterotrigonosigmoidostomy
ureteroureteral
ureteroureterostomy
ureterouterine
ureterovaginal
ureterovesical
ureterovesicoplasty
ureterovesicostomy
urethra
    bulbous u.
    external u. orifice
    internal u. orifice
    meatal stenosis, u.
    muliebris, u.
    prostatic u.
    sphincter muscle of u.
    stricture, u.
    trigonitis, u.
    virilis, u.
urethral
    orifice, u.
    stricture, u.
    valve, u.
urethritis
    nongonococcal u.
    nonspecific u.
    petrificans, u.
    simple u.
    specific u.
    venerea u.
urethroblenorrhea
urethrobulbar
urethrocele
urethrocystitis
urethrocystogram
urethrocystography
urethrocystopexy
urethrogram
    retrograde u.
urethrography
    retrograde u.
urethropenile
urethroperineal
urethroperineoscrotal
urethropexy
urethrophyma
urethrorectaal
urethrorrhagia
urethrorrhaphy
urethroscope
urethroscrotal
urethrospasm
urethrostenosis
urethrotome
    Maisonneuve's u.
urethrovaginal fistula
urethrovesical
    angle, u.
uric acid nephropathy
uricosuria
urinary
    bladder, u.
    conduit, u.
    excretion, u.
    stasis, u.
    tract, u.
urine
    Bence Jones u.
    black u.
    chylous u.
    cloudy u.
    curde u.
    diabetic u.
    dyspeptic u.
    effluxing clear u.
    febrile u.
    gouty u.
    milky u.
    nebulous u.
    residual u.
    straw-colored u.
urinocryoscopy
urinogenital

Additional Entries __________

urinogenous
urinoma
urocele
urochrome
urocyst
urocystitis
urogenital
 apparatus, u.
 diaphragm, u.
 fold, u.
 organs, u.
 ostium, u.
 sinus, u.
Urografin
urogram
urography
 ascending u.
 cystoscopic u.
 descending u.
 excretion u.
 excretory u.
 intravenous u.
 oral u.
 retrograde
urokinase (thrombolytic)
 protocol, u.
urokinetic
urokymography
urolith
urolithiasis
uronoscopy
uropathy
 obstructive u.
uropyoureter
uroradiology
urorectal
 septum, u.
uroscopy
urticaria
 bullous u.
 giant u.
 hemorrhagica, u.

urticaria *(continued)*
 medicamentosa, u.
 papular u.
 pigmentosa, u.
 solar u.
U.S. Catheter and Instrument Corporation
U-shaped cartilaginous rings
uteri
 adenomyosis u.
 corpus u.
 fibromyomata u.
 leiomyoma u.
 myomata u.
uterine
 artery, u.
 atony, u.
 bleeding, u.
 cavity, u.
 corpus, u.
 dysfunctional u. bleeding
 fibroid, u.
 fundus, u.
 glands, u.
 musculature, u.
 myomectomy, u.
 plexus, u.
 procidentia, u.
 prolapse, u.
 reflection, u.
 segment, u.
 suspension, u.
uteroabdominal
uterocervical
utero-ovarian
uteroplacental
uterorectal
uterosacral
 ligaments, u.
uterosalpingography
uteroscope
uterotubography

Additional Entries

uterovaginal
uteroventral
uterovesical
uterus
    anteflexed u.
    anteverted u.
    arcuate u.
    bicornuate u.
    boggy u.
    cervix of u.
    double u.
    fibroid u.
    fundus of u.
    gravid u.
    infantile u.
    inversion of u.
    involution of u.
    isthmus of u.
    masculinus u.
    palmate folds of u.
    rudimentary u.
    septate u.
    subinvolution of u.

uterus *(continued)*
    T-shaped u.
utricle
    prostatic u.
    vestibule, u. of
utricular
utriculi
utriculitis
utriculosaccular
utriculus
U-tube
U turn of right coronary artery
uvea
uveitis
uveoneuraxitis
uveoparotid
uveoscleritis
uvula
    bladder, u. of
    cerebellum, u. of
    palatine u.
    vesicae, u.

Additional Entries

V

V (vanadium)
V (volt)
vacuolated
vacuum
  degeneration, v.
  disk, v.
  joint, v.
  tube, v.
vagal
vagi
vagina
vaginae
  mucosae, v.
vaginal
  artery, v.
  bulb, v.
  cuff, v.
  flora, v.
  folds, v.
  fornices, v.
  fornix, v.
  inclusion cyst, v.
  orifice, v.
  outlet, v.
  plexus, v.
  process, v.
  vault, v.
  wall, v.
vaginoabdominal
vaginocele
vaginography
vaginolabial
vaginomycosis
vaginopathy
vaginoperineal
vaginoperitoneal
vaginopexy
vaginoplasty
vaginoscope
vaginovesical
vagoaccessorius
vagoglossopharyngeal
vagogram
vagolytic
vagotomy
vagus
  nerve, v.
  pulse, v.
  reflex, v.
  stimulation, v.
valence
  bone, v.
  state, v.
Valentin's corpuscles
Valentine's position
valgus
  deformity, v.
  hallux v. deformity
  pes v.
  strain, v.
  talipes v.
vallate
vallecula
valleculae
Valleix's points
Valsalva's
  anomaly, V.
  maneuver, V.
  sinus, V.
Valsuani's disease
valva
valve
  anal v.
  aortic v.
  artificial v.
  atrioventricular v.
  attenuation v.
  auriculoventricular v.
  Beraud's v.
  bicuspid v.

Additional Entries ____________________

valve *(continued)*
cardiac v.
colic v.
coronary sinus, v. of
dehiscence, v.
eustachian v.
flair v.
Hasner's v.
heart v.
Heister's v.
Houston's v.
ileocecal v.
incompetent v.
inferior vena cava, v. of
Kerckring's v.
leaflet, v.
lymphatic v.
mitral v.
mitral v. prolapse
prosthesis, v.
pulmonary v.
pyloric v.
right and left venous v.
semilunar aortic v.
thesbesian v.
tricuspid v.
ureteral v.
Varolius v.
vegetation, v.
veins, v. of
Vieussens v.
valvula (pl. valvulae)
valvular
anomaly, v.
atresia, v.
disease, v.
incompetence, v.
pulmonary stenosis, v.
regurgitation, v.
rheumatic v. disease
stenosis, v.
valvulae conniventes
valvulitis
rheumatic v.
valvuloplasty
valvulotome
vanadium (V)
Van Brunn's nests
van Buren's disease
Vance dilator
Van de Graaff accelerator
van den Bergh's disease
van Hoorne's canal
Van Sonnenberg sump
Vaquez's disease
variable enhancement
Varian
Clinac 2500 accelerator, V.
Clinic 2500 accelerator, V.
4–MeV accelerator, V.
simulator, V.
varices
esophageal v.
gastric v.
varicocele
varicography
varicoid
varicophlebitis
varicose
ulcer, v.
varicosities
superficial v.
tortuous v.
varicosity
varix
anastomotic v.
aneurysmal v.
aneurysmoid v.
esophageal v.
isolated esophageal v.
papillary vv.
Varolius' valve

Additional Entries

varum
genu v.
varus
deformity, v.
hallux v.
pes v.
vas
deferens, v.
vasal
Vascoray
vascular
calcification, v.
capsule, v.
cystic lesion, v.
deformity, v.
dissection, v.
Doppler, v.
ectasia, v.
enlargement, v.
enteric fistula, v.
flow imaging, v.
groove, v.
insult, v.
laceration, v.
lake, v.
malformation, v.
markings, v.
narrowing, v.
occlusion, v.
phenomena, v.
pseudoaneurysm, v.
ring, v.
stenosis, v.
system, v.
territory, v.
tunic, v.
vascularity
vascularize
vasculature
vasculitic
vasculitis
vasculolymphatic
vasculopathy
vasoactive
vasoconstrictor
vasocorona
vasodepression
vasodilation
vasodilator
vasoepididymography
vasoepididymostomy
vasoformative
cells, v.
vasoganglion
vasogenic
vasography
vasomotor
vasoneuropathy
vasoparesis
vasopressin
vasopuncture
vasospasm
vasospastic
vasotrophic
vasotropic
vasovagal
attack, v.
syncope, v.
vasovesiculitis
Vater's ampulla
Vater-Pacini corpuscles
vault
defect, v.
vaginal v.
V configuration
VCUG (voiding cystourethrogram)
vector
vectorcardiogram
spatial v.
vectorcardiograph
vectorcardiography

Additional Entries

vectorscope
vegetative
  endocarditis, v.
Veillon tube
vein (s)
  accompanying v.
  accompanying (hypoglossal nerve) v.
  adrenal v's.
  afferent v's.
  allantoic v's.
  anastomotic (inferior) v.
  anastomotic (superior) v.
  angular v.
  anonymous v's.
  antebrachial (median) v.
  appendicular v.
  aqueous v's.
  arciform v's.
  arcuate (kidney) v's.
  arterial v.
  arterial (Soemmering) v.
  ascending (Rosenthal) v's.
  Ascher's v's.
  auditory (internal) v's.
  auricular (anterior) v's.
  auricular (posterior) v.
  axillary v.
  azygos v.
  azgos (left) v.
  azygos (lesser superior) v.
  basal v.
  basilic v.
  basilic (median) v.
  basivertebral v's.
  brachial v's.
  brachiocephalic v's.
  Breschet's v's.
  bronchial v's.
  Browning's v.

vein (s) *(continued)*
  Burow's v.
  cardiac v's.
  cardiac (anterior) v's.
  cardiac (great) v.
  cardiac (middle) v.
  cardiac (small v.
  cardiac (smallest) v's.
  cardinal v's.
  carotid (external) v.
  cavernous (penis) v's.
  central v.
  central (hepatic lobules) v's.
  central (liver) v's.
  central (retina) v.
  central (suprarenal gland) v.
  cepahlic v.
  cephalic (accessory) v.
  cephalic (median) v.
  cerebellar (inferior) v's.
  cerebellar (superior) v's.
  cerebral v's.
  cerebral (anterior) v.
  cerebral (great) v.
  cerebral (inferior) v's.
  cerebral (internal) v's.
  cerebral (middle, deep) v.
  cerebral (middle, superficial) v.
  cerebral (superior) v's.
  cervical (deep) v.
  cervical (transverse) v's.
  choroid v.
  ciliary v's.
  circumflex foemoral (lateral) v's.
  circumflex femoral (medial) v's.
  circumflex iliac (deep) v.

Additional Entries ______

vein (s) *(continued)*
circumflex iliac (superficial) v.
colic (left) v.
(colic (middle) v.
colic (right) v.
conjunctival v's.
coronary v.
costoaxillary v's.
cubital (median) v.
cutaneous v.
cutaneous (ulnar) v.
cystic v.
deep (clitoris) v's.
deep (penis) v's.
deep (thigh) v.
deep (tongue) v.
digital (palmar) v's.
digital (plantar) v's.
digital (foot, common) v's.
digital (foot, dorsal) v's.
diploic v's.
diploic (frontal) v.
diploic (occipital) v.
diploic (temporal, anterior) v.
diploic (temporal, posterior) v.
dorsal (clitoris, deep) v.
dorsal (clitoris, superficial) v's.
dorsal (penis, deep) v.
dorsal (clitoris, superficial) v's.
dorsal (penis, deep) v.
dorsal (penis, superficial) v's.
dorsal (tongue) v's.
dorsispinal v's.
duodenal v's.
emissary v.

vein (s) *(continued)*
emissary (condylar) v.
emissary (mastoid) v.
emissary (occipital) v.
emissary (parietal) v.
emulgent v.
epigastric (inferior) v.
epigastric (superficial) v.
epigastric (superior) v's.
episcleral v's.
esophageal v's.
ethmoidal v's.
facial
facial (anterior) v.
facial (common) v.
facial (deep) v.
facial (posterior) v.
facial (transverse) v.
femoral v.
femoral (deep) v.
femoropopliteal v.
fibular v's.
frontal v's.
Galen's v's.
gastric (left) v.
gastric (right) v.
gastric (short) v's.
gastroepiploic (left) v.
gastroepiploic (right) v.
genicular v's.
gluteal (inferior) v's.
gluteal (superior) v's.
hemiazygos v.
hemiazygos (accessory) v.
hemorrhoidal (inferior) v's.
hemorrhoidal (middle) v's.
hemorrhoidal (superior) v.
hepatic v's.

Additional Entries

vein (s) *(continued)*
- hypogastric v.
- hypophyseoportal v's.
- ileal v's.
- ileocolic v.
- iliac (common)
- iliac (external) v.
- iliac (internal) v.
- iliolumbar v.
- innominate v's.
- intercapital v's.
- intercapitular (of foot) v's.
- intercapitular (of hand) v's.
- intercostal (anterior) v's.
- intercostal (highest) v.
- intercostal (posterior, IV-XI) v's.
- intercostal (superior, left) v.
- intercostal (superior, right) v.
- interlobar (of kidney) v's.
- inteerlobular (of kidney) v's.
- interlobular (of liver) v's.
- interosseous (of foot, dorsal) v's.
- interosseous metacarpal (dorsal) v's.
- intervertebral v.
- jejunal v's.
- jugular (anterior) v.
- jugular (anterior horizontal) v.
- jugular (external) v.
- jugular (internal) v.
- Kohlrausch v's.
- Krukenberg's v's.

vein (s) *(continued)*
- Kuhnt's postcentral v.
- Labbe's v.
- labial (anterior) v's.
- labial (posterior) v's.
- labial (superior) v.
- lacrimal v.
- laryngeal (inferior) v.
- laryngeal (superior) v.
- lingual v.
- lingual (deep) v.
- lingual (dorsal) v's.
- lumbar I and II v's.
- lumbar III and IV v's.
- lumbar (ascending) v.
- mammary (external) v's.
- mammary (internal) v.
- Marshall's oblique v.
- masseteric v's.
- maxillary v's.
- median elbow v.
- median forearm v.
- median neck v.
- mediastinal v's.
- meningeal v's.
- meningeal (middle) v's.
- mesenteric (inferior) v.
- mesenteric (superior) v.
- metacarpal (dorsal) v's.
- metacarpal (palmar) v's.
- metatarsal (dorsal) v's.
- metatarsal (plantar) v's.
- muscular v's.
- musculophrenic v's.
- nasal (external) v's.
- nasofrontal v.
- oblique (left atrium)
- obturator v's.
- occipital v.
- oesophageal v's.
- of aqueduct of vestibule, v.

Additional Entries

vein (s) *(continued)*
of bulb of penis, v.
of bulb of vestibule, v.
of canaliculus of cochlea, v.
of cochlear canal, v.
of kidney, v's.
of Marshall, v.
of pterygoid canal, v.
of Sappey, v's.
of septum pellucidum, v.
of sylvian fossa, v.
of Thebesius, v's.
of vertebral column (external) v's.
of Vieussens, v's.
omphalomesenteric v's.
ophthalmic (inferior) v.
ophthalmic (superior) v.
ophthalmomeningeal v.
ovarian (left) v.
ovarian (right) v.
palatine (external) v.
palpebral v's.
palpebral (inferior) v's.
palpebral (superior) v's.
pancreatic v's.
pancreaticoduodenal v's.
paraumbilical v's.
parietal Santorini v.
parotid v's.
parotid (anterior) v's.
parotid (posterior) v's.
parumbilical v's.
perforating v's.
pericardiac v's.
pericardiacophrenic v's.
peroneal v's.
pharyngeal v's.
phrenic (inferior) v's.
phrenic (superior) v's.
popliteal v.

vein (s) *(continued)*
portal v.
postcardinal v's.
posterior left ventricle v.
precardinal v's.
prepyloric v.
primary head v's.
pudendal (external) v's.
pudendal (internal) v.
pulmonary v's.
pulmonary (inferior, left) v.
pulmonary (inferior, right) v.
pulmonary (superior, left) v.
pulmonary (superior, right) v.
pulp v's.
pyloric v's.
radial v's.
radial (external of Soemmering) v.
ranine v.
rectal (inferior) v's.
rectal (middle) v's.
rectal (superior) v.
renal v's.
retromandibular v.
Retzius's v's.
Rosenthal's v.
Ruysch's v's.
sacral (lateral) v's.
sacral (middle) v.
salvatella v.
saphenous (accessory) v.
saphenous (great) v.
saphenous (small) v.
scrotal (anterior) v's.
scrotal (posterior) v's.
sigmoid v's.
small heart v.

Additional Entries

vein (s) *(continued)*
spermatic v.
spinal v's.
spiral modiolus v.
splenic v.
stellate kidney v's.
Stensen's v's.
sternocleidomastoid v.
striate v.
stylomastoid v.
subcardinal v's.
subclavian v.
subcostal v.
subcutaneous abdomen v's.
sublingual v.
sublobular v's.
submental v.
supracardinal v's.
supraorbital v.
suprarenal (left) v.
suprarenal (right) v.
suprascapular v.
supratrochlear v's.
sylvian v.
temporal (deep) v's.
temporal (middle) v.
temporal (superficial) v's.
temporomandibular articular v's.
terminal v.
testicular (left) v.
testicular (right) v.
thalamostriate v.
thebesian v's.
thoracic (internal) v's.
thoracic (lateral) v's.
thoracoacromial v.
thoracoepigastric v's.
thymic v's.
thyroid (inferior) v.

vein (s) *(continued)*
thyroid (middle) v's.
thyroid (superior) v.
tibial (anterior) v's.
tibial (posterior) v's.
trabecular v's.
tracheal v's.
transverse (face) v.
transverse (neck) v's.
Trolard's v.
tympanic v's.
ulnar v's.
umbilical v.
umbilical (left) v.
uterine v's.
varicose v.
vertebral v.
vertebral (accessory) v.
vertebral (superficial) v's.
vesalian v.
vesical v's.
vestibular v's.
vidian v's.
vitelline v's.
vorticose v's.

vela
velamen
velamenta
cerebri, v.
velamentous
insertion of umbilical cord, v.
velamentum
Vella's fistula
velocity
light, v. of
motor nerve conduction v.
velopharyngeal
velum
velopharyngeal

Additional Entries

velopharyngeal *(continued)*
- closure, v.
- function, v.
- structures, v.

Velpeau cast

vena cava
- inferior v.c.
- superior v.c.

vena
- advenhentes, vv.
- anastomotica inferior, v.
- anastomitica superior, v.
- angularis, v.
- anonymae (dextra et sinistra), vv.
- appendicularis, v.
- aqueductus vestibuli, v.
- arciformes renis, vv.
- arcuatae renis, vv.
- articulares mandibulae, vv.
- articulares temporomandibulares, vv.
- auditivae internae, vv.
- auriculares anteriores, vv.
- auricularis posterior, v.
- axillaris, v.
- azygos, v.
- basalis, v.
- basalis, v.
- basilica, v.
- basivertebrales, vv.
- brachiales, vv.
- brachiocephalicae (dextra et sinistra), vv.
- bronchiales, vv.
- bronchiales anteriores, vv.
- bronchiales posteriores, vv.
- bulbi penis, v.
- bulbi vestibuli, v.

vena *(continued)*
- canaliculi cochleae, v.
- canalis pterygoidei, v.
- canalis pterygoidei, v.
- cavae, vv.
- cava inferior, v.
- cava superior, v.
- cavernosae penis, vv.
- centralis glandulae suprarenalis, v.
- centrales hepatis, vv.
- centralis retinae, v.
- cephalica, v.
- cephalic accessoria, v.
- cerebelli inferiores, vv.
- cerebelli superiores, vv.
- cerebri, vv.
- cerebri anterior, v.
- cerebri inferiores, vv.
- cerebri internae, vv.
- cerebri magna, v.
- cerebri magna, v.
- cerebri media, v.
- cerebri media profunda, v.
- cerebri media superficialis, v.
- cerebri superiores, vv.
- cervicalis profunda, v.
- choroidea, v.
- choroideae oculi, vv.
- ciliares, vv.
- ciliares anteriores, vv.
- ciliares posteriores, vv.
- circumflexae femoris laterales, vv.
- circumflexae femoris mediales, vv.
- circumflexa ilium profunda, v.
- circumflexa ilium superficialis, v.
- colica dextra, v.

Additional Entries

vena *(continued)*
colica media, v.
colica sinistra, v.
comitans, v.
comitantes arteriae femoralis, vv.
comitans nervi hypoglossi, v.
conjunctivales, vv.
conjunctivales anteriores, vv.
conjunctivales posteriores, vv.
cordis, vv.
cordis anteriores, vv.
cordis magna, v.
cordis media, v.
cordis minimae, vv.
cordis parva, v.
conaria ventriculi, v.
costoaxillares, vv.
cutanea, v.
cystica, v.
digitales communes pedis, vv.
digitales dorsales pedis, vv.
digitales palmares, vv.
digitales pedis dorsales, vv.
digitales plantares, vv.
digitales volares communes, vv.
digitales volares propriae, vv.
diploicae, vv.
diploica frontalis, v.
diploica occipitalis, v.
diploica temporalis anterior, v.
diploica temporalis posterior, v.

vena *(continued)*
dorsalis clitoridis profunda, v.
dorsales clitoridis superficiales, vv.
dorsales linguae, vv.
dorsalis penis profunda, v.
dorsales penis subcutaneae, vv.
dorsales penis superficiales, vv.
duodenales, vv.
emissaria, v.
emissaria condylaris, v.
emissaria mastoidea, v.
emissaria occipitalis, v.
emissaria parietalis, v.
epigastrica inferior, v.
epigastrica superficialis, v.
epigastricae superiores, vv.
episclerales, vv.
esophageae, vv.
ethmoidales, vv.
ethmoidalis anterior, v.
ethmoidalis posterior, v.
facialis, v.
facialis anterior, v.
facialis communis, v.
facialis posterior, v.
faciei profunda, v.
femoralis, v.
femoropoplitea, v.
fibulares, vv.
frontales, vv.
gastricae breves, vv.
gastrica dextra, v.
gastrica sinistra, v.
gastroepiploica dextra, v.

Additional Entries

vena *(continued)*
gastroepiploica sinistra, v.
genus, vv.
glutaeae inferiores, vv.
glutaeae superiores, vv.
gluteae inferiores, vv.
gluteae superiores, vv.
haemorrhoidales inferiores, vv.
haemorrhoidalis media, v.
haemorrhoidalis superior, v.
hemiazygos, v.
hemiazygos accessoria, v.
hepaticae, vv.
hepaticae dextrae, vv.
hepaticae mediae, vv.
hepaticae sinistrae, vv.
hypogastrica, v.
ileocolica, v.
iliaca communis, v.
iliaca externa, v.
iliaca interna, v.
iliolumbalis, v.
inferior v. cava, v.
intercapitalares, vv.
intercapitulares manus, vv.
intercapitulares pedis, vv.
intercostales, vv.
intercostales anteriores, vv.
intercostales posteriores IV-XI, vv.
intercostalis superior dextra, v.
intercostalis superior sinistra, v.

vena *(continued)*
intercostalis suprema, v.
interlobares renis, vv.
interlobulares hepatis, vv.
interlobulares renis, vv.
intervertebralis, vv.
intestinales, vv.
jejunales et ilei, vv.
jugularis anterior, v.
jugularis externa, v.
jugularis interna, v.
labiales anteriores, vv.
labiales inferiores, vv.
labiales posteriores, vv.
labialis superiores, v.
labyrinthi, vv.
lacrimalis, v.
laryngea inferior, v.
laryngea superior, v.
lienalis, v.
lingualis, v.
lumbales, vv.
lumbales vv.
lumbales, vv.
lumbalis ascendens, v.
mammaria interna, v.
massetericae, vv.
maxillares, vv.
mediana antibrachii, v.
mediana basilica, v.
mediana cephalica, v.
mediana colli, v.
mediana cubitii, v.
mediastinales, vv.
mediastinales anteriores, vv.
meningeae, vv.
meningeae mediae, vv.
mesenterica inferior, v.
mesenterica superior, v.

Additional Entries

vena *(continued)*
metacarpeae dorsales, vv.
metacarpeae palmares, vv.
metacarpeae volares, vv.
metatarseae dorsales, vv.
metatarseae plantares, vv.
musculares, vv.
musculophrenicae, vv.
nasales externae, vv.
nasofrontalis, v.
obliqua atrii sinistri, v.
obliqua atrii sinistri, v.
obturatoriae, vv.
occipitalis, v.
oesophageae, vv.
ophthalmica inferior, v.
ophthalmica superior, v.
ophthalmomeningea, v.
ovarica, v.
ovarica dextra, v.
ovarica sinistra, v.
palatina, v.
palatina externa, v.
palpebrales, vv.
palpebrales inferiores, vv.
palpebrales superiores, vv.
pancreaticae, vv.
pancreaticoduodenales, vv.
paraumbilicales, vv.
parotideae, vv.
parotideae anteriores, vv.
parotideae posteriores, vv.
parumbilicales, vv.
pectorales, vv.

vena *(continued)*
perforantes, vv.
perforantes femoris, vv.
pericardiacae, vv.
pericardiacophrenicae, vv.
peroneae, vv.
pharyngeae, vv.
phrenicae inferiores, vv.
phrenicae superiores, vv.
poplitea, v.
portae, v.
posterior ventriculi sinistri cordis, v.
prepylorica, v.
profundae, vv.
profundae clitoridis, vv.
profunda femoris, v.
profunda linguae, v.
profundae penis, vv.
pudendae externae, vv.
pudenda interna, v.
pulmonales, vv.
pulmonales dextrae, vv.
pulmonalis inferior dextra, v.
pulmonalis inferior sinistra, v.
pulmonales sinistrae, vv.
pulmonalis superior dextra, v.
pulmonalis superior sinistra, v.
radiales, vv.
rectales inferiores, vv.
rectales mediae, vv.
rectalis superior, v.
renales, vv.
renis, vv.
retromandibularis, v.
revehentes, vv.
sacrales latrerales, vv.

Additional Entries

vena *(continued)*
sacralis media, v.
sacralis mediana, v.
saphena accessoria, v.
saphena magna, v.
saphena parva, v.
scapularis dorsalis, v.
scrotales anteriores, vv.
scrotales posteriores, vv.
septi pellucidi, v.
sigmoideae, vv.
spermatica, v.
spinales, vv.
spinales externae anteriores, vv.
spinales externae posteriores, vv.
spinales internae, vv.
spiralis modioli, v.
stellatae renis, vv.
sternocleidomastoidea, v.
striata, v.
stylomastoidea, v.
subclavia, v.
subcostalis, v.
subcutaneae abdominis, vv.
sublingualis, v.
submentalis, v.
superior v. cava, v.
supraorbitalis, v.
suprarenales, vv.
suprarenalis dextra, v.
suprarenalis sinistra, v.
suprascapularis, v.
supratrochleares, vv.
temporalis media, v.
temporales profundae, vv.
temporales superficiales, vv.

vena *(continued)*
terminalis, v.
testicularis, v.
testicularis dextra, v.
testicularis sinistra, v.
thalamostriata, v.
thoracalis lateralis, v.
thoracicae internae, vv.
thoracica lateralis, v.
thoracoacromialis, v.
thoracoepigastricae, vv.
thymicae, vv.
thyreoidea ima, v.
thyreoideae inferiores, vv.
thyreoideae superiores, vv.
thyroidea inferior, v.
thyroideae mediae, vv.
thyroidea superior, v.
tibiales anteriores, vv.
tibiales posteriores, vv.
tracheales, vv.
transversae colli, vv.
transversa faciei, v.
transversa scapulae, v.
tympanicae, vv.
ulnares, vv.
umbilicalis, v.
umbilicalis sinistra, v.
uterinae, vv.
vasorum, vv.
vertebralies, v.
vertebralis accessoria, v.
vertebralis anterior, v.
vesicales, vv.
vestibulares, vv.
vorticosae, vv.

vena cava
time-activity curve, v.c.
tumor, v.c.

venacavogram

Additional Entries

venacavography
venae
veniplex
venipuncture
venisection
venisuture
venoatrial
venofibrosis
venogram
    isotope v.
venography
    dural v.
    hepatic (wedged) v.
    portal v.
    selective v.
venomotor
veno-occlusive
venoperitoneostomy
venopressor
venosclerosis
venosinal
venostasis
venous
    angiography, v.
    arches, v.
    central v. catheter
    central v. pressure
    collaterals, v.
    insufficiency, v.
    jugular v. distention (JVD)
    jugular v. pulse (JVP)
    lacunae of dura mater, v.
    lake, v.
    line, v.
    mesocardium, v.
    occlusion, v.
    ovarian plexus, v.
    pampiniform plexus, v.
    pharyngeal plexus, v.
    phase, v.

venous *(continued)*
    plexus, v.
    portal v. flow
    pterygoid plexus, v.
    pudendal plexus, v.
    pulmonary v. congestion
    sampling, v.
    scan, v.
    shunt, v.
    sinuses, v.
    spermatic plexus, v.
    spread, v.
    stasis, v.
    thrombosis, v.
    umbrella, v.
    uterine plexus, v.
    vaginal plexus, v.
    valves, v.
    vesical plexus, v.
ventilation
    holes, v.
    perfusion scan, v. (VPS)
    perfusion mismatch, v.
    pulmonary v.
    quantification (VQ) scan, v.
    scan, v.
ventilator
ventrad
ventral
    aorta, v.
    cochlear nucleus, v.
    fissure, v.
    hernia, v.
    lamina, v.
    mesogastrium, v.
    psalterium, v.
    pulmonary nerves, v.
    spinal artery, v.
    spinothalamic fasciculus, v.
ventralward

Additional Entries

ventricle (s)
brain, v. of
cerebrum, v. of
floor of third v.
fornix, v. of
horns of lateral v.
mid-brain, v. of
spinal cord, v. of
Sylvius, v. of
terminal, v. of
ventricular
aneurysm, v.
angiography, v.
arrhythmia, v.
bigeminy, v.
block, v.
chambers, v.
contraction, v.
decompensation, v.
defect, v.
defibrillation, v.
depression, v.
diastolic pressure, v.
dysfunction, v.
ectopic activity, v.
ejection, v.
ejection fraction, v.
end-diastolic pressure, v.
end-systolic count, v.
ependyma, v.
escape, v.
extrasystole, v.
failure, v.
fibrillation, v.
flutter, v.
folds, v.
gallop, v.
heart failure, v.
hypertrophy, v.
injection, v.
inversion, v.
ligament, v.
ventricular *(continued)*
myocardium, v.
outflow tract stenosis, v.
premature beat, v.
premature contraction, v.
pressure, v.
rate, v.
response, v.
septal aneurysm, v.
septal defect, v.
septum, v.
standstill, v.
strain, v.
stroke volume, v.
system, v.
systole, v.
tachycardia, v.
ventriculi
ventriculitis
ventriculoatrial (V-A) shunt
ventriculoatriostomy
ventriculocaval shunt
ventriculocisternal shunt
ventriculocisternostomy
ventriculocordectomy
ventriculogram
isotope v.
ventriculography
bubble v.
central v.
gas v.
positive contrast v.
ventriculomegaly
ventriculometry
ventriculomyotomy
ventriculoperitoneal (V-P) shunt
ventriculopleural shunt
ventriculopuncture
ventriculoscope
ventriculoscopy

Additional Entries

ventriculostomy
ventriculosubarachnoid
ventriculotomy
ventriculvenostomy
ventriculovenous
ventriculus
  dexter, v.
  laryngis, v.
  lateralis, v.
  quartus, v.
  sinister,v.
  tertius, v.
ventriduct
ventriduction
ventriflexion
ventrimesal
ventrocystorrhaphy
ventrodorsad
ventrodorsal
ventrofixation
ventroinguinal
ventrolateral
ventromedian
  fissure of medulla oblongata, v.
ventroposterior
ventroscopy
ventrovesicofixation
venula
venulae
venular
venule
Veraguth's fold
Verga's lacrimal groove
verge
  anal v.
  rectal v.
vermian
  fossa, v.
  tumor, v.
vermiform
  appendix, v.

vermiform *(continued)*
  process, v.
vermilion
  border, v.
vermis
  cerebellum, v. of
vermography
Verneuil's canals
Verocay bodies
verruca (pl. verrucae)
  acuminata v.
  vulgaris v.
verruciform
verrucosis
verrucous
  endocarditis, v.
verruga
  peruana, v.
vertebra (pl. vertebrae)
vertebral
  artery, v.
  beaks, v.
  body, v.
  canal, v.
  collapse, v.
  column, v.
  compression fracture, v.
  fascia, v.
  foramen, v.
  gouging, v.
  groove, v.
  malalignment, v.
  notches, v.
  ribs, v.
  rotation, v.
  veins, v.
  venous plexus, v.
vertebrate
vertebrated catheter
vertebrobasilar
vertebrochondral
vertebrocostal

Additional Entries

vertebrodidymus
vertebrofemoral
vertebroiliac
vertebromammary
vertebrophrenic
    angle, v.
vertebrosacral
vertebrosternal
vertex
vertical
    beam projection, v.
    beam technique, v.
    Bucky, V.
    cassette holder, v.
    cassette stand, v.
    dense trabeculations, v.
    lingualis muscle, v.
    plane, v.
verticosubmental position
vertiginous
vertigraphy
verumontanum
vesica (pl. vesicae)
    fellea, v.
    urinaria, v.
vesical
    artery, v.
    neck, v.
    plexus, v.
    reflex, v.
    trabeculation, v.
vesication
vesicle
    auditory v.
    germinal v.
    lens v.
    optic v.
    otic v.
    seminal v.
    umbilical v.
vesicoabdominal
vesicocavernous
vesicocele
vesicocervical
vesicocolic fistula
vesicocolonic
vesicoenteric fistula
vesicofixation
vesicointestinal
vesicoperineal
vesicoprostatic
    plexus of veins, v.
vesicopustule
vesicorectal fistula
vesicorenal
vesicosigmoid
vesicosigmoidostomy
vesicospinal
vesicostomy
vesicoumbilical
    ligaments, v.
vesicoureteral reflux
vesicoureterogram
vesicourethral
vesicouterine
    excavation, v.
vesicovaginal fistula
vesicovaginorectal
vesicula
vesiculae
    seminales, v.
vesicular
    ovarian follicles, v.
vesiculectomy
vesiculiform
vesiculitis
vesiculobronchial
vesiculocavernous
vesiculogram
vesiculography
vesiculopapular
vesiculopustular
vesiculotubular
vesiculotympanic

Additional Entries

vessel
vestibula
vestibular
    arteries, v.
    bulb, v.
    fissure, v.
    ganglion, v.
    glands, v.
    lip, v.
    membrane, v.
    nerve, v.
vestibule
    aortic v.
    internal ear, v. of
    labyrinth, v. of
    larynx, v. of
    mouth, v. of
    nasal cavity, v. of
    omental bursa, v. of
    vagina, v. of
vestibulogenic
vestibulo-ocular
vestibuloplasty
vestibulospinal
    fasciculus, v.
vestibulourethral
vestibulum
vestige
vestigial
    Marshall, v.fold of
    pericardium, v. fold of
vestigium
viable
vibrocardiogram
vibrometer
vibrophone
vibrophonocardiograph
Vicq d'Azyr
    band, V.
    bundle, V.
Victoreen R-meter
Vidal's disease
videofluoroscopy
video study
vidian
    artery, v.
    canal, v.
    nerve, v.
Vieussens
    ansa, V.
    ring, V.
    valve, V.
Vignal's cells
vignetting distortion
Villard's button
villi
    arachnoid v.
    chorion, v. of
    intestine, v. of
villiferous
villitis
villoma
villonodular
    synovitis, v.
villositis
villous
    adenoma, v.
villus
Vim-Silverman needle
Vincent's angina
vincula
    tendinum, v.
    fingers, v. of
    toes, v. of
vinculum
violet
    gential v.
viral pneumonitis
Virchow's angle
Virchow-Robin spaces
viroplasm
virulent
viruliferous
viscera

Additional Entries

visceral
- aortography, v.
- arches, v.
- nervous system, v.
- receptors, v.
- veins, v.

viscerocranium
visceromegaly
visceroparietal
visceroperitoneal
visceropleural
visceroptosis
viscerosensory
visceroskeletal
viscerotrophic
viscerotropic
viscosity
viscous
- bile, v. (sludge)

viscus (any large interior organ)
Vistec sponge
visual
- acuity, v.
- area, v.
- centers, v.
- display, v.
- evoked potential, v.
- evoked response, v.
- purple v.

visuoauditory
visuopsychic
- area, v.

visuosensory
- area, v.

vital rays
vitelline
- circulation, v.
- duct, v.
- fluid, v.
- membrane, v.
- veins, v.

vitellus
vitreous
- body, v.
- cavity, v.
- chamber, v.
- detachment, v.
- floater, v.
- hemorrhage, v.
- humor, v.
- opacity, v.
- strand, v.
- stroma, v.

vitreum
vivid enhancement
vocal
- cords, v.
- folds, v.
- process, v.

Vogt's
- angle, V.
- point, V.
- syndrome, V.

Vogt-Hueter point
voiding
- cystogram, v.
- cystourethrogram, v. (VCUG)
- cystourethrography, v.

Voigt's boundary lines
Voillemier's point
Voit's nucleus
vola
volar
- arches, v.
- branch, v.
- carpal artery, v.
- carpal ligament, v.
- network, v.
- digital arteries, v.
- digital nerves, v.
- interosseous artery, v.
- interosseous nerve, v.

Additional Entries

volar *(continued)*
metacarpal arteries, v.
metacarpal veins, v.
venous arches, v.
Volkmann's
canal, V.
contracture, V.
volt (V)
voltage waveform
Voltolini's disease
volume
averaging, v.
blood v.
determinations, v.
distribution, v. of
end-diastolic v.
expiratory reserve v.
extracellular fluid v.
forced expiratory v.
imaging, v.
implant, v.
inspiratory reserve v.
left ventricular end-diastolic v.
left ventricular stroke v.
loss, v.
mean corpuscular v.
minute v.
overload, v.
right ventricular end-diastolic v.

volume *(continued)*
studies, v.
total air v.
volvulus
vomer
vomerobasilar
vomeronasal
cartilage, v.
organs, v.
Von Gierke disease
von Hippel-Lindau disease
von Recklinghausen's disease
vortex (of heart)
Vossius lenticular ring
voxel
size, v.
VPB (ventricular premature beat)
VPS (ventilation/perfusion) scan
VQ (ventilation/quantification) scan
intermediate VQ
match VQ
match and mismatch VQ
negative VQ
positive VQ
V-shape demarcation
Vulpian's atrophy
vulva

Additional Entries

W

W (tungsten)
w (watt)
Wachendorf's membrane
Wader and Andrews tongue depressor
Wagner's
- corpuscles, W.
- disease, W.

Wagstaffe's fracture
waist apron
Waldenstrom's disease
Waldenstrom's macroglobulinemia
Waldeyer's
- fluid, W.
- germinal epithelium, W.
- odontoblasts, W.
- ring, W.
- zona vasculosa, W.

wall (s)
- beaded w.
- nonparallel w.

Wallenberg's
- bundle, W.

Wallerian degeneration
wall-less detector
Walthard's islets
Walther's ducts
wandering
- pacemaker, w.

Wangensteen tube
Warbug's coenzyme
warfarin
wart
- mosaic w.
- plantar w.
- venereal w.

Wartenberg's disease
washings
- bronchial w.

washings *(continued)*
- gastric w.
- nasopharyngeal w.

wash-in phase
washout phase
Wassilieff's disease
water
- bag, w.
- bath, w.
- filled vessel, w.
- range, w.
- soluble contrast agent, w.
- soluble solution, w.

watershed
- infarct, w.

Waters projection
Waterston shunt
Waters view
Watson-Crick helix
watt (w.)
wattage
watt-second
wave
- alpha w.
- beta w.
- delta w.
- form, w.
- guide applicator, w.
- length, w.
- light w.
- like behavior, w.
- mechanics, w.
- P w.
- percussion w.
- peristaltic w.
- Q w.
- R w.
- radio w.
- sound w.

Additional Entries ______________________________

wave *(continued)*
- standing w.
- ST-T w.
- T w.
- theta w.
- U w.

wax
- ledge, w.
- pencil, w.
- waxy appearance, w.

WB (weightbearing)

weak
- echo, w.
- interactions, w.

web
- esophageal w.
- like, w. (one word)
- pharyngeal w.
- space, w.

Weber's
- disease, W.
- glands, W.

Weber-Christian disease

wedge
- angle, w.
- biopsy, w.
- factor, w.
- filter, w.
- isodose angle w.
- liver biopsy w.
- pair arrangement, w.
- port w.
- pulmonary w. position
- pulmonary w. pressure
- resection, w.
- shaped, w.
- shaped foam pad, w.
- shaped lesion, w.
- type osteotomy, w.

wedged
- field, w.
- pair of fields, w.

wedging

Wegener's granulomatosis

Wegner's disease

weightbearing

weight/volume (w/v)

Weil's basal layer

Weil's disease

Weil's stain

Weisbach's angle

Weitbrecht's cord

Welcker's basal angle

well-circumscribed

well-collimated megavoltage radiation beam

well-defined
- flow study, w-d
- fluid, w-d
- halo, w-d
- water density, w-d

well-demarcated lytic lesion

well-marginated

Wenckebach's disease

Werdnig-Hoffmann disease

Werlhof's disease

Wermer syndrome

Werner-His disease

Wernicke's
- aphasia, W.
- area, W.
- center, W.

Wernicke-Mann hemiplegia

Wertheim radical hysterectomy

Westberg's space

Westermark sign

Westphal's nucleus

Westphal-Strumpell disease

wet lung

wet reading

WFR/Aquaplast Corporation

Wharton's
- duct, W.

Additional Entries

Wharton's *(continued)*
jelly, W.
Whipple's
disease, W.
procedure, W.
resection, W.
whistle-tip catheter
whistling-face syndrome
Whitaker test
white
blood cells, w.
lead markers, w.
light, w.
matter, w.
substance of Schwann, w.
whole-body
image, w-b
irradiation, w-b
retention, w-b
scan, w-b
Whytt's disease
Wickham's striae
Widal-Abrami disease
wide-field
external beam irradiation, w-f
radiation technique, w-f
widening
carina, w. of
fusiform w. of abdominal aorta
mediastinum, w. of
suture, w.of
widespread
internal echoes, w.
metastases, w.
width
Wilde's cords
Wildermuth's ear
Willis'
antrum, W.

Willis' *(continued)*
circle, W.
Willock's respiratory jacket
Wilms' tumor
Wilson-Mikity syndrome
Wilson's
degeneration, W.
disease, W.
muscle, W.
Winchester-type disc
windblown
window
antral w.
aortic w.
level, w. (WL)
oval w.
round w.
width, w. (WW)
windowing
windpipe
wing
scapula, w. of
winged catheter
winged scapula
Winkler's disease
Winslow, foramen of
Winthrop Laboratories
wire
electrodes, w.
guide, w.
hook, w.
-loop lesion, w.
mesh implant, w.
monitoring, w.
monofilament w.
pacing electrode w.
stainless steel w.
suture, w.
Wirsung's
canal, W.
duct, W.
wisdom teeth

Additional Entries

Wiskott-Aldrich syndrome
WL (window level)
Wolfe mammographic parenchymal pattern
Wolfenden's position
wolffian
body, W.
duct, W.
tubules, W.
Wolff-Parkinson-White syndrome
Wolfring's glands
Wolfe's classification
womb
Wood's light
Wood's preparation
wool coil
wool-tailed coil
wormian bones
wound breakdown
W quantity
Wrisberg's
cardiac ganglion, W.
cartilages, W.
ligament, W.
nerve, W.
w/v (weight/volume)
WW (window width)

Additional Entries

X

- xanthelasma
- xanthemia
- xanthine
- xanthochromia
- xanthocyte
- xanthogranuloma
  - juvenile, x.
- xanthogranulomatous pyelonephritis
- xanthoma
  - diabetic x.
  - disseminatum, x.
  - eruptive x.
  - generalized x.
  - multiplex, x.
  - palpabrarum, x.
  - planar x.
  - plane x.
  - tuberosum, x.
  - tuberous x.
- xanthomatosis
  - bulbi, x.
- xanthomatous
- xanthous
- X-axis
- X-body
- Xe (xenon)
  - 133 Xe gas
  - 133 Xe inhalation method
  - 133 Xe-in-saline
  - 127 Xe radioaerosol
  - 133 Xe ventilation study
  - 133 Xe washout
- xenograft
- xenography
- xenon-133 (Xe-133) radioisotope
- xeroderma
- xeroderma *(continued)*
  - pigmentosum, x.
- xeromammogram
- xeromammography
- xerophthalmia
- xeroradiographic (XR) plate
- xeroradiographic pneumoencephalogram
- xeroradiography
- xerosialography
- xerosis
- xerostomia
- xerotomography
- xiphisternal node
- xiphisternum
- xiphocostal
- xiphoid
  - appendix, x.
  - bone, x.
  - cartilage, x.
  - process, x.
  - pubis, x. to
- x-radiation
- x-ray
  - absorption, x.
  - bath, x.
  - beam, x.
  - contamination, x.
  - couch, x.
  - escape peak, x.
  - field, x.
  - film, x.
  - generator, x.
  - jacket, x.
  - output, x.
  - peak, x.
  - picture, x.
  - production, x.
  - table, x.

Additional Entries

x-ray *(continued)*
- target, x.
- treatment beam, x.
- tube, x.

x-ray *(continued)*
- tube anode, x.

Xylocaine
xy plane

Additional Entries

Y

Y (yttrium)
  90 Y isotope, plaque
  synchondroses, Y
Yb (ytterbium)
  169 Yb-DTPA
Yankauer type suction tube
Y-axis
yoke
Young tongue forceps
Y-shaped
  acetabulum, Y.
  cartilage, Y.
  ligament of Bigelow, Y.
ytterbium (Yb)
  169 Yb-DTPA
yttrium (Y)
  90 Y isotope
  synchondroses

Additional Entries

Z

Z (atomic number)
Zahn's lines
Zang's space
Z-axis
zeisian gland
Z element
Zellwegger syndrome
Zenker's
  crystals, Z.
  degeneration, Z.
  diverticulum, Z.
  fluid, Z.
  pharyngoesophageal diverticulum, Z.
zero field splitting
zero time
zestocautery
zeugmatography
Ziehen-Oppenheimn disease
Ziemssen's motor points
zeugmatography
Zimmerlin's atrophy
Zimmermann's arch
zinc (Zn)
  chloride Zn 65
Zinn's
  anulus, Z.
  artery, Z.
  ligament, Z.
  zonule, Z.
zirconium (Zr)
Z-line of esophagus
Zn (zinc)
Zollinger-Ellison syndrome
Zollner's lines
zona (pl. zonae)
zone
  ciliary z.
  comfort z.
  epileptogenic z.

zone *(continued)*
  erogenous z.
  Lissauer's marginal z.
  looser z. (pseudofracture)
  transitional z.
zonifugal
zonipetal
zonogram
zonography
zonula
  ciliaris, z.
zonule
  ciliary
  Zinn, z. of
zonulitis
zoom
  function, z.
  lens, z.
Z pulse
Zr (zirconium)
Zuckerkandl's
  body, Z.
  organs, Z.
zygapophyseal joint
zygoma
zygomatic
  arch, z.
  bone, z.
  branch, z.
  muscle, z.
  nerve, z.
  process, z.
zygomaticofacial
  foramen, z.
  nerve, z.
zygomaticofrontal
  suture, z.
zygomaticomaxillary
zygomatico-orbital

Additional Entries ______________________________

____

____

zygomatico-orbital *(cont'd)*
 foramina, z.
zygomaticosphenoid
zygomaticotemporal
 foramen, z.
zygomaticotemporal *(cont'd)*
 nerve, z.
 suture, z.
zygomaxillare
zygomaxillary

Additional Entries